AF292276

Mental Health Promotion for Refugees and Other Culturally and/or Linguistically Diverse Migrant Populations

Mental Health Promotion for Refugees and Other Culturally and/or Linguistically Diverse Migrant Populations

Editors

Shameran Slewa-Younan
Greg Armstrong

MDPI • Basel • Beijing • Wuhan • Barcelona • Belgrade • Manchester • Tokyo • Cluj • Tianjin

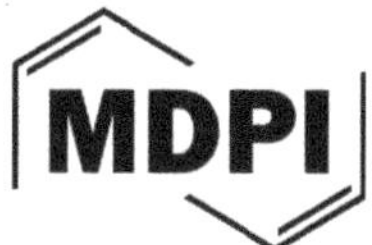

Editors
Shameran Slewa-Younan
Mental Health, School of
Medicine
Western Sydney University
Sydney
Australia

Greg Armstrong
Nossal Institute for Global
Health, Melbourne School of
Population and Global Health
Melbourne University
Melbourne, Victoria
Australia

Editorial Office
MDPI
St. Alban-Anlage 66
4052 Basel, Switzerland

This is a reprint of articles from the Special Issue published online in the open access journal *International Journal of Environmental Research and Public Health* (ISSN 1660-4601) (available at: www. mdpi.com/journal/ijerph/special_issues/Refugee_Mirgant_Populations).

For citation purposes, cite each article independently as indicated on the article page online and as indicated below:

LastName, A.A.; LastName, B.B.; LastName, C.C. Article Title. *Journal Name* **Year**, *Volume Number*, Page Range.

ISBN 978-3-0365-4714-5 (Hbk)
ISBN 978-3-0365-4713-8 (PDF)

Contents

About the Editors

Shameran Slewa-Younan

Shameran Slewa-Younan is the Associate Professor in Mental Health at the School of Medicine, Western Sydney University and Honorary Senior Research Fellow, Centre for Mental Health, University of Melbourne. She is also a board member of South Western Sydney Local Health District (2015 onwards), NSW Health.

Associate Professor Slewa-Younan has been practicing as a cross-cultural bilingual psychologist since 2001 when she joined the NSW Transcultural Mental Health Service and currently practices in Fairfield, Sydney, an area of high need with high numbers of refugees. Her focus has always been on providing optimal psychological care for resettling refugees, in this practice, she offers psychological assessment and treatment utilising a Cognitive Behavioural approach that is informed from a bilingual and bicultural perspective. Additionally, A/Prof Slewa-Younan is well known within the South Western Sydney community and is frequently called upon to provide psycho-education to community members, leaders and treatment providers. She has provided talks on mental health topics at community forums and initiatives. She has well-regarded reputation within the local community, evidenced by her ongoing referrals and clinical waitlist.

Since 2014, she has gained a reputation as one of the leading scholars on the mental health literacy of refugees and other cross-cultural populations, evidenced by her significant research output and collaborations with multiple institutions both domestic and international. She has published over 70 peer-reviewed publications including several invited articles and has appeared on ABC news regarding the mental health outcomes of Iraqi refugees in Australia and was awarded significant contribution prize by Australian Psychological Society for her teaching, research and clinical cross-cultural work (2018).

Greg Armstrong

Dr Gregory Armstrong is a multidisciplinary public health researcher and mental health social worker with a PhD in International Health from The University of Melbourne. He is a Senior Research Fellow with the Melbourne School of Population and Global Health at The University of Melbourne and has undertaken cross-cultural public health research and consultancies in Australia and in low and middle-income countries (LMICs) over the past 12 years with specialisations in mental health, suicide prevention and program evaluation. He has a passion for evidence-based training interventions in the area of community mental health and has developed and/or evaluated mental health training programs for social workers and First Nations Peoples in Australia and lay health workers in India. Gregory sits on the Research Advisory Committees for the Australian Association of Social Workers and Beyond Blue. He is Deputy Editor of International Journal of Mental Health Systems and also supports teaching in the Master of Public Health and Master of Social Work courses.

Preface to "Mental Health Promotion for Refugees and Other Culturally and/or Linguistically Diverse Migrant Populations"

Mental health promotion is a wide ranging concept influenced by cultural, socio-economic and political factors. Nonetheless, the goal of mental health promotion is to positively influence the determinants of mental health by undertaking effective multi-level interventions across numerous sectors, settings and environments. Within populations such as refugee groups, exposure to pre-migratory traumatic events combined with stressors during their travel and following migration and resettlement can lead to a higher risk of the development of psychological distress and mental ill-health. As such, mental health promotion efforts are needed to ensure that systems are in place to support refugees to maintain good mental health, to enhance understanding and engagement with mental health care where it is needed and to provide mental health services that are effective for such heterogeneous populations.

This Special Issue of *IJERPH* sought to invite researchers in mental health, public health and policy and social sciences to submit high quality research that focuses on improving our understanding of how to promote mental health and best care practices for refugees and other culturally and/or linguistically diverse migrant populations. A total of 11 papers were accepted following peer-review and are reflective of the broad spectrum of work encompassing mental health promotion for these target populations. Issues discussed included mental health screening, working with interpreters, differing cultural understanding of mental health and help-seeking including the impact of stigma and interventional programs focused on promoting mental wellbeing and physical health. We hope this Special Issue will assist in building the knowledge base to inform mental health promotion activities and initiatives for refugees and other culturally and/or linguistically diverse migrant populations.

Shameran Slewa-Younan and Greg Armstrong
Editors

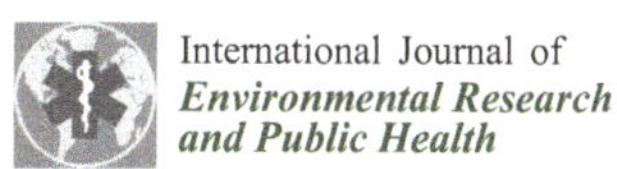
International Journal of
Environmental Research and Public Health

Review

How Are Non-Medical Settlement Service Organizations Supporting Access to Healthcare and Mental Health Services for Immigrants: A Scoping Review

Ayesha Ratnayake [1,*], Shahab Sayfi [2], Luisa Veronis [3], Sara Torres [4], Sihyun Baek [5] and Kevin Pottie [6,7]

[1] Faculty of Health Sciences, University of Ottawa, Ottawa, ON K1N 6N5, Canada
[2] Faculty of Science, University of Ottawa, Ottawa, ON K1N 6N5, Canada; ssayf086@uottawa.ca
[3] Department of Geography, Environment and Geomatics, University of Ottawa, Ottawa, ON K1N 6N5, Canada; lveronis@uottawa.ca
[4] School of Social Work, Laurentian University, Sudbury, ON P3E 2C6, Canada; storres@laurentian.ca
[5] Faculty of Medicine, University of Ottawa, Ottawa, ON K1N 6N5, Canada; sbaek040@uottawa.ca
[6] C.T. Lamont Primary Health Care Research Centre, University of Ottawa, Ottawa, ON K1N 6N5, Canada; kpottie@uwo.ca
[7] Department of Family Medicine, Western University, London, ON N6A 3K7, Canada
* Correspondence: aratn084@uottawa.ca

Abstract: Following resettlement in high-income countries, many immigrants and refugees experience barriers to accessing primary healthcare. Local non-medical settlement organizations, such as the Local Immigration Partnerships in Canada, that support immigrant integration, may also support access to mental health and healthcare services for immigrant populations. This scoping review aims to identify and map the types and characteristics of approaches and interventions that immigrant settlement organizations undertake to support access to primary healthcare for clients. We systematically searched MEDLINE, Social Services Abstracts, CINAHL, and PsycInfo databases from 1 May 2013 to 31 May 2021 and mapped research findings using the Social-Ecological Model. The search identified 3299 citations; 10 studies met all inclusion criteria. Results suggest these organizations support access to primary healthcare services, often at the individual, relationship and community level, by collaborating with health sector partners in the community, connecting clients to health services and service providers, advocating for immigrant health, providing educational programming, and initiating community development/mobilization and advocacy activities. Further research is needed to better understand the impact of local non-medical immigrant settlement organizations involved in health care planning and service delivery on reducing barriers to access in order for primary care services to reach marginalized, high-need immigrant populations.

Keywords: immigrants; refugees; primary healthcare access; settlement service organizations; health equity

Citation: Ratnayake, A.; Sayfi, S.; Veronis, L.; Torres, S.; Baek, S.; Pottie, K. How Are Non-Medical Settlement Service Organizations Supporting Access to Healthcare and Mental Health Services for Immigrants: A Scoping Review. *Int. J. Environ. Res. Public Health* **2022**, *19*, 3616. https://doi.org/10.3390/ijerph19063616

Academic Editors: Shameran Slewa-Younan and Greg Armstrong

Received: 31 January 2022
Accepted: 14 March 2022
Published: 18 March 2022

Publisher's Note: MDPI stays neutral with regard to jurisdictional claims in published maps and institutional affiliations.

1. Introduction

Given the growing numbers of culturally and linguistically diverse newcomers settling in Canada annually, pressure is being placed on provincial and federal governments to involve local non-medical immigrant settlement organizations in the development of accessible equitable healthcare and welfare services to meet the complex needs of expanding marginalized populations such as immigrants and refugees [1,2]. Asylum seekers also often have significant healthcare needs, due to premigration and post-migration experiences, yet tend to have low participation in primary healthcare systems [3,4]. Further, there is a growing need to support migrants' access to mental health services, as research has shown that they are at a higher risk for mental health problems compared to the general population but are less likely to seek care [5].

The focus on access to quality primary healthcare services is important, since these populations may be vulnerable and often experience considerable barriers to accessing quality primary healthcare, including limited English language proficiency, culturally inappropriate care and varying health beliefs, transportation difficulties, a general lack of social support, health system and health literacy issues, and high service costs [2,6–9]. Additionally, many health professionals report increased complexity on their end when serving migrant and refugee clients, relating to factors such as language interpretation difficulties, social determinants of health that require a multi-sector response, as well as difficulties for clients in understanding various health service entitlements [10]. Since the COVID-19 pandemic reduced community settlement services, primary care practitioners reported a corresponding reduction in access to primary healthcare for refugees and newcomers [11].

Local non-medical immigrant settlement organizations that support immigrant integration can facilitate collaborative efforts to increase access to mental health and healthcare services for migrants. They can also support information sharing by acting as a platform to connect various actors horizontally across sectors and vertically within sectors. These partnerships create a social space where civil society, businesses, private-sector stakeholders, local municipalities, and other stakeholders can discuss priority issues [12]. Variations of local immigrant settlement organizations and partnerships can be found globally; for example, the Strategic Migration Partnership in London, Local Immigration Partnerships (LIPs) in Canada, and the Mayor's Offices for Immigrant Affairs in Chicago, are a few well-established groups [12]. In Canada, LIPs play an essential role in immigrant settlement and integration [13,14]. Led by municipal or regional governments, or community organizations, LIPs are broad, cross-sectoral convening bodies that integrate newcomer needs into a city's community planning [13]. The LIPs play a central role in supporting immigrant populations by increasing local stakeholders' engagement in newcomers' integration processes, supporting community-level research and planning, and improving service coordination [15].

There has been some mixed-methods research, conducted with providers, refugees and interpreters, to gain insight into how these non-medical immigrant settlement organizations collaborate with the health sector [16]; however, to the best of our knowledge, the ways and opportunities through which these non-medical immigrant settlement organizations are supporting immigrants' access to mental health and other healthcare services have not been thoroughly examined or defined [17]. We aimed to address this knowledge gap by establishing how these "untapped resource" organizations contribute to improving immigrant access to primary health care services to create more health-enhancing environments for communities and marginalized populations. To guide our review, we asked the following research question: How do non-medical, local immigrant settlement organizations support access to healthcare services (i.e., primary healthcare services and/or specialized healthcare services) for immigrant populations in high-income countries? Our objectives were to identify and to map the types of approaches and interventions that non-medical immigrant settlement organizations use to support primary care access for immigrants. To inform our analysis and mapping approach, we adopted the social-ecological model [18].

2. Materials and Methods

2.1. Protocol

We developed a protocol for this scoping review using Arksey and O'Malley's 2005 five-stage methodological framework [19], and refined stage 5 as per recommendations made by the Joana Briggs Institute [20]. This scoping review included the following five key stages: (1) identifying the research question; (2) identifying relevant studies; (3) study selection; (4) charting the data; and (5) collating, summarizing, and reporting the results. To map and organize our data, we used an Excel data extraction sheet informed by the social-ecological model [18]. To report our findings, we replaced Arksey and O'Malley's approach with the Preferred Reporting Items for Systematic Reviews and Meta-Analyses Scoping

Review (PRISMA-ScR) checklist (see Additional File S1 in Supplementary Materials) [21]. The final version of the protocol is available upon request.

2.2. Data Sources and Search Strategy

In consultation with an expert health sciences librarian (LS), we developed a strategy to systematically search—using keywords, MeSH terms, major subject headings and/or the thesaurus functions—the following four electronic databases from 1 May 2013 to 31 May 2021: MEDLINE, Social Services Abstracts, PsycInfo, and Cumulative Index to Nursing and Allied Health Literature (CINAHL). An expert social sciences research librarian (PL) reviewed our social services abstracts search strategy, which consisted of terms such as refugee, immigrant, asylum seeker, local, community, partnership, organization, collaboration, primary health care, clinical care, health services accessibility, mental health services, Canada, United States, and Australia; the search terms were combined using Boolean operators (see Additional File S2 in Supplementary Materials for complete search strategy). Moreover, the search query was tailored to the specific requirements of each database. Lastly, we scanned references of the included articles for any relevant studies.

2.3. Eligibility Criteria

We included articles that met the following criteria: (1) included refugee, asylum seeker, or immigrant populations; (2) described local non-medical immigrant settlement-type organizations that support immigrant access to primary or clinical health care services; and (3) were conducted in industrialized countries with demographic, economic, political, and social characteristics comparable to those of Canada, and that are ranked on healthcare system performance by the Commonwealth Fund (see Table 1 for full inclusion criteria) [22]. Moreover, we used the United Nations High Commissioner for Refugees (UNHCR) definitions for asylum seekers and refugees as criteria for paper inclusion, while relying on Statistics Canada's definition for the term immigrant [23–25]. Specifically, we included studies that focused on refugees, asylum seekers, and immigrants 16 years of age and older; those that examined populations of any other age were excluded due to methodological challenges around the design, conduct and reporting of pediatric systematic reviews. For feasibility reasons, studies on undocumented migrants, transient migrant workers, foreign temporary workers, and foreign students were excluded. Organizations that did not conduct settlement-type work for immigrant populations, were not local, or were medical organizations were excluded. Lastly, countries that were not ranked by the Commonwealth Fund on healthcare system performance were excluded [22].

Table 1. Selection Criteria for studies included in the review.

Inclusion Criteria	Description	Exclusion Criteria
Population	Asylum seeker (16 years and older) "Someone whose request for sanctuary has yet to be processed" [23]. Refugee (16 years and older) "Someone who is unable or unwilling to return to their country of origin owing to a well-founded fear of being persecuted for reasons of race, religion, nationality, membership of a particular social group, or political opinion" [24]. Immigrant (16 years and older) "Immigrant refers to a person who is, or who has ever been, a landed immigrant or permanent resident. Such a person has been granted the right to live in Canada permanently by immigration authorities. Immigrants who have obtained Canadian citizenship by naturalization are included in this group." [25].	All populations other than immigrants, refugees and asylum seekers of all ages. Exclude for feasibility reasons the following: undocumented migrants, transient migrant workers, foreign temporary workers, and foreign students.

Table 1. *Cont.*

Inclusion Criteria	Description	Exclusion Criteria
Intervention/ Phenomena of Interest	Non-medical (nonclinical) local immigrant settlement organizations that support immigrant population's access to healthcare services (i.e., healthcare being primary health care or clinical care services)	All other organizations
Context	Industrialized countries with demographics and/or country characteristics comparable to Canada that are ranked on health care system performance by the Commonwealth Fund: Australia, Canada, France, Germany, Netherlands, New Zealand, Norway, Sweden, Switzerland, UK, USA [22,26].	All other countries
Research Type	Research publications (methods, data and analysis) quantitative, qualitative, or mixed-method documents published in peer-reviewed publications	Exclude literature reviews, gray literature
Year of Publication	Last 8 years (since March 2013)	Prior to the last 8 years
Language of Publication	All languages	No exclusion

Due to resource constraints, we applied restrictions to select articles that were most relevant. Literature reviews were excluded since, by nature, they are not primary data research publications; gray literature was excluded because the diverse formats and audiences of these texts can present a significant challenge in a systematic search for peer-reviewed evidence. We also excluded studies that were published prior to the last 8 years after reviewing Waleed M. Sweileh et al.'s 2018 paper "Bibliometric analysis of global migration health research in peer-reviewed literature (2000–2016)" in BMC Public Health, since it analyzed peer-reviewed literature in global migration health published worldwide [27]. Based on two key findings from the Bibliometrics, we applied the assumption that much of the global migration health research performed from 2014 onwards has taken into consideration prior research in earlier years; these key findings are as follows: the Bibliometrics' Figure 1 analysis demonstrates an up-tick in global migration health publications from 2014–2016 (approximately one third of the retrieved documents in the analysis were published in the last 3 years of the study); and the Bibliometric reference list includes publications that focused on access to healthcare services and community organization support for migrants that were published between 2015–2017—for example, Taylor J.'s 2017 systematic review of social determinants of health on access to healthcare [28]. Therefore, since this "explosion" of migrant access to healthcare research occurs around 2014, we decided to limit our study's search to publications from 2013 and onwards.

2.4. Study Selection Process

Search results were imported into COVIDENCE, an online systematic review software [29]. The inclusion criteria were used for screening titles and abstracts during level 1 screening and reviewing full-text articles during level 2 screening. Two reviewers (AR and SS) independently screened the title and abstract of each article for inclusion. Reviewers connected with one another throughout the screening process to resolve conflicts and discuss any uncertainties that arose during the selection process. All articles deemed relevant after title and abstract screening were included for full-text screening. Using the same process, the two reviewers (AR and SS) subsequently screened the full text of potentially relevant articles to determine eligibility. Disagreements were resolved through discussion between the two reviewers. Once agreement was reached, the full-text articles chosen for inclusion in the study were reviewed for data extraction.

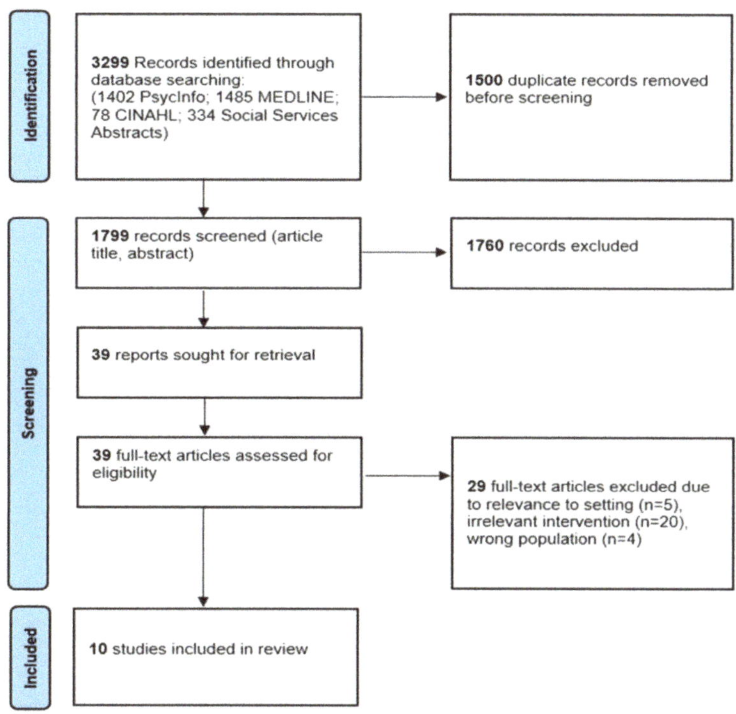

Figure 1. The Preferred Reporting Items for Systematic Reviews and Meta-Analyses (PRISMA) study flow diagram.

2.5. Data Extraction

A standardized data extraction template, informed by framework analysis using the social-ecological model, was developed with input from the entire review team [18]. We chose the social-ecological model because it is a commonly used population health framework to conceptualize health broadly, taking into consideration that health is affected by dynamic interactions among various personal and environmental factors [18]. At minimum, results for our study were extracted as they applied to the framework analysis (individual level, relationship level, community level, societal level) and study criteria. For all of the articles included in the final analysis, data were extracted on the following variables: (1) author and year of publication, (2) source origin (i.e., country where the study took place), (3) aim/purpose of the study, (4) list of organizations that participated in the study, (5) study population/sample size/study participant description (i.e., participant characteristics), (6) methodology, (7) intervention type, (8) concepts or phenomena of interest, (9) outcomes measured, and (10) key findings/author conclusions/implications. In order to ensure the validity of the data extraction form, it was piloted by two reviewers (SS and SB), and accuracy of the content was reviewed by a third reviewer (AR). For all articles, two reviewers extracted data in duplicate and independently (SS and SB). Results were compared and disagreements were resolved by discussion or with help from a third reviewer (AR).

2.6. Methodological Quality Appraisal

We did not appraise the methodological quality or risk of bias of the included articles, which is consistent with guidance on scoping review conduct [20]. As a scoping review, the purpose of this study was to aggregate the findings and present a mapping of the research rather than to evaluate the quality of the individual studies [19]. Therefore, a critical appraisal of the methods for the strength of the evidence was not performed.

2.7. Data Mapping and Synthesis

As Carroll et al., 2013 recommended, we used a framework analysis method to structure our results [30]. Specifically, the theoretical social-ecological model was applied to map and group findings into themes and identify and explain outliers [18]. Results are presented in a table summarizing the characteristics of included studies with narrative descriptions. We discuss the application of findings to the broader context and discussion on non-medical immigrant settlement organizations supporting access to healthcare service and provide conclusions/implications for policy research and practice. We also identify and discuss strengths and limitations of the scoping review.

3. Results

3.1. Literature Search

A total of 3299 records were identified through database searching. After removal of duplicate citations, 1799 records were screened by title and abstract. Title abstract screening resulted in the exclusion of 1760 records, leaving 39 potentially relevant full-text articles that were sought for retrieval and assessed for eligibility using the inclusion criteria. Figure 1 presents the details of the search process. From these, 29 full-text articles were further excluded due to relevance to setting, irrelevant intervention or wrong population. The remaining 10 articles were included in this review: Chadwick and Collins, 2015 (study 1) [31]; Cheng et al., 2019 (study 2) [32]; Frost et al., 2018 (study 3) [33]; Isaacs et al., 2013 (study 4) [34]; Isaacs et al., 2013 (study 5) [35]; Koehn et al., 2019 (study 6) [36]; McMurray et al., 2014 (study 7) [37]; Salami et al., 2019 (study 8) [38]; Torres et al., 2013 (study 9) [39]; and Torres et al., 2014 (study 10) [7]. Characteristics of included studies are summarized in Table 2.

Table 2. Characteristics of included studies.

Study #	Authors/Year	Source Origin	Study Design	Local Non-Medical Settlement Organization	Study Population	Outcome: Approach to Support Access to Primary Healthcare Services for Immigrants	Social-Ecological Model Level
1	Chadwick et al., 2015	Canada	quantitative survey analysis; qualitative interviews	settlement service organizations	recent immigrants in large or small urban centers	connects to healthcare services/collaborates with health sector institutions (via resources to services such as appointment accompaniment and referrals to external community service providers, delivery of group programs)	Individual, relationship, community
2	Cheng et al., 2019	Australia	community-based intervention development	local settlement support agencies	asylum seekers newly released from detention in South Eastern Melbourne	connects to healthcare services/collaborates with health sector institutions (via the development of the asylum integrated healthcare pathway)	relationship, community
3	Frost et al., 2018	United States	exploratory, post hoc, single-group only research design with interviews	local refugee resettlement agency	Burmese-speaking refugee women in Houston Texas	provides health promotion programs (via health education program)	individual

Table 2. *Cont.*

Study #	Authors/Year	Source Origin	Study Design	Local Non-Medical Settlement Organization	Study Population	Outcome: Approach to Support Access to Primary Healthcare Services for Immigrants	Social-Ecological Model Level
4	Isaacs et al., 2013a	Canada	qualitative case study includes survey and interviews	community-based organization	recent immigrant families in an urban center in Atlantic Canada	connects to healthcare services/collaborates with health sector institutions (via role as broker organization)	community
5	Issacs et al., 2013b	Canada	qualitative case study includes surveys and interviews	community-based organization	recent immigrants and/or families in an urban community in Atlantic Canada	connects to healthcare services/collaborates with health sector institutions (via cultural competence trust with network)	relationship
6	Koehn et al., 2019	Canada	qualitative case study includes focus groups and interviews	immigrant-serving agencies	Punjabi and Korean-speaking older immigrants	connects to healthcare services/collaborates with health sector institutions (via capacity to connect with services and provide culturally responsive health information and navigational support)	relationship
7	McMurray et al., 2014	Canada	before/after repeated survey design	local receiving center	government-assisted refugees (primarily coming from Northwest Africa, the Middle East, and Southeast Asia) in Ontario	connects to healthcare services/collaborates with health sector institutions (via partnership between a dedicated health clinic, a local reception center, and community providers)	individual, relationship, community
8	Salami et al., 2019	Canada	qualitative descriptive design includes interviews, focus groups	immigrant-serving agencies	immigrants, refugees in Alberta	connects to healthcare services/collaborates with health sector institutions (by identifying client needs, referring clients to specialized mental health services)	individual
9	Torres et al., 2013	Canada	qualitative and quantitative case study includes direct observation, interviews, document and database analysis	community-based organization	at-risk immigrant and refugee women and their families in Edmonton	provides health promotion programs (e.g., perinatal program intervention through innovative Multicultural Health Brokers Co-op); undertakes community capacity building and policy advocacy activities (e.g., perinatal program intervention through innovative Multicultural Health Brokers Co-op)	individual, relationship, community, society

Table 2. *Cont.*

Study #	Authors/Year	Source Origin	Study Design	Local Non-Medical Settlement Organization	Study Population	Outcome: Approach to Support Access to Primary Healthcare Services for Immigrants	Social-Ecological Model Level
10	Torres et al., 2014	Canada	qualitative and quantitative case study includes direct observation, interviews, document and database analysis	community-based organization	new immigrants, refugees, and their families in Edmonton	connects to healthcare services/collaborates with health sector institutions (via role as cultural health broker through innovative Multicultural Health Brokers Co-op); provides health promotion programs (via educational outreach on disease management through innovative Multicultural Health Brokers Co-op); provides 'on the ground' assistance to clients (e.g., transport to clinics, accompanies clients to doctors appointments when language difficulties are present)	individual, relationship, community

Note: Studies 4 and 5 derive from the same research and research team but have different objectives. Studies 9 and 10 derive from the same research but also have different objectives.

3.2. Study Characteristics

Of the 10 articles, eight were carried out in Canada (study 1, 4–10), one was in the USA (study 3), and one was in Australia (study 2). Three studies were published in 2019 (study 2, 6, 8), one in 2018 (study 3), one in 2015 (study 1), two in 2014 (study 7, 10), and three in 2013 (study 4, 5, 9). Study designs included qualitative interviews (study 1, 3–6, 8–10), qualitative surveys (study 4, 5), quantitative survey analysis (study 1), intervention development/piloting (study 2), before/after repeated survey design (study 7), focus groups (study 6, 8), and other research methods such as direct observation, document/database analysis (study 9, 10). Local non-medical immigrant settlement organizations in the 10 studies were described as settlement service organizations (study 1), local settlement support agencies (study 2), local refugee resettlement agency (study 3), community-based organizations (study 4, 5, 9, 10), immigrant-serving agencies (study 6, 8), and local receiving center (study 7).

In the 10 articles reviewed, the local non-medical immigrant settlement organizations' priority populations served included recent immigrants in small or large urban centers (study 1); asylum seekers newly released from detention (study 2) (note: 93% of the clients were men, 54% of clients were aged between 22 and 34 years, countries of origin included Afghanistan (30.4%), Sri Lanka (25.3%), Iran (19.2%), Pakistan (10.7%), Other (6%), Stateless (3.7%), Vietnam (3.3%), and Iraq (1.4%)); Burmese-speaking refugee women (study 3), recent immigrant families in urban centers (study 4, 5); Punjabi and Korean-speaking immigrants (study 6); government-assisted refugees (study 7) (note: study population included males (50.9%) and females (49.1%) with a large percentage under the age of 18 (49.2%), primarily coming from Northwest Africa, the Middle East, and Southeast Asia); immigrants and refugees (study 8); and at-risk immigrant and refugee women and their families (study 9, 10).

3.3. Approaches to Support Access to Primary Healthcare Services for Immigrants

The findings from our study are presented below according to the various levels of the Social-Ecological Model [18]. The first level, individual, identifies personal and biological factors that directly or indirectly impact health outcomes, while the second level, relationships, consists of close social environment factors that may influence the health outcomes of an individual. The community level of the Social-Ecological Model refers to the various factors associated with the setting in which a person goes about their daily life. Lastly, the societal level looks at broad social, economic, and political factors that influence a person's health status [18].

3.3.1. Individual Level

Two studies fell under this theme. Study 3 evaluated a pilot health education intervention delivered to Burmese-speaking refugee women, clients at a resettlement agency in Houston, Texas. Developed in partnership with the University of Texas Health Science Center, the intervention provided learning events to develop new skills to navigate health services, held discussions on health topics and question and answer (Q&A) sessions with medical providers, and disseminated health education resources. The increased opportunities to practice English and develop vocabulary allowed participants to be more confident in executing skills such as calling a doctor's office to make appointments or taking the bus. The study noted that lack of compatibility and agency buy-in were two main barriers to creating a feasible and sustainable intervention.

Next, study 8 focused on service providers' perceptions of immigrant and refugee access to and use of mental health services. Findings showed that immigrant-serving agencies played a significant role in identifying clients experiencing a crisis or struggling with mental health conditions and connecting these individuals to mental health services. Further, these providers also evaluated the fit of an interpreter or cultural broker (brokers provide education and cultural translation support) with a client. In terms of challenges, the participants noted a desire for increased mental health training on identifying client needs and referring clients to specialized mental health services.

3.3.2. Relationship Level

Relationship level was examined in two studies. In study 5, the focus was on community-based organizations' trust in the cultural competency of other local service providers and its influence on meeting the complex healthcare needs of recent immigrant families. Cultural competency in this study refered to the ability and preparedness of a service organization to understand and respond to the health needs of immigrant families. Competence trust among service organizations was key for families to have access to healthcare services, whereas a lack of trust led to constrained workflow within the system, more avoidance behavior, and less interaction. The study found settlement service organizations to be exemplars of cultural competency.

Study 6 explored immigrant-serving agencies' roles as partner organizations to dementia service institutions and in facilitating access to dementia diagnosis and care services and supports provided by dementia service institutions. Findings from focus groups with older immigrant adults showed that the immigrant-serving agency connected with immigrant clients and was able to engender trust and provide culturally responsive health information as well as support in navigating the health system. The immigrant-serving agency lacked specific knowledge on dementia (a barrier to aligning their messages with clients' perceptions).

3.3.3. Community Level

Study 4 addressed community-level relations by uncovering the role of settlement service organizations as broker organizations supporting a network of community-based services that meet the primary healthcare needs of immigrants. For example, settlement services in this study function as brokers by acting as a hub for health information for immigrant clients, by being a source of referral to primary care services for immigrant families, and by fostering collaboration in service delivery to high-needs immigrant families while building system competencies with partners. Further, compared to other service-sector organizations, immigrant settlement services in this study were found to have the greatest numbers of strong ties to partners in their community network. Barriers for settlement service organizations to assume the broker role included funding issues or capacity-building resource issues.

3.3.4. Multiple Levels

While no study examined relations solely at the society level, a total of five studies addressed healthcare issues at multiple levels. Study 1 covers individual, relationship and community levels. Specifically, it examined the relationship between recent immigrants' self-perceived mental health and social supports available for them. Findings revealed that each settlement service organization provided social support by engaging in private meetings with clients or providing referrals to community agencies, local organizations for psychological/clinical counseling, or community group programs. Settlement service organizations in small urban centers offered more tangible social supports compared to those in large urban settings; these included resources to primary healthcare services such as appointment accompaniment and additional referrals to healthcare service providers outside the clients' community. A limiting factor to being able to provide these social supports was the amount of dedicated staff time needed.

Study 10 explored the successes of community health workers at the individual, relationship and community levels in facilitating access to healthcare for recent immigrants and refugees through a case study of a Multicultural Health Broker Co-op collaborating with a health services public health unit. Findings from this study show the complementary role that multicultural health brokers and community health workers fill within the health system. Multicultural health brokers and community health workers work towards breaking down barriers (such as language, economic conditions, systematic discrimination) to accessing healthcare services for immigrant and refugee families. For example, multicultural health brokers/community health workers accompany clients to appointments or clinics, organize community development initiatives, and offer educational outreach programs on chronic disease prevention and management. A challenge for these community health workers and multicultural health brokers is not being formally recognized as part of the human health resource workforce.

As another study considering the individual, relationship, and community levels, study 7 assessed the impact of a refugee health clinic's partnership with a local refugee receiving center and community providers on referrals and wait times. The refugee health clinic model uses integrating mechanisms to deliver culturally appropriate and responsive primary care. Within this partnership model, gateway services are provided by the local receiving center's case workers/settlement workers and professionals from the family practice (e.g., nurse, resident physician). The health clinic delivers comprehensive care via family physicians; interpreters (if needed) are funded by the refugee receiving center. The model also includes ancillary services that are delivered in a community setting by providers willing to treat government-assisted refugees. Study findings demonstrated a 30% decrease in wait times for an appointment with a healthcare provider; an 18% increase in government-assisted refugees securing a permanent family doctor within a year after arrival; and almost a doubling of referrals to non-physician primary healthcare providers (e.g., dentists, optometrists). The study notes that this partnership model is built on goodwill; no formal contracts or funding beyond regular settlement services support was pursued.

Study 2 describes the Asylum Seeker Integrated Healthcare Pathway, an intervention influencing factors on the relationship and community levels, created to improve linkage to health services for asylum seekers newly released from detention. The Pathway consists of settlement support agencies in partnership and collaboration with local primary and emergency healthcare services in Melbourne. The Pathway intervention embeds a clinical health screening and triage process, facilitated by settlement support agencies, into existing community orientation programs for asylum seekers. Findings showed agencies supporting the coordination of healthcare appointments; assisting clients to appointments; and linking clients with culturally responsive care options. Through this initiative, clients had timely access to services. The study noted that an ongoing consideration for the success of this intervention is the capacity of the primary healthcare practices to meet the unique health needs of asylum seekers.

Study 9 addressed individual, relationship, community, and society levels. It discussed the community health worker role in a Multicultural Health Broker Co-op (MCHB Co-op) that supports at-risk immigrant refugee women and their families by contributing to their settlement and integration into communities. The study aimed to better understand the health promotion functions and programs of the MCHB Co-op model and health brokers practice and found that both are able to offer a variety of supports to immigrant and refugee families; the Co-op provides educational support to help them realize their rights in order to overcome access to care barriers as patients (e.g., asking doctors for health information), as program users (e.g., seeking services from the health system), and as citizens (e.g., voicing their concerns to policy decision-makers). Two factors that could have negative implications on the community capacity-building programs and the services delivered by the MCHB Co-op were unstable funding and heavy caseloads.

4. Discussion

Findings from this scoping review show that local non-medical immigrant settlement organizations in the 10 articles had established approaches/interventions to support immigrants' access to primary healthcare services. Further, most of the studies show that mental health support was an important component of the established approaches/interventions. These include: connecting to healthcare services and/or collaborating with health sector institutions; providing health promotion programs; undertaking community capacity-building and policy advocacy activities; and providing 'on the ground' assistance to clients. Using the social-ecological model to map these approaches [18], we found that most occurred at multiple levels (individual, relationship, community, and/or society) (study 1, 2, 7, 9, 10); two studies applied approaches/interventions that influence factors to access healthcare services at the individual level (study 3, 8); two studies applied approaches/interventions that influence factors to access healthcare services at the relationship level (study 5, 6); one study applied approaches/interventions that influence factors to access healthcare services at the community level (study 4); and no studies applied approaches/interventions at solely the society level (this may be because societal factors that favor or impair healthcare access, such as health/economic/social policies, require significant intersectoral action to reduce socioeconomic inequalities to healthcare service access).

Out of the 10 studies included in this review, eight were Canadian; this highlights the uniqueness of the Canadian settlement model and long experience of the settlement sector in collaborating and partnering with organizations both within the sector and across other sectors. A case in point is the creation and deployment of LIPs since 2008, and the work they have done to coordinate service provision, for example, by launching numerous innovative initiatives, some focused on primary healthcare, during Canada's Syrian Refugee Resettlement Initiative in 2015–2016 [15].

As seen in this scoping review, local non-medical immigrant settlement organizations support immigrant access to primary healthcare; however, the scope and quality of services available to immigrants may not be uniform across settlement organizations. Settlement service organizations in Canada receive funding from multiple sources including the federal and provincial governments [40], which can influence or limit a settlement organization's mandate and/or resources. Further, a lack of responsive and forward-planning federal policy coordinating the provision of settlement services can also lead to disparities in the quality and range of settlement service organization programming between regions where settlement organizations operate [41,42]. Although community-based organizations often enjoy functioning with less bureaucratic control and with organizational structures that can be adapted to social/economic/political contexts to allow for more tailored programming to address inequities and specific marginalized population needs within their communities, these organizations often face challenges of overextended staff with limited resources/funding [43]. Despite the challenges, these organizations are uniquely positioned 'on the ground', where they are able to identify the healthcare needs of immigrant populations within the community and closely work with clients (e.g., via community health workers) to address health concerns (e.g., education programming internal to the settlement organization), support healthcare system navigation, provide referrals to health services, and partner/collaborate with health sector institutions to delivery health programs and initiatives [44]. These functions and roles are consistent with literature outlining successful organizational 'building blocks' to improve access to primary healthcare for marginalized populations [45].

Local non-medical immigrant settlement organizations may not be structurally or financially able to take on extensive activities to increase access to primary healthcare themselves, however, they have a place in the health system. Consistent with previous literature, community-based organizations are increasingly recognized for their importance in primary healthcare; their unique closeness to immigrant populations and their ability to understand and respond to these populations makes them a valuable partner, source of knowledge, and gateway to marginalized populations for primary healthcare providers and institutions [3,46]. Health systems and services could benefit from including these community-based organizations in their future plans to address the health needs of immigrant populations. There is a need for in-depth research on community collaboration for health equity.

4.1. Implications for Research

This scoping review contributes to the literature by making visible the work that local non-medical immigrant settlement organizations do to advance health equity. Nevertheless, more international consensus is needed on terms for community settlement programs and more research on the collaborative relationships that exist or do not exist between community programs and community primary healthcare clinics to explore the impact on health outcomes for immigrant populations. Future research and development in this area is needed to better understand the impact of local non-medical immigrant settlement organizations involved in healthcare planning and service delivery on reducing barriers to access in order for primary care services to reach marginalized, high-need immigrant populations. Further studies could also look at what local non-medical immigrant settlement organizations do to advance health equity in areas linked to the determinants of health, which influence the health outcomes of individuals. This work requires multi-sector response, including but not limited to dealing with migration status, food security, and discrimination. Lastly, it would be beneficial for future research to build on this review by specifically considering the addition of gray literature from different countries and their local non-medical immigrant settlement organizations; gray literature can be very current, detailed, geographically specific, and in essence provide a rich and balanced picture of approaches/interventions to complement these foundational review findings.

4.2. Strengths and Limitations of This Scoping Review

Strengths of this scoping review include its methodological approach—that is, using a predefined protocol aligned with Arksey and O'Malley's framework and the JBI guidance, along with the use of predefined eligibility criteria by two reviewers when selecting the articles [19,20]. There also are a number of limitations, however, that ought to be noted: reviewers did not appraise the quality of the evidence; the scoping review was limited to published peer-reviewed studies; the broad concept of local non-medical immigrant settlement organizations may not have captured all organizations that perform local settlement work with immigrants; the language and terms used in the search may not have been internationally used, and thus, we predominantly identified Canadian-only publications; and many of the studies lacked details on organizational structure, capacity, and programming, which would have been useful to better understand how these organizations are able to support access to primary care.

5. Conclusions

Using a social-ecological approach, this scoping review mapped and highlighted current approaches/interventions relating to how local non-medical immigrant settlement organizations support access to primary healthcare services for immigrant populations. Although these findings may not be globally representative and, therefore, not generalizable, they suggest that these organizations are able to support access to primary healthcare services by collaborating with health sector partners in the community network, connecting clients to health services and service providers, advocating for immigrant health, providing educational programming, and also taking on community development/mobilization and advocacy activities to promote access to healthcare. Including these local non-medical immigrant settlement organizations in healthcare planning and service delivery may provide more scope to respond to and reach marginalized, high-need immigrant populations. Strategies to encourage the involvement of local non-medical immigrant settlement organizations in healthcare planning, implementation, and service delivery are needed. Although most of the articles in this review were Canadian, other countries may consider adapting the approaches and interventions identified to their context and needs. As a next step, we recommend a critical assessment of each identified approach/intervention to better understand the feasibility to implement the necessary elements (e.g., human resources required, cost, acceptability of approach), and the extent of its effectiveness. A critical assessment can help relevant stakeholders decide if the identified approaches/interventions in this review are worth adapting.

Supplementary Materials: The following supporting information can be downloaded at: https://www.mdpi.com/article/10.3390/ijerph19063616/s1. The following are available upon request from the corresponding author: File S1: Preferred Reporting Items for Systematic reviews and Meta-Analyses extension for Scoping Reviews (PRISMA-ScR) Checklist; File S2: Search Strategies for all Databases; File S3: Data Extraction Sheet.

Author Contributions: Conceptualization, A.R., L.V., S.T. and K.P.; Methodology, A.R., L.V., S.T., K.P.; Software, A.R.; Validation, A.R., L.V., S.T. and K.P.; Formal Analysis, A.R.; Investigation, A.R.; Resources, A.R.; Data Curation, A.R., S.S., S.B.; Writing—Original Draft Preparation, A.R.; Writing—Review and Editing, A.R., S.S., S.B., L.V., S.T. and K.P.; Visualization, A.R.; Supervision, L.V. and K.P.; Project Administration, A.R.; Funding Acquisition, A.R. All authors have read and agreed to the published version of the manuscript.

Funding: This research received funding from Bruyère Research Institute, Ottawa, ON, Canada.

Institutional Review Board Statement: Not applicable.

Informed Consent Statement: Not applicable.

Data Availability Statement: The Supplementary Excel File (S3) holds information extracted from studies used in this review.

Acknowledgments: We would like to acknowledge the expert librarian services of Lindsey Sikora and Patrick Labelle at the University of Ottawa.

Conflicts of Interest: The authors declare no conflict of interest.

References

1. Ma, M.C.K. Local Immigration Partnerships: How Is Peterborough Engaged with Immigrant Integration? In *Canadian Perspectives on Immigration in Small Cities*; Bonifacio, G., Drolet, J., Eds.; Springer International Publishing: Cham, Switzerland, 2017; pp. 55–74. [CrossRef]
2. Pottie, K.; Greenaway, C.; Feightner, J.; Welch, V.; Swinkels, H.; Rashid, M.; Narasiah, L.; Kirmayer, L.J.; Ueffing, E.; MacDonald, N.E.; et al. Evidence-based clinical guidelines for immigrants and refugees. *Can. Med. Assoc. J.* **2011**, *183*, E824–E925. [CrossRef] [PubMed]

3. Cheng, I.H.; Wahidi, S.; Vasi, S.; Samuel, S. Importance of community engagement in primary health care: The case of Afghan refugees. *Aust. J. Prim. Health* **2015**, *21*, 262–267. [CrossRef] [PubMed]
4. Legido-Quigley, H.; Pocock, N.; Teng Tan, S.; Pajin, L.; Suphanchaimat, R.; Wickramage, K.; McKee, M.; Pottie, K. Health care is not universal if undocumented migrants are excluded. *BMJ* **2019**, *366*, 1–5. [CrossRef]
5. Lu, J.; Jamani, S.; Benjamen, J.; Agbata, E.; Magwood, O.; Pottie, K. Global Mental Health and Services for Migrants in Primary Care Settings in High-Income Countries: A Scoping Review. *Int. J. Environ. Res. Public Health* **2020**, *17*, 8627. [CrossRef]
6. Beiser, M. The Health of Immigrants and Refugees in Canada. *Can. J. Public Health* **2005**, *96*, S30–S44. [CrossRef]
7. Torres, S.; Labonté, R.; Spitzer, D.L.; Andrew, C.; Amaratunga, C. Improving health equity: The promising role of community health workers in Canada. *Healthc. Policy* **2014**, *10*, 73–85. [CrossRef] [PubMed]
8. Spitzer, D. In Visible Bodies: Minority Women, Nurses, Time, and the New Economy of Care. *Med. Anthropol. Q.* **2004**, *18*, 490–508. [CrossRef] [PubMed]
9. Long, K.M.; Vasi, S.; Westbury, S.; Shergill, S.; Guilbert-Savary, C.; Whitelaw, A.; Cheng, I.H.; Russell, G. Improving access to refugee-focused health services for people from refugee-like backgrounds in south-eastern Melbourne through the education sector. *Aust. J. Prim. Health* **2021**, *27*, 93–101. [CrossRef] [PubMed]
10. Ziersch, A.; Freeman, T.; Javanparast, S.; Mackean, T.; Baum, F. Regional primary health care organisations and migrant and refugee health: The importance of prioritisation, funding, collaboration and engagement. *Aust. N. Z. J. Public Health* **2020**, *44*, 152–159. [CrossRef]
11. Arya, N.; Redditt, V.J.; Talavlikar, R.; Holland, T.; Brindamour, M.; Wright, V.; Saad, A.; Beukeboom, C.; Coakley, A.; Rashid, M.; et al. Caring for refugees and newcomers in the post–COVID-19 era. *Can. Fam. Physician* **2021**, *67*, 575–581.
12. Papademetriou, D.G. Migration's Local Dividends How Cities and Regions Can Make the Most of Immigration. Available online: http://www.migrationpolicy.org/research/migrations-local-dividends-how-cities-and-regions-can-make-most-immigration-transatlantic (accessed on 9 August 2020).
13. Citizenship and Immigration Canada (CIC). Local Immigration Partnerships: Outcomes 2008–2013. Available online: http://p2pcanada.ca/files/2014/07/Local-Immigration-Partnerships-Outcomes-2008-2013.pdf (accessed on 9 August 2020).
14. Walton-Roberts, M.; Veronis, L.; Wayland, S.; Dam, H.; Cullen, B. Syrian refugee resettlement and the role of Local Immigration Partnerships in Ontario, Canada. *Can. Geogr. Le Géographe Can.* **2019**, *63*, 347–359. [CrossRef]
15. Veronis, L. Building intersectoral partnerships as place-based strategy for immigrant and refugee (re)settlement: The Ottawa Local Immigration Partnership. *Can. Geogr. Le Géographe Can.* **2019**, *63*, 391–404. [CrossRef]
16. Dubus, N.; LeBoeuf, H.S. A qualitative study of the perceived effectiveness of refugee services among consumers, providers, and interpreters. *Transcult. Psychiatry* **2019**, *56*, 827–844. [CrossRef] [PubMed]
17. Burr, K. Local Immigration Partnerships: Building Welcoming and Inclusive Communities through Multi-Level Governance. Available online: http://ontario.p2pcanada.ca/wp-content/blogs.dir/1/files/2011/10/Local-Immigration-Partnerships-Building-Welcoming-and-Inclusive-Communities.pdf (accessed on 9 August 2020).
18. Agency for Toxic Substances and Disease Registry. Models and Frameworks for the Practice of Community Engagement. Available online: https://www.atsdr.cdc.gov/communityengagement/pce_models.html (accessed on 2 January 2022).
19. Arksey, H.; O'Malley, L. Scoping studies: Towards a methodological framework. *Int. J. Soc. Res. Methodol.* **2005**, *8*, 19–32. [CrossRef]
20. Peters, M.D.; Godfrey, C.M.; Khalil, H.; McInerney, P.; Parker, D.; Soares, C.B. Guidance for conducting systematic scoping reviews. *Int. J. Evid-Based Healthc.* **2015**, *13*, 141–146. [CrossRef] [PubMed]
21. Tricco, A.C.; Lillie, E.; Zarin, W.; O'Brien, K.K.; Colquhoun, H.; Levac, D.; Moher, D.; Peters, M.; Horsley, T.; Weeks, L.; et al. PRISMA Extension for Scoping Reviews (PRISMA-ScR): Checklist and Explanation. *Ann. Intern. Med.* **2018**, *169*, 467–473. [CrossRef]
22. Commonwealth Fund. NEW INTERNATIONAL STUDY: U.S. Health System Ranks Last Among 11 Countries; Many Americans Struggle to Afford Care as Income Inequality Widens. Available online: https://www.commonwealthfund.org/press-release/2021/new-international-study-us-health-system-ranks-last-among-11-countries-many (accessed on 2 January 2022).
23. United Nations High Commissioner for Refugees. Asylum-Seekers. Available online: https://www.unhcr.org/asylum-seekers.html (accessed on 2 January 2022).
24. United Nations High Commissioner for Refugees. What Is a Refugee? Available online: https://www.unhcr.org/what-is-a-refugee.html (accessed on 2 January 2022).
25. Statistics Canada. Immigrant. Available online: https://www23.statcan.gc.ca/imdb/p3Var.pl?Function=Unit&Id=85107 (accessed on 2 January 2022).
26. Schneider, E.C.; Sarnak, D.O.; Squires, D.; Shah, A.; Doty, M.M. Mirror, Mirror 2017: International Comparison Reflects Flaw and Opportunities for Better, U.S. Health Care. Available online: https://australiangpalliance.com.au/wp-content/uploads/2018/05/Schneider_mirror_mirror_2017.pdf (accessed on 2 January 2022).
27. Sweileh, W.M.; Wickramage, K.; Pottie, K.; Hui, C.; Roberts, B.; Sawalha, A.F.; Zyoud, S. Bibliometric analysis of global migration health research in peer-reviewed literature (2000–2016). *BMC Public Health* **2018**, *18*, 777. [CrossRef]
28. Taylor, J.; Lamaro Haintz, G. Influence of the social determinants of health on access to healthcare services among refugees in Australia. *Aust. J. Prim. Care* **2017**, *24*, 14–28. [CrossRef]

29. Veritas Health Innovation. *Covidence Systematic Review Software*; Covidence: Melbourne, Australia, 2020; Available online: www.covidence.org (accessed on 2 January 2022).
30. Carroll, C.; Booth, A.; Leaviss, J.; Rick, J. "Best fit" framework synthesis: Refining the method. *BMC Med. Res. Methodol.* **2013**, *13*, 37. [CrossRef]
31. Chadwick, K.A.; Collins, P.A. Examining the relationship between social support availability, urban center size, and self-perceived mental health of recent immigrants to Canada: A mixed-methods analysis. *Soc. Sci. Med.* **2015**, *128*, 220–230. [CrossRef]
32. Cheng, I.H.; McBride, J.; Decker, M.; Watson, T.; Jakubenko, H.; Russo, A. The Asylum Seeker Integrated Healthcare Pathway: A collaborative approach to improving access to primary health care in South Eastern Melbourne, Victoria, Australia. *Aust. J. Prim. Care* **2019**, *25*, 6–12. [CrossRef]
33. Frost, E.L.; Markham, C.; Springer, A. Refugee health education:evaluating a community-based approach to empowering refugee women in Houston, Texas. *Adv. Soc. Work.* **2018**, *18*, 949–964. [CrossRef]
34. Isaacs, S.; Valaitis, R.; Newbold, K.B.; Black, M.; Sargeant, J. Brokering for the primary healthcare needs of recent immigrant families in Atlantic, Canada. *Prim. Health Care Res. Dev.* **2013**, *14*, 63–79. [CrossRef] [PubMed]
35. Isaacs, S.; Valaitis, R.; Newbold, B.; Black, M.; Sargeant, J. Competence trust among providers as fundamental to a culturally competent primary healthcare system for immigrant families. *Prim. Health Care Res. Dev.* **2013**, *14*, 80–89. [CrossRef] [PubMed]
36. Koehn, S.D.; Donahue, M.; Feldman, F.; Drummond, N. Fostering trust and sharing responsibility to increase access to dementia care for immigrant older adults. *Ethn. Health* **2019**, *27*, 83–99. [CrossRef]
37. McMurray, J.; Breward, K.; Breward, M.; Alder, R.; Arya, N. Integrated Primary Care Improves Access to Healthcare for Newly Arrived Refugees in Canada. *J. Immigr. Minor. Health* **2014**, *16*, 576–585. [CrossRef] [PubMed]
38. Salami, B.; Salma, J.; Hegadoren, K. Access and utilization of mental health services for immigrants and refugees: Perspectives of immigrant service providers. *Int. J. Ment. Health Nurs.* **2019**, *28*, 152–161. [CrossRef] [PubMed]
39. Torres, S.; Spitzer, D.L.; Labonté, R.; Amaratunga, C.; Andrew, C. Community health workers in Canada: Innovative approaches to health promotion outreach and community development among immigrant and refugee populations. *J. Ambul. Care Manag.* **2013**, *36*, 305–318. [CrossRef] [PubMed]
40. Saddiq, K.D. *The Two-Tier Settlement System: A Review of Current Newcomer Settlement Services in Canada*; CERIS working paper, no. 34; CERIS—The Ontario Metropolis Centre: Toronto, ON, Canada, 2004.
41. Simich, L.; Beiser, M.; Stewart, M.; Mwakarimba, E. Providing social support for immigrants and refugees in Canada: Challenges and directions. *J. Immigr. Health* **2005**, *7*, 259–268. [CrossRef] [PubMed]
42. Stewart, M.; Anderson, J.; Beiser, M.; Mwakarimba, E.; Neufeld, A.; Simich, L.; Spitzer, D. Multicultural meanings of social support among immigrants and refugees. *Int. Migr.* **2008**, *46*, 123–159. [CrossRef]
43. Flanagan, S.M.; Hancock, B. Reaching the Hard to Reach'—Lessons Learned From the VCS (Voluntary and Community Sector). A Qualitative Study. *BMC Health Serv. Res.* **2010**, *10*, 92–100. [CrossRef] [PubMed]
44. Najafizada, S.A.; Bourgeault, I.L.; Labonte, R.; Packer, C.; Torres, S. Community health workers in Canada and other high-income countries: A scoping review and research gaps. *Can. J. Public Health/Rev. Can. De Sante Publique* **2015**, *106*, e157–e164. [CrossRef] [PubMed]
45. Smithman, M.A.; Descôteaux, S.; Dionne, É.; Richard, L.; Breton, M.; Khanassov, V.; Haggerty, J.L.; IMPACT Research Team. Typology of organizational innovation components: Building blocks to improve access to primary healthcare for vulnerable populations. *Int. J. Equity Health* **2020**, *19*, 174. [CrossRef] [PubMed]
46. Vasquez Guzman, C.E.; Hess, J.M.; Casas, N.; Medina, D.; Galvis, M.; Torres, D.A.; Handal, A.J.; Carreon-Fuentes, A.; Hernandez-Vallant, A.; Chavez, M.J.; et al. Latinx/@ immigrant inclusion trajectories: Individual agency, structural constraints, and the role of community-based organizations in immigrant mobilities. *Am. J. Orthopsychiatr.* **2020**, *90*, 772–786. [CrossRef] [PubMed]

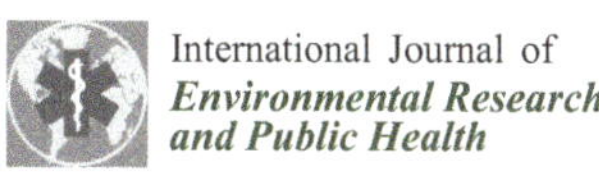

International Journal of
*Environmental Research
and Public Health*

MDPI

Review

Mental Health Screening Approaches for Resettling Refugees and Asylum Seekers: A Scoping Review

Olivia Magwood [1,2], Azaad Kassam [3,4,5], Dorsa Mavedatnia [6], Oreen Mendonca [1], Ammar Saad [1,7,8], Hafsa Hasan [1,9], Maria Madana [6], Dominique Ranger [1], Yvonne Tan [1,10] and Kevin Pottie [1,11,*]

1 C.T. Lamont Primary Care Research Center, Bruyère Research Institute, 85 Primrose Avenue, Ottawa, ON K1R 7G5, Canada; omagwood@bruyere.org (O.M.); oreenmend@gmail.com (O.M.); ammar.saad@uottawa.ca (A.S.); hafsa.hsnn@gmail.com (H.H.); dominiqueranger.730@gmail.com (D.R.); yvonnetann@yahoo.com (Y.T.)
2 Interdisciplinary School of Health Sciences, Faculty of Health Sciences, University of Ottawa, 25 University Private, Ottawa, ON K1N 7K4, Canada
3 Department of Psychiatry, University of Ottawa, 75 Laurier Ave E, Ottawa, ON K1N 6N5, Canada; a.kassam@pqchc.com
4 Pinecrest-Queensway Community Health Centre, 1365 Richmond Rd #2, Ottawa, ON K2B 6R7, Canada
5 Ottawa Newcomer Health Centre, 291 Argyle, Ottawa, ON K2P 1B8, Canada
6 Faculty of Medicine, University of Ottawa, 451 Smyth Road, Ottawa, ON K1H 8M5, Canada; dmave060@uottawa.ca (D.M.); mmada042@uottawa.ca (M.M.)
7 School of Epidemiology and Public Health, University of Ottawa, 600 Peter Morand Crescent, Ottawa, ON K1G 5Z3, Canada
8 Children's Hospital of Eastern Ontario Research Institute, Ottawa, ON K1H 5B2, Canada
9 Institute of Health Policy, Management and Evaluation, University of Toronto, 155 College St, Toronto, ON M5T 3M6, Canada
10 Faculty of Arts and Sciences, Queen's University, 99 University Ave, Kingston, ON K7L 3N6, Canada
11 Department of Family Medicine, Western University, London, ON N6A 3K7, Canada
* Correspondence: kpottie@uwo.ca

Citation: Magwood, O.; Kassam, A.; Mavedatnia, D.; Mendonca, O.; Saad, A.; Hasan, H.; Madana, M.; Ranger, D.; Tan, Y.; Pottie, K. Mental Health Screening Approaches for Resettling Refugees and Asylum Seekers: A Scoping Review. *Int. J. Environ. Res. Public Health* **2022**, *19*, 3549. https://doi.org/10.3390/ijerph19063549

Academic Editors: Greg Armstrong and Shameran Slewa-Younan

Received: 27 January 2022
Accepted: 8 March 2022
Published: 16 March 2022

Publisher's Note: MDPI stays neutral with regard to jurisdictional claims in published maps and institutional affiliations.

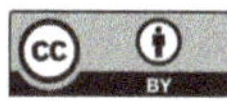

Abstract: Refugees and asylum seekers often face delayed mental health diagnoses, treatment, and care. COVID-19 has exacerbated these issues. Delays in diagnosis and care can reduce the impact of resettlement services and may lead to poor long-term outcomes. This scoping review aims to characterize studies that report on mental health screening for resettling refugees and asylum seekers pre-departure and post-arrival to a resettlement state. We systematically searched six bibliographic databases for articles published between 1995 and 2020 and conducted a grey literature search. We included publications that evaluated early mental health screening approaches for refugees of all ages. Our search identified 25,862 citations and 70 met the full eligibility criteria. We included 45 publications that described mental health screening programs, 25 screening tool validation studies, and we characterized 85 mental health screening tools. Two grey literature reports described pre-departure mental health screening. Among the included publications, three reported on two programs for women, 11 reported on programs for children and adolescents, and four reported on approaches for survivors of torture. Programs most frequently screened for overall mental health, PTSD, and depression. Important considerations that emerged from the literature include cultural and psychological safety to prevent re-traumatization and digital tools to offer more private and accessible self-assessments.

Keywords: refugee; asylum seeker; mental health; resettlement; migration; screening; health assessment

1. Introduction

Approximately 79.5 million people around the world have been forced to leave their homes, and nearly 26 million are considered refugees [1]. The COVID-19 pandemic has also created unprecedented delays in resettlement [2]. In 2022, a projected 1.47 million refugees will need urgent resettlement [3]. "Resettlement" is the selection and transfer of refugees from a state in which they have sought temporary protection to a third state that has agreed to admit them as refugees with permanent residence status [4]. This status ensures protection against refoulement and provides a resettled refugee and their family or dependents with access to civil, political, economic, social, and cultural rights [1]. Conversely, an asylum seeker is someone whose claim for protection and resettlement has not yet been finally decided on by the country in which the claim is submitted [5].

Providing refugees and asylum seekers appropriate and timely mental health services is a global challenge [6]. Most recently, the COVID-19 pandemic has dramatically reduced programs and delayed refugee resettlement, thereby increasing uncertainty and isolation [2,7]. Early screening and care for common mental health disorders is now recognized as a priority for resettlement programs [8,9]. However, there is a risk that screening for mental health can lead to re-traumatization [10]. Therefore, screening approaches should incorporate safety, comfort, physical care, ensure access to basic needs, and use culturally appropriate tools and clinical assessments [11].

Refugees encounter many risk factors for poor mental health outcomes before, during, and after migration and resettlement [6]. Such factors include exposure to traumatic violence, genocide, and economic hardship; experience of physical harm and separation; and poor socioeconomic conditions once resettled, such as social isolation, racism, and unemployment [12,13]. Refugees are at risk of developing common mental health disorders including depression, anxiety, posttraumatic stress disorder (PTSD), and related somatic health symptoms [6,14,15]. Epidemiological studies indicate that the age-standardized point prevalence of PTSD and major depression in conflict-affected populations is estimated to be 12.9% and 7.6%, respectively [16]. As a comparison, it has been estimated that approximately 4.4% of the world's population suffers from major depression [17] and 3.3% from PTSD [18]. However, the true prevalence of common mental disorders among refugees could be higher since there is no systematic or consistent approach to diagnose mental disorders in this population [12].

Pre-departure overseas health assessments and screening represent a potential, but often underdeveloped, component of the migration health screening process for resettling refugees. A health assessment is a medical examination, usually conducted by a registered medical practitioner (or "panel physician") based on criteria set by the resettlement state [19]. Health assessments are conducted as a measure to limit or prevent the transmission of diseases of public health importance to their host populations and to avert potential costs and burdens on local health systems [19]. These assessments support the health of migrating populations as well as protect domestic public health, promote collaboration with international health partners, and strengthen understanding of the health profiles of diverse arriving populations [20]. For example, health assessment results may be communicated to local resettlement agencies so that appropriate health services can be arranged for the refugees on arrival [21]. However, if refugee health assessment processors are to meaningfully contribute to the public health good, then they need to overcome exclusionary approaches, be linked to the national health systems, and be complemented by health promotion measures to enhance the health-seeking behaviour of refugees [19]. Currently, there are 24 official resettlement states (See Supplementary File S1) for whom pre-departure mental health screening approaches for refugees could be beneficial.

Current health assessments do not routinely screen for common mental health concerns. Providing early care for treatable mental health conditions could help refugees benefit from resettlement, language, cultural and employment training programs, develop positive relationships, reduce intergenerational trauma, gain access to employment, and ultimately lead to more meaningful and productive lives [8]. Developing early common mental health screening and treatment programs is therefore an important first step when integrating refugees into local primary healthcare services [22].

The majority of synthesized literature on refugee mental health to date focuses on the prevalence of mental illness (for example, [23–25]); access to mental health services (for example, [26,27]); and tailored programs and interventions (for example, [28–30]).

There is limited available evidence which characterizes screening tools and procedures specific to assessing mental health among refugee and asylum-seeking populations during resettlement. One existing systematic review identified only seven screening tools for trauma and mental health assessment in refugee children [31]. Older reviews suggest that more tools have been used among adult populations; however, the authors concluded that existing tools had limited or untested validity and reliability in refugees [32,33].

2. Research Objectives

The objective of this scoping review is to identify and characterize mental health screening approaches for refugees and asylum seekers. This review aims to inform and catalyze country-level resettlement policies and practices regarding the identification of mental health conditions and linkage to care by addressing the following research question:

What are the characteristics of existing and emerging approaches to mental health screening for resettling refugees and asylum seekers? (See Box 1).

Box 1. Research sub-questions

➢ In what setting(s) has refugee mental health screening been conducted?
➢ At what point in time during the migration pathway is screening conducted and for what purpose?
➢ What tools have been used in the refugee population, and what conditions do they screen for?
➢ In which language(s) and formats are mental health assessments delivered?
➢ Have any of these tools been adapted, validated, or evaluated specifically for use among refugees?
➢ What approaches are used to screen vulnerable subgroups?
➢ What are the professional characteristics and training of individuals who administer mental health assessments?
➢ What are the lessons learned from pilots/approaches that have been tried on the ground?

3. Methods

We registered the methods of this scoping review on the Open Science Framework (DOI: 10.17605/OSF.IO/RWVBE) and published an open-access protocol [34]. We reported our review according to the PRISMA extension for scoping reviews (PRISMA-ScR; [35]) [Supplementary File S2]. We reported our search strategy according to the PRISMA Statement for Reporting Literature Searches in Systematic Reviews (PRISMA-S; [36]) [Supplementary File S3]. We created a logic model to outline the conceptual framework involved in the mental health screening process (Figure 1).

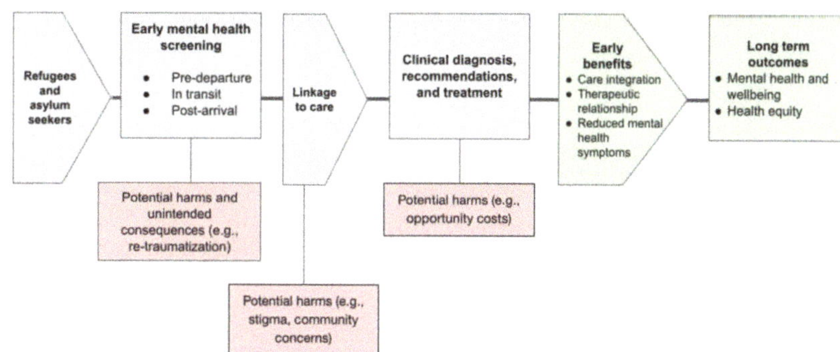

Figure 1. Logic model of mental health screening along the resettlement pathway.

4. Eligibility Criteria

We identified eligible studies using the SPIDER acronym (Table 1). We included publications of quantitative, qualitative, or mixed-methods evidence that evaluated approaches to the early screening of mental health disorders among resettling refugees and asylum seekers of all ages. We defined the resettling period as 6 months prior to travel and 12 months after arrival in the resettlement country. We excluded qualitative publications that focused on patient experiences rather than characteristics of early screening approaches. By "approach", we mean the process from the assessment of mental health to the transfer of results to the patient, immigration officials, or healthcare providers, including the development of the assessment tool itself if it included pilot-testing and validation among refugees. We considered documents published in any language. We restricted the year of publication from 1995 to 2020 to coincide with the creation of the Annual Tripartite Consultations on Resettlement (ATCR) and subsequent UNHCR Resettlement Handbook [37].

Table 1. Eligibility criteria.

SPIDER	Inclusion Criteria	Exclusion Criteria
Sample	Refugees and asylum seekers of all ages	All populations other than refugees and asylum seekers
Phenomenon of Interest	Pre-settlement overseas screening approaches or post-arrival (<12 months) approaches for mental health	Screening for other health conditions Routine screening after 1 year post-arrival
Design	Experimental and quasi-experimental studies Observational studies Program evaluations Resettlement handbooks and manuals Policy documents Development & validation studies Clinical assessment studies	Systematic reviews Scoping reviews Literature reviews Commentaries/opinion Theoretical papers
Evaluation	Characteristics of screening approaches	Estimates of effect Experiences/views
Research type	Quantitative, qualitative, or mixed-method documents published in peer-reviewed or grey literature	N/A
Other		
Year of publication	1995–2020	Prior to 1995
Language of publication	All languages eligible	N/A

5. Search Methods

We developed our search strategies in consultation with a health sciences librarian. We searched the following databases, individually, from 1995 to 2020: EMBASE (Ovid; 1995 to 24 December 2020); Medline (Ovid; 1995 to 21 December 2020); PsycINFO (Ovid; 1995 to December Week 3 2020); Cochrane Central Register of Controlled Trials (CENTRAL) (Ovid; 1995 to January Week 2 2021); Cumulative Index to Nursing and Allied Health Literature (CINAHL) (Ebsco; January 1995 to January Week 2 2021). We used a combination of keywords and subject headings. Complete search strategies for each database are available in Supplementary File S4.

In addition to searching bibliographic databases, we conducted a focused grey literature search. We searched the government websites from the 24 countries listed in Supplementary File S1 and the International Organization for Migration (IOM). We contacted an immigration policy researcher from each country of the Immigration and Refugee Health Working Group (Australia, Canada, New Zealand, United Kingdom, United States of America) and other experts to identify any missing literature.

6. Screening and Selection

We used Covidence software [38] and a two-part study selection process: (1) a title and abstract review, and (2) full-text review. Two review authors independently assessed all potential studies and documents against a priori inclusion and exclusion criteria (Table 1). We resolved any disagreements through discussion, or we consulted a third review author.

7. Data Extraction and Management

We developed a standardized extraction sheet. Pairs of reviewers extracted data in duplicate and independently. They compared results and resolved disagreements by discussion or with help from a third reviewer. To ensure the validity of the data extraction form, we piloted this form with two reviewers and the accuracy of the content was confirmed with a third reviewer. Reviewers extracted all variables identified in our protocol [34].

8. Synthesis of Results

We summarized the data according to the setting, timing, and purpose of the assessment, as well as the characteristics of screening tools and administrators. We narratively described approaches for special populations and implementation lessons learned, as described by the study authors. As a scoping review, the purpose of this study is to present an overview of the research rather than to evaluate the quality of the individual studies; therefore, we did not conduct an overall assessment or appraisal of the strength of the evidence.

9. Results

Our systematic search identified 25,857 citations. After the removal of duplicates, we screened 14,607 citations by title and abstract. We retained 315 for full text review. Of these, 66 met full eligibility criteria. Reasons for exclusion are presented in Figure 2 and Supplementary File S5. Additionally, our grey literature search identified two additional publications for inclusion. Two studies were brought forward by immigration representatives and other subject matter experts, for a total of 70 included studies.

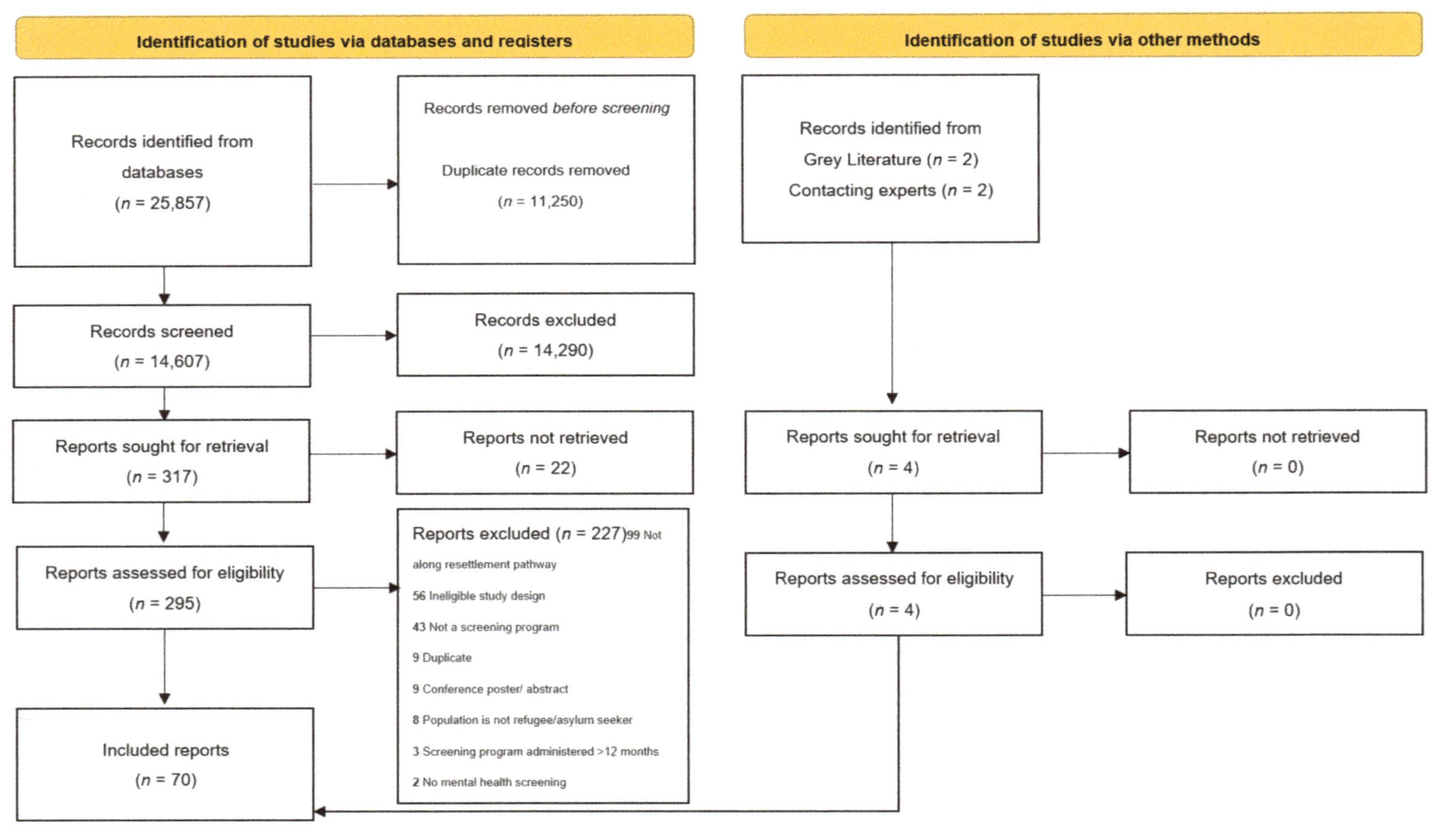

Figure 2. PRISMA Flow Diagram.

10. Characteristics of Included Studies

We summarized the characteristics of all included publications of refugee mental health screening approaches (see Table 2). This included 45 publications which described screening programs, and 25 validation studies conducted in 13 different resettlement countries. Most assessments (90% of included studies) occurred within the first 12 months post-arrival to the resettlement country (see Figure 3). We identified two reports of pre-departure screening prior to resettlement [4,39]. Post-arrival assessments were most common in the USA, Switzerland, and Australia (See Figure 4). While some assessments were conducted in tertiary care settings (i.e., hospitals), most refugees sought health assessments in primary care clinics or interdisciplinary refugee health clinics (see Figure 5). Assessments were also held in community or public health centres or other settings such as detention centres, national intermediary centres, independent medical examinations, and torture treatment centres. One study reported that mental health screening was most effective when completed during a home visit [40]. Among publications which included asylum seeker populations (18/70), the majority conducted screening at reception centres and asylum accommodations.

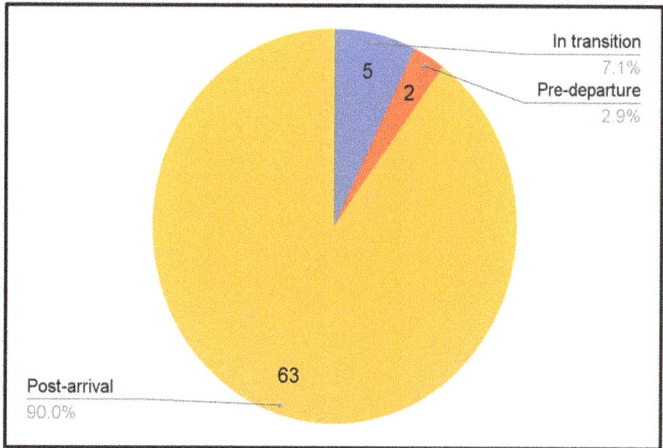

Figure 3. Timing of mental health assessments.

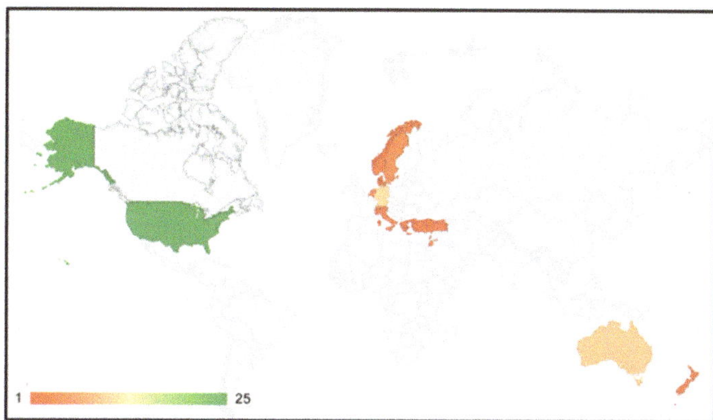

Figure 4. Global distribution of mental health assessments for refugees and asylum seekers according to setting of screening. To note: we identified one publication on pre-departure screening conducted in Lebanon prior to departure to the UK.

Table 2. Characteristics of included studies ($n = 70$).

Study	Design	Setting	Timing of Assessment	Population	Mental Health Condition Assessed and Assessment Tool	Administration Details
Al-Obaidi (2015) [41]	Screening program	Refugee health care programs USA	Post-arrival	Refugees Burma, Haiti, Sudan, Iraq, Afghanistan, Somalia, and Cuba	Mental health assessment was not widely practiced (6/16 refugee-serving organizations). Assessment conducted by asking a few basic questions, e.g., for adults, any history of sleep problems, loss of energy, loss of appetite, feeling depressed, torture; and asking about the story of the refugee's journey; for children, any history of seizures, learning problems, and head injuries In Denver, screening includes a DSM-based, non-validated questionnaire designed to detect major depression and PTSD The Seattle and New Mexico programs offer the Refugee Health Screener-15 (RHS-15) [PTSD, Depression, Anxiety]	In Denver, the mental health screening is conducted by a master's level social worker Screening using the RHS-15 administered by health care providers. Clients themselves can complete the form if they have the appropriate level of education Interpreter not present Oral interview Assessment time not reported
Arnetz (2014) [42]	Validation study	Community centees USA	Post-arrival	Refugees Age 18–69 years, M = 33.41, SD = 11.29 54% male Iraq	Pre-immigration trauma exposure: Trauma section of Harvard Trauma Questionnaire (HTQ) PTSD: Civilian version of the PTSD Checklist (PCL-C) Depression: Hospital Anxiety and Depression Scale (HADS)	Administered by trained Arabic-speaking research personnel Interpreter present Self-assessment survey 120 min
Baird (2020) [43]	Screening program	Nurse-managed urban primary care safety-net clinic USA	Post-arrival	Refugees Mean age 32.8 years, SD = 13.6, Range = 17–72; 46% male. Country of origin not reported	Emotional distress including anxiety, depression, and PTSD: Refugee Health Screener-15 (RHS-15)	Administered by trained Doctor of Nursing Practice (DNP) family nurse practitioners Interpreter present Likert Scale, oral interview 60 min
Barbieri (2019) [44]	Validation study	Outpatient clinic and reception centre Italy	Post-arrival	Refugees and asylum seekers Age 18 and older (M = 25.1 years, SD = 6.7); 86% male Participants were from 19 African countries, mainly West Africa	PTSD: Posttraumatic Stress Disorder Checklist (PCL-5) CPTSD: International Trauma Questionnaire (ICD-11)	Administered by cultural mediator, a medical doctor, and a clinical psychologist Interpreter present Oral interview 60–90 min

Table 2. *Cont.*

Study	Design	Setting	Timing of Assessment	Population	Mental Health Condition Assessed and Assessment Tool	Administration Details
Barnes (2001) [40]	Screening program	Local health department not affiliated with a hospital, combined with home visits USA	Post-arrival	Refugees Age 18–74 46.4% male Vietnam, Cuba, Bosnia, and African countries	Depression: DSM-IV criteria psychiatric interview	Administered by psychiatric residents with multi-national immigrant backgrounds (Africa and India) Interpretation provided by a paid interpreter (Vietnamese), administrative assistant (Bosnian), or nurse (Spanish). Family members also acted as interpreters (e.g., Farsi) Oral interview Assessment time not reported
Bertelsen (2018) [45]	Screening program	Primary care torture treatment centre USA	Post-arrival	Asylum seekers Mean age of 36.6 years (SD10.2) 66.2% male Majority from Sub-Saharan Africa (Guinea, Burkina Faso, and Democratic Republic of Congo being the most represented). Minority from Asia (with the Nepal and Tibet accounting for the majority of these)	PTSD: Harvard Trauma Questionnaire (HTQ) Major depressive disorder: Patient Health Questionnaire-9 (PHQ-9)	Administered by mental health professionals Interpreter present Oral interview Assessment time not reported
Bjarta (2018) [46]	Validation study	Asylum accommodations and health and service centres Sweden	Post-arrival	Refugees and asylum seekers aged 18 years and older; 72% male Afghanistan, Syria, Iraq, Iran, Eritrea, and Somalia	PTSD, depression, anxiety: Refugee Health Screener (RHS-13) Depression: Patient Health Questionnaire 9 (PHQ-9) Generalized anxiety: Generalized Anxiety Disorder 7 (GAD-7) PTSD: Primary Care PTSD-4 (PC-PTSD-4) Quality of life: World Health Organization Quality of Life–Brief Version (WHOQOL-BREF)	Self-assessment facilitated by bilingual administration staff Interpreter (bilingual staff) present Tablet. Audio support was available in Arabic, Dari, Farsi, and Tigrinya for individuals with low reading proficiency Assessment time not reported
Boyle (2019) [47]	Screening program	Refugee antenatal clinic Australia	Post-arrival	Refugees of childbearing age (below 35 years old) 100% female Afghanistan, Myanmar, Iraq, the Republic of South Sudan, and Sri Lanka.	Depression and anxiety: Edinburgh Postnatal Depression Scale (EPDS) Perinatal mental health: Monash Psychosocial Screening Tool	Self-assessment. Clinic staff available for assistance Interpreter present if needed Electronic via tablet 6–10 min

Table 2. *Cont.*

Study	Design	Setting	Timing of Assessment	Population	Mental Health Condition Assessed and Assessment Tool	Administration Details
Brink (2016) [48]	Validation study	Primary care clinic USA	Post-arrival	Karen Refugees Aged 18–80 (M = 38.09, SD 13.82) 30% male Burma	PTSD and MDD: PTSD and MDD portions of the structured clinical interview for DSM disorders (SCID-CV for DSM-IV)	A physician with mental health training and a Karen interpreter administered the measures Oral interview and Likert-scale questionnaire Assessment time not reported
Buchwald (1995) [49]	Screening program	Ten refugee public health clinics USA	Post-arrival	Refugees Aged 16–85 yo (average age 31) 95% male Vietnam	Depression: Vietnamese Depression Scale	Administered by trained community health nurse Interpreter present Self-assessment 5 min
Churbaji (2020) [50]	Validation study	University hospital Germany	Post-arrival	Refugees Mean age 33.5 yo 75% male Syria, Iraq, Palestine	Depression and PTSD: Mini International Neuropsychiatric Interview (MINI) Depression: Patient Health Questionnaire, 9 (PHQ-9) PTSD: Harvard Trauma Questionnaire (HTQ)	Not reported
Cook (2015) [51]	Screening program	Primary care clinic USA	Post-arrival	Arabic-speaking Karen refugees Aged 18 yo and over (mean age: 35 (SD 14.6) 51% male	Four semi-structured items which asked retrospectively about lifetime experiences of primary and secondary war trauma and torture	Administered by trained research assistants (social work trainees) Interpreter present Oral interview Assessment time not reported
Di Pietro (2021) [52]	Validation study	Second-line reception centre Italy	Post-arrival	Unaccompanied migrant minors Age 12–18 yo 100% male Bangladesh, Egypt, Gambia, Senegal, Benin, Tunisia, Guinea Bissau, Morocco	Overall psychological needs: Unaccompanied Migrant Minors Questionnaire (AEGIS-Q)	Interpreter not present Self-administered with cultural mediator 20 min
Durieux-Paillard (2006) [53]	Validation study	Migrant health centre (University Hospital) Switzerland	Post-arrival	Asylum seekers Age 16 years or older	MDD and PTSD: Mini International Neuropsychiatric Interview (MINI)	Nurses without mental health training Interpreter present Oral interview 45 min

Table 2. *Cont.*

Study	Design	Setting	Timing of Assessment	Population	Mental Health Condition Assessed and Assessment Tool	Administration Details
El Ghaziri (2019) [54]	Screening program	Centre for primary care and public health Switzerland	Post-arrival	Refugee families Members over age 8 yo 40–60% female Syria	Risk behaviours: ASSIST Support: Multidimensional Scale of Perceived Social Support (MSPSS) Parent-child relationship: Family Peer Relationship Questionnaire, Arabic version (A-FPRQ) Adults: major depressive disorder, panic disorder, posttraumatic stress disorder, generalized anxiety: Mini International Neuropsychiatric Interview (MINI) Children: major depressive disorder, panic disorder, separation anxiety, posttraumatic stress disorder: Mini International Neuropsychiatric Interview for Kids (MINI Kid)	Research assistant Interpreter present (research assistant) Administration mode not reported Assessment time not reported
Eytan (2007) [55]	Validation study	Primary care clinic Switzerland	In transition	Refugees Mean age 30 yo 75% male 33 countries, mostly Africa and Central or Eastern Europe	Major depressive episodes and PTSD: Mini International Neuropsychiatric Interview (MINI)	Administered by trained nurse Interpreter present Oral interview Assessment time not reported
Eytan (2002) [56]	Screening program	IME assessment Switzerland	In transition	Refugees, median age 24 yo 72% male Kosovo	MDD and PTSD: Mini International Neuropsychiatric Interview (MINI)	Administered by trained nurse Interpreter present Oral interview Assessment time not reported
Geltman (2005) [57]	Screening program	Unaccompanied Refugee Minors Program (URMP) sites USA	Post-arrival	Refugee minors, mean age 17.6 yo 84% male Sudan	PTSD: Harvard Trauma Questionnaire (HTQ) and Child Health Questionnaire (CHQ)	Administered by staff Interpreter not present Oral interview and self-assessment Assessment time not reported
Green (2021) [58]	Screening program	Primary care "office" USA	Post-arrival	Refugees, age 4–18 yo 56% male Bhutan, Burma, Democratic Republic of Congo/Burundi, Iraq, Somalia	PTSD, depression, trauma: Strengths and Difficulties Questionnaire (SDQ)	Administered by interpreters Interpreter present Oral interview Assessment time not reported
Hanes (2017) [59]	Screening program	Hospital refugee health service Australia	Post-arrival	Refugees Age 2–16 yo mean age 9.4 yo 49% male Top 7 countries: Burma, Afghanistan, Sudan, Ethiopia Congo, Somalia, Iran	Adverse childhood experiences: Strengths and Difficulties Questionnaire (SDQ)	Interpreter present Self-administered Assessment time not reported

Table 2. *Cont.*

Study	Design	Setting	Timing of Assessment	Population	Mental Health Condition Assessed and Assessment Tool	Administration Details
Hauff (1995) [60]	Screening program	n/a Norway	Post-arrival	Refugees Age over 15 yo 79% male Vietnam	Psychiatric disorders: Symptom Checklist 90 (SCL-90) and Present State Examination (PSE)	Researcher Interpreter present Oral interview Assessment time not reported
Heenan (2019) [61]	Screening program	Specialist immigrant health service within a children's hospital Australia	Post-arrival	Refugee children Age 7 months to 16 years old 64.8% male Syria, Iraq	Mental health (including PTSD) and development screening was conducted, but no assessment tool is described	Refugee health program nurses Primary care health assessment Assessment time not reported
Hirani (2018) [62]	Screening program	Tertiary refugee health service Australia	Post-arrival	Adolescent refugees Age 12–17 years old (mean age 14; 49% male) 15 countries (Middle East, Africa, Asia)	Psychosocial assessment: Home, Education/Eating, Activities, Drugs, Sexuality, Suicide/mental health' (HEADSS) Questionnaire	Interviewer Interpreter present Oral interview 25–60 min
Hobbs (2002) [63]	Screening program	Public health hospital New Zealand	Post-arrival	Asylum seekers Age 0–60+ years old 68.1% male Middle Eastern countries	Symptoms, or history of symptoms, of psychological illness: Auckland Public Health Protection Asylum Seekers Screening	Clinic staff Health screening Assessment time not reported
Hocking (2018) [64]	Validation study	Asylum seeker welfare centre Australia	Post-arrival	Refugees 19–82 yo, median age 33 69.8% male Mostly from countries in Africa and Asia	Major depressive disorder (MDD) and post-traumatic stress disorder (PTSD): Mental Health Screening Tool for Asylum seekers and Refugees (STAR-MH)	Administered by trained non-mental health workers Interpreter present Oral interview 6 min
Hollifield (2013) [65]	Validation study	Public health centre USA	Post-arrival	Refugees Age over 14 yo 50% male Bhutan, Burma, and Iraq	Anxiety, depression, PTSD: Refugee Health Screener-15 (RHS-15)	Administered by physicians or public health clinic staff Interpreter present Oral interview 4–12 min
Hollifield (2016) [66]	Validation study	Public health centre USA	Post-arrival	Refugees Age over 14 yo 50% male Bhutan, Burma, and Iraq	Anxiety and depression: Hopkins Symptom Checklist 25 (HSCL-25) PTSD: Posttraumatic Symptom Scale- Self Report (PSS-SR) Anxiety, depression, PTSD: Refugee Health Screener-15 (RHS-15)	Administered by trained public health nurses Interpreter not present Oral interview Assessment time not reported

Table 2. *Cont.*

Study	Design	Setting	Timing of Assessment	Population	Mental Health Condition Assessed and Assessment Tool	Administration Details
Hough (2019) [39]	Screening program	Refugee clinic Lebanon	Pre-departure	Refugees 18 years and above 50% male Syria	General mental health: Global Mental Health Assessment Tool (GMHAT)	Administered by healthcare professionals (psychiatrist, general physician, pediatrician, and two nurses) Administrators served as translators Computerized tool 15–20 min
International Organization for Migration (IOM) (2020) [4]	Screening program	IOM migration health assessment clinics Lebanon, Turkey, and Jordan	Pre-departure	Refugees: majority younger than 30 (67.1%), with the highest number in the under-10 age group 51.2% male	Not described	Not described
Jakobsen (2017) [67]	Validation study	Setting not reported Norway	Post-arrival	Unaccompanied adolescent asylum seekers Age 15–18 years old (mean: 16.2) 100% male Afghanistan, Somalia	PTSD, anxiety, and depression: combined Hopkins Symptom Checklist-25 (HSCL-25) and Harvard Trauma Questionnaire (HTQ- IV)	Interpreter present Self-administered via laptop computer Assessment duration not reported
Javanbakht (2019) [68]	Screening program	Primary care clinic USA	Post-arrival	Refugees Age 18–65 yo 52.9% male Syria	PTSD: PTSD Checklist Civilian version (PCL-C) Anxiety and depression: Hopkins Symptom Checklist 25 items (HSCL-25)	Research assistant Interpreter present (research assistant) Self-assessment 20 min (5–10 min per tool)
Johnson-Agbakwu (2014) [69]	Screening program	Refugee women's health clinic with a behavioural health partnership USA	Post-arrival	Refugees Age 18 years and older 100% female Iraq, Burma, Somalia	Anxiety, depression, PTSD: Refugee Health Screener-15 (RHS-15)	Cultural health navigator (served as interpreter) Oral interview 5–10 min
Kaltenbach (2017) [70]	Validation study	Refugee accommodation Germany	In transition	Refugees Age over 12 yo, median age 28.79 yo Majority from Syria, minority from Afghanistan, Albania, Kosovo, Serbia, Iraq, Macedonia, Somalia, Georgia	PTSD, depression, anxiety: Refugee Health Screener-15 (RHS-15) Semi-structured interview: PTSD: Post-traumatic Stress Disorder Checklist-5 (PCL-5) Depression: Refugee Health Screener (RHS-15)—only the first 13 questions Trauma exposure: Life Events Checklist (LEC-5) Psychological distress: semi-structured interview via Brief Symptom Inventory -18	RHS Self-administered Interpreter present if needed 10–30 min Semi-structured interview by a clinical psychologist Interpreter present Oral interview 90 min

Table 2. *Cont.*

Study	Design	Setting	Timing of Assessment	Population	Mental Health Condition Assessed and Assessment Tool	Administration Details
Kennedy (1999) [71]	Screening program	Primary care clinic (University Hospital) USA	Post-arrival	Adult refugees and their children	Depression, anxiety, and PTSD: A set of questions about history of imprisonment, trauma, or torture + a 25-item, self-administered symptom checklist that surveys for symptoms of depression, anxiety, and PTSD. The checklist was developed by Dawn Noggle, PhD, of the International Rescue Committee in Arizona. In addition, parents are asked standard questions about their children's adjustment and symptoms of stress or depression	Administered by nurse or physician Interpreter present Self-assessment symptom checklist Assessment time not reported
Kleijn (2001) [72]	Validation study	Psychiatric clinic Netherlands	Post-arrival	Refugees 81% male Arabic, Farsi, or Serbo-Croatian speaking regions	PTSD: The Harvard Trauma Questionnaire (HTQ) Depression and Anxiety: Hopkins Symptoms Checklist-25(HSCL-25)	Administered by psychologist or psychiatrist Interpreter present Self-assessment Assessment time not reported
Kleinert (2019) [73]	Screening program	Primary care centre within a reception centre Germany	Post-arrival	Refugee and asylum seekers median age of all patients was 26 years, SD 18.529 51% of asylum-seeker patients and 49% of resettlement-refugee patients were female Iraq, Syria, Afghanistan, Georgia, Iran	Mental and behavioural disorders classified by ICD 10: Digital Communication Assistance Tool (DCAT)	General practitioners and nurses Digital Communication Assistance Tool (DCAT) via tablet No interpreter present Self-assessment Assessment time not reported
Kroger (2016) [74]	Screening Program	Reception centre Germany	Post-arrival	Refugees and asylum seekers Average age 30.5 88.2% male Balkan States, Middle East, Northern Africa, rest of Africa	PTSD: Post-traumatic Diagnostic Scale-8 (PDS-8) Depression: Patient Health Questionnaire (PHQ-8)	Administered by psychological psychotherapist, medical assistant, or psychology undergraduate students Interpreter present Oral interview 15–90 min
LeMaster (2018) [75]	Screening program	Local resettlement agencies USA	Post-arrival	Refugees Mean age 33.4 Iraq	PTSD: civilian version of the PTSD Checklist (PCL-C) and Harvard Trauma Questionnaire (HTQ) Depression: Hospital Anxiety and Depression Scale	Administered by a trained Arabic-speaking interviewer Interpreter present Oral interview 120 min
Lillee (2015) [76]	Screening program	Humanitarian entrant health service Australia	Post-arrival	Refugees Age 18–70 48.7% male Africa, South-Eastern and South-Western Asia	Non-specific psychological distress: The Kessler Psychological Distress Scale (K10) PTSD: PTSD treatment screener	Administered by physicians Interpreter present Oral interview or self-assessment 10–15 min

Table 2. *Cont.*

Study	Design	Setting	Timing of Assessment	Population	Mental Health Condition Assessed and Assessment Tool	Administration Details
Loutan (1999) [77]	Screening program	University Hospital Switzerland	Post-arrival	Refugees Median age 27 67% male Yugoslavia, Somalia, Angola, Sri-Lanka	Physical and psychological symptoms and previous exposure to traumatic events: No name; short questionnaire developed and tested at the Policlinic	Administered by trained nurses (who were multilingual) Interpreter not present Oral interview 15 min
Masmas (2008) [78]	Screening program	Reception centre Denmark	Post-arrival	Asylum seekers, average age 32 years (16–73 years) 71% male Afghanistan, Iraq, Iran, Syria, and Chechnya	PTSD: International Classification of Disease Codes (ICD-10) Overall psychological health: WHO's General Health Questionnaire	Administered by trained health care professionals Translator available if needed Oral interview 60 min
McLeod (2005) [79]	Screening program	Refugee resettlement centre medical clinic New Zealand	Post-arrival	Refugees: majority 20–34 years old 53.2% male, 34 different nationalities, majority Iraqi, Somali, Ethiopian	Psychosocial assessment—screening tool not reported	Administered by trained health care professionals Administration details not reported
Mewes 2018 [80]	Validation study	Asylum accommodation or at meeting points for asylum seekers Germany	Post-arrival	Asylum seekers Aged 18 years and older (M = 31.9 years SD 7.8), 67% male Most participants came from Iran, Afghanistan, Syria, or African countries	PTSD and depression: Process of Recognition and Orientation of Torture Victims in European Countries to Facilitate Care and Treatment (PROTECT) Questionnaire PTSD: Posttraumatic Diagnostic Scale (PDS) Depression: Patient Health Questionnaire-9 (PHQ9)	Self-assessment The software 'MultiCasi' was used via a laptop with touchscreen Interpreter present Assessment time not reported
Morina (2017) [81]	Screening program	Clinical setting outpatient clinic Switzerland	Post-arrival	Refugees Aged 28–64 (mean 50.07, SD 8.65) 77% male Afghanistan, Sri Lanka, Iraq, Turkey, Sudan	PTSD: Posttraumatic Diagnostic Scale based on DSM-5 (PDS) Depression: Hopkins Symptom Checklist-25 (HSCL-25) Quality of Life: EUROHIS-QoL Questionnaire	Interview with therapist Interpreter present Oral interview Assessed in 24 min or Computer assisted self-interviews using multi-adaptive psychological screening software (MAPSS) Tablet Assessed in 9 min

Table 2. *Cont.*

Study	Design	Setting	Timing of Assessment	Population	Mental Health Condition Assessed and Assessment Tool	Administration Details
Nehring (2021) [82]	Validation study	Reception camp Germany	Post-arrival	Refugee children Age 4–14 years (mean: 8.9 years (SD: 2.8)) tijana59.0% male Syria	PTSD: Child Behaviour Checklist (CBCL)	Child and adolescent psychiatrists Interpreter and native speaking doctors were present Oral interview with parents and children The duration of all examinations lasted 1–2 days for one family
Nikendei (2019) [83]	Screening program	Outpatient clinic Germany	Post-arrival	Asylum seekers Age over 18 yo Asia, Africa, Eastern Europe	PTSD: Primary Care PTSD Screen for DSM-5 (PC-PTSD-5) Depression: Patient Health Questionnaire-2 (PHQ-2) General anxiety: Generalized Anxiety Disorder (GAD-2) Panic symptoms: PHQ-PD Social well-being: World Health Organization- Five Well-Being Index (WHO-5) Alcohol and drug addiction: three screening questions derived from the screening questions from the SCID (Structured Clinical Interview)	Research assistant Interpreter available Self-assessment Assessment time not reported
Ovitt (2003) [84]	Screening program	Resettlement office or at participants' homes USA	Post-arrival	Refugees Ages 29–72 yo 50% male Bosnia	Anxiety and depression: The Hopkins Symptom Checklist-25 (HSCL-25) and a client questionnaire	Psychiatrist or medical doctor Interpreter not present Oral interview Assessment time not reported
Polcher (2016) [85]	Screening program	Community health centre USA	Post-arrival	Refugees Ages 18 yo or older tijana41% male Bhutan, Iraq, Somalia, Congo, Sudan, Burma, Iran, and Eritrea	Anxiety, depression and PTSD: Refugee Health Screener–15 (RHS-15)	Administered by trained interpreters and medical assistants Interpreter present Oral interview 10–15 min
Poole (2020) [86]	Validation study	Refugee camp Greece	In transition	Refugees Mean age 30 years, range 18–61. 59% male Syria	Major Depressive Disorder (MDD): Patient Health Questionnaires (PHQ-2 and PHQ-8)	Administered by research personnel Arabic-English interpreter present Oral interview Assessment time not reported
Rasmussen (2015) [87]	Validation study	Primary care clinic USA	Post-arrival	Asylum seekers Mean age 34.9 yo 59% male West Africa, Himalayan Asia, and Central Africa	PTSD: Harvard Trauma Questionnaire (HTQ)	Administered by trained interpreters Interpreter present Oral interview Assessment time not reported

Table 2. *Cont.*

Study	Design	Setting	Timing of Assessment	Population	Mental Health Condition Assessed and Assessment Tool	Administration Details
Richter (2015) [88]	Screening program	Central reception facilities Germany	Post-arrival	Asylum seekers Mean age 31.9 years old, SD 10.6 66.8% male Iran, Russia, Afghanistan, and Iraq	General psychiatric assessment: Structured diagnostic interview MINI-International Neuropsychiatric Interview (MINI-Plus) Essen Trauma Inventory (ETI) Brief Symptom Inventory (BSI) Montgomery-Asberg Depression Scale (MADRS) WHO-5 Pittsburgh Sleep Quality Index (PSQI)	Administered by a physician Interpreter present Oral interview 3 h (two 1.5 h sessions)
Salari (2017) [89]	Validation study	Primary care clinic Sweden	Post-arrival	Refugees Ages 9–18 97.6% male Majority from Afghanistan. Others from Iran, Syria, Iraq, Pakistan, Somalia, Eritrea, Ethiopia, Libya, and Lebanon	PTSD: Children's Revised Impact of Event Scale (CRIES-8)	Clinicians and nurses Interpreter present if needed Self-assessment Assessment time not reported
Savin (2005) [90]	Screening program	Primary care clinic USA	Post-arrival	Refugees Ages 18 years old and over (mean age 27.4) 51.5% male 24 countries of origin: most frequently Bosnia, Russia, Ukraine, Sudan, Somalia, Ethiopia, Afghanistan, Burma, Vietnam, Iran, and Iraq	PTSD, anxiety, depression: 25-item psychiatric symptom checklist derived from the Diagnostic and Statistical Manual of Mental Disorders, Fourth Edition (DSM-IV)	Administered by a team composed of a case manager from a publicly funded resettlement agency, a primary care nurse experienced with culturally diverse populations, a primary care physician, and if needed, a psychologist or psychiatrist. Nurses primarily administered the screening tool Interpreter present Oral interview Assessment time not reported
Schweitzer (2011) [91]	Screening program	Settlement service Australia	Post-arrival	Refugees Mean age 34.13 yo (range 18–80 yo) 43.9% male Burma	Pre-migration trauma: HTQ Depression, anxiety, somatization: Hopkins Symptom Checklist-37 (HSCL-37) Post-migration stressors: Post-migration Living Difficulties Checklist	Researchers and counsellors Interpreter present Oral interview 2–3 h

Table 2. *Cont.*

Study	Design	Setting	Timing of Assessment	Population	Mental Health Condition Assessed and Assessment Tool	Administration Details
Seagle (2019) [92]	Screening program	Outpatient clinics USA	Post-arrival	Administrative sample, 64% refugees Age 14 years and older 42.6% male Cuba, Burma, Afghanistan, Bhutan, Iraq, Somalia, Iran, Ethiopia, Syria	Not reported; however, the authors state that clinicians may consider the use of the Refugee Health Screener-15 (RHS-15), Harvard Trauma Questionnaire (HTQ), Vietnamese Depression Scale (VDS), New Mexico Refugee Symptom Checklist 121 (NMRSCL-121), and the Hopkins Symptom Checklist 25 (HSCL-25) Georgia public health officials recommend use of the RHS-15	Administered by clinicians Interpreter present Self-assessment and oral interview Time of assessment was variable
Shannon (2015) [93]	Screening program	Primary care clinic USA	Post-arrival	Refugees Mean age 35.27 51.4% male Burma	PTSD, distress, somatic complaints, depression: unspecified 32-item questionnaire	Administered by trained research staff Interpreter present Self-assessment 45 min
Sondergaard (2001) [94]	Screening program	Reception centre Sweden	Post-arrival	Refugees Ages 18–48, mean age 35 yo 63% male Iraq	PTSD: Questionnaire developed uniquely for this study, based on the Holmes-Rahe Life Event Questionnaire	Assessor background not reported Interpreter not present Self-assessment Assessment duration not reported
Sondergaard (2003) [95]	Validation study	Reception centre Sweden	Post-arrival	Refugees Ages 18–48, mean age 35 yo 63% male Iraq	Mental health screen using Health Leaflet: Harvard Trauma Questionnaire (HTQ), Impact of Event Scale (IES-22), General Health Questionnaire (GHQ-28), Hopkins Symptoms Checklist (HSCL-25) PTSD: Structured Clinical Interview for DSM Disorders (SCID) or Clinician Administered PTSD Scale for DSM-5 (CAPS) Depression: Hopkins Symptoms Checklist (HSCL-25)	Administered by case manager Interpreter not present Self-assessment Assessment time not reported
Stingl (2019) [96]	Screening program	Reception centre (RC) & communal accommodation (CU) Germany	Post-arrival	Refugees Mean age 25.6 (RC), 28.9 (CU) 92.9% (RC), 69.8% (CU) male Afghanistan, Algeria, Ethiopia, Eritrea, Iraq, Iran, Somalia, Syria	Depression, anxiety, and PTSD: Refugee Health Screener (RHS-15)	Administered by doctorate students and a linguist Interpreter present Written Likert-scale 4–12 min

Table 2. *Cont.*

Study	Design	Setting	Timing of Assessment	Population	Mental Health Condition Assessed and Assessment Tool	Administration Details
Sukale (2017) [97]	Screening program	Clearing and pre-clearing institution Germany	Post-arrival	Refugee minors Age 16.24 years, SD 1.03 100% male Syria, Afghanistan, Iran, Somalia, Sudan, Iraq	Providing Online Resource and Trauma Assessment (PORTA) screening tool, which comprises of disorder-specific questionnaires: Trauma: CATS Depression and Anxiety: Refugee Health Screener (RHS-15) + Patient Health Questionnaire-9 (PHQ-9) Behavioural problems: Strengths and Difficulties Questionnaire Self harm and suicidality: SITBI	Self-administered Interpreter present if needed Online questionnaire via computer (PORTA) 30–90 min
Tay (2013) [98]	Screening program	Reception centre Australia	In transition	Asylum seekers Mean age 39 65% male 18 countries- majority from Iran, Ghana, Zimbabwe, Afghanistan, and China	PTSD and depression: Structured Clinical Interview for DSM-IV (SCID) PTSD: Harvard Trauma Questionnaire (HTQ) Depression: Hopkins Symptoms Checklist (HSCL-25)	Assessment by psychologists Interpreter present Oral interview 120 min
Thulesius (1999) [99]	Validation study	Asylum centre (refugees) and Healthcare clinic (Swedish comparison group) Netherlands	Post-arrival	Refugees Mean age 33.7 58% male Bosnia-Herzegovina	PTSD and depression: Modified Posttraumatic Symptom Scale (PTSS-10-70)	Assessor background not reported Interpreter not present Self-assessment Assessment time not reported
van Os (2018) [100]	Screening program	National intermediary organizations Netherlands	Post-arrival	Refugees and asylum seekers—16 unaccompanied children (15–18 years) and 11 accompanied children (4–16 years) 63% male 44% from Afghanistan	Well-being and child development: Best Interests of the Child (BIC-Q), Strengths and Difficulties Questionnaire (SDQ) Stressful life events: Stressful Life Events (SLE) PTSD: Reactions of Adolescents on Traumatic Stress (RATS)	Assessment by trained professionals Interpreter present Self-assessment and oral interview 180–240 min
Van Dijk (1999) [101]	Validation study	Psychiatric hospital Netherlands	Post-arrival	Refugees Mean age 35.7 years, range 17–70 67% male Diverse nationalities (country not specified)	PTSD: Harvard Trauma Questionnaire (HTQ), Hopkins Symptom Check List-90 (HSCL-90), DSM-IV	Administered by psychiatrists and psychological assistants Interpreter present Oral interview Assessment time not reported

Table 2. *Cont.*

Study	Design	Setting	Timing of Assessment	Population	Mental Health Condition Assessed and Assessment Tool	Administration Details
Vergara (2003) [102]	Screening program	Refugee health program USA	Post-arrival	26,374 refugees, or 38.1% of all refugees, resetting in the United States during fiscal year 1997 No additional characteristics reported	3/9 sites offered mental status examinations during the domestic refugee health assessment. Specific mental health conditions and assessment tools not reported	Not reported
Weine (1998) [103]	Screening program	Primary care clinic USA	Post-arrival	Refugees Ages 13–59 yo 50% male Bosnia	PTSD: PTSD Symptoms Scale, the Communal Traumatic Experiences Inventory, the Global Assessment of Functioning (DSM-IV), and the Symptoms Checklist 90 (SCL-90-R)	Administered by mental health professionals Interpreter present Oral interview 60–120 min
Willey (2020) [104]	Screening program	Refugee antenatal clinic Australia	Post-arrival	Women from a refugee background or considered refugee-like, i.e., arrived in Australia on a spousal visa from a refugee-source country such as Afghanistan	Depression and anxiety: Edinburgh Postnatal Depression Scale (EPDS) Perinatal mental health: Monash Psychosocial Screening Tool	Administered by maternal care staff (midwives, bi-cultural workers) Interpreter present Electronic tablet 10 min
Wulfes (2019) [105]	Validation study	Refugee accommodations Germany	Post-arrival	Refugee and asylum seekers Ages 17–90 yo, average age 32.9 64.4% male Syria, Iraq, Afghanistan, Iran, Sudan	1. Posttraumatic stress screening: PQ 2. Traumatic events: a list of events that was modified from those included in the Posttraumatic Diagnostic Scale (PDS) 3. Posttraumatic stress symptoms: PDS-8 4. Depression: Patient Health Questionnaire 9 (PHQ-9) 5. Axis I disorders: Structured Clinical Interview for DSM Disorders (SCID)	Administered by staff without medical or psychological health training I interpreter not present Self-assessment Assessment time not reported
Yalim (2021) [106]	Screening program	Refugee resettlement agency/home visit USA	Post-arrival	Refugees Aged 18 years and older (mean age 36.38 years, SD 12.5) Majority from Democratic Republic of Congo, Iraq, Syria, and Eritrea	PTSD, depression, anxiety: Refugee Health Screener (RHS-15)	Administered by research personnel Interpreter present Oral interview or self-assessment, depending on the literacy level of the participant 20–30 min
Young (2016) [107]	Screening program	Detention centres Australia	Post-arrival	Asylum seekers and refugees (detainees) All ages 73% male	Depression, anxiety, and PTSD: Self-rated Kessler 10 (K-10) The Harvard Trauma Questionnaire (HTQ) The Clinician-rated Health of the Nation Outcome Scores (HoNOS) The Clinician-rated Health of the Nation Child and Adolescent Outcome Scores (HoNOSCA)	Administered by mental health professionals (nurse or psychologist) Interpreter present Self-assessment Assessment time not reported

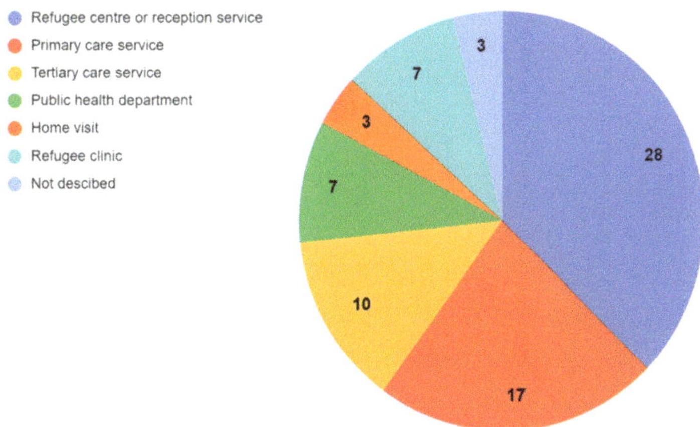

Figure 5. Setting of mental health assessments.

11. Conditions and Mental Health Screening Tools

A total of 85 mental health screening tools were identified (Table 3). Several of these tools are available in multiple languages and are either self-administered or administered by various trained professionals such as primary care providers (PCPs), mental health specialists (MHSs), or community health workers (CHWs). Several tools could also be administered by a lay person without clinical training [46,64,80]. The most common tools were the Harvard Trauma Questionnaire (HTQ), the Hopkins Symptom Checklist-25 (HSCL-25), the Mini International Neuropsychiatric Interview (MINI), and the Refugee Health Screener-15 (RHS-15). The most common screened mental health conditions were overall mental health, PTSD, depression, and anxiety (see Figure 6).

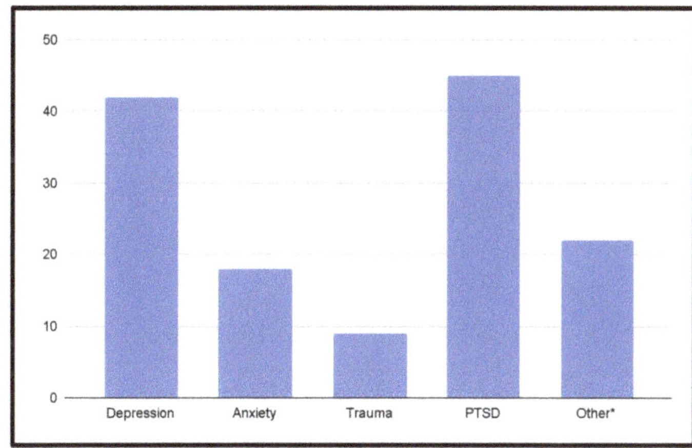

Figure 6. Overview of mental health conditions assessed among refugees and asylum seekers. * NB: Any mental health assessments that did not include depression, anxiety, trauma, or PTSD were categorized as 'Other' (e.g., general mental health, panic disorders, adverse childhood events, etc.)

Table 3. Mental Health Screening Tool Characteristics.

	Screening Tool	Studies	Mental Health Conditions Assessed	Administrator	Languages
1	Family Peer Relationship Questionnaire, Arabic version (A-FPRQ)	El Ghaziri 2019	OTHER	unspecified	unspecified
2	Unaccompanied Migrant Minors Questionnaire (AEGIS-Q)	Di Pietro 2020	OTHER	unspecified	unspecified
3	Al-Obaidi et al. DSM-based non-validated questionnaire	Al-Obaidi 2015	Depression, PTSD	Master's level social worker	unspecified
4	Arab Acculturation Scale	LeMaster 2018	PTSD, Depression, OTHER	unspecified	unspecified
5	Alcohol, Smoking and Substance Involvement Screening Test (ASSIST)	El Ghaziri 2019	Substance Use Disorder	unspecified	unspecified
6	Best Interests of the Child (BIC-Q)	van Os 2018	Disruptive Behaviour Disorders, Depression	unspecified	Arabic, Dari, Farsi, Somali
7	Brief Symptom Inventory-18 (BSI-18)	Kaltenbach 2017 Richter 2015	Depression, PTSD, Somatoform Disorders	unspecified	Albanian, Arabic, Farsi, Kurdish, Russian, Serbian, Somali
8	Child Behaviour Checklist (CBCL)	Nehring 2021	PTSD	MHS	German
9	Child Health Questionnaire (CHQ)	Geltman 2005	OTHER	Community health worker (CHW)	English
10	Children's Revised Impact of Event Scale (CRIES-8)	Salari 2017	PTSD	Primary care provider (PCP)	Arabic, Dari, Farsi, Kurdish/Sorani, Swedish
11	Communal Traumatic Experiences Inventory (CTEI)	Weine 1998	PTSD, Depression	Mental health specialist (MHS), PCP, lay person (LAY)	Croatian
12	Cook et al. author-developed interview	Cook 2015	OTHER	Research assistants trained Master's or Ph.D. level social work students	unspecified
13	Digital Communication Assistance Tool (DCAT)	Kleinert 2019	PTSD, Depression, Anxiety, Substance Use Disorder, Disruptive Behaviour Disorders, Somatoform Disorders, OTHER	Self-assessment, PCP	Modern Standard Arabic, Arabic Syrian, Arabic Egyptian, Arabic Tunisian, Arabic Moroccan, Turkish, Persian, Kurdish Sorani, Kurdish Kurmanji, Kurdish Feyli, Pashto Kandahari, Pashto Mazurka
14	Edinburgh Postnatal Depression Scale (EPDS)	Boyle 2019 Willey 2020	Depression	MHS, PCP, CHW, LAY	unspecified
15	Essen Trauma Inventory (ETI)	Richter 2015	Trauma	MHS	German
16	Eytan et al. (2002) author-developed interview	Eytan 2002	Health Conditions, Presence of Symptoms and Previous Exposure to Trauma	Nurses	French, German, Italian, Spanish, Portuguese, English
17	Family Assessment Device (FAD)	El Ghaziri 2019	OTHER	unspecified	unspecified
18	Geltman et al. author-developed ad-hoc assessment	Geltman 2005	Emotionally Traumatic Exposures	Staff from local URMO agencies	English
19	Generalized Anxiety Disorder 7 (GAD-7)	Bjarta 2018	Anxiety	MHS, PCP, CHW	Arabic, Dari
20	GB	El Ghaziri 2019	OTHER	unspecified	unspecified
21	General Health Questionnaire (GHQ-28)	Sondergaard 2003	Depression	Self-rating	unspecified
22	Global Assessment of Functioning Scale (DSM-IV)	Weine 1998	OTHER	MHS, PCP, CHW	Croatian

Table 3. *Cont.*

	Screening Tool	Studies	Mental Health Conditions Assessed	Administrator	Languages
23	Global Mental Health Assessment Tool (GMHAT)	Hough 2019	Anxiety, Depression, Substance Use Disorders, Disruptive Behaviour Disorders	PCP, MHS	English, Arabic
24	Hospital Anxiety and Depression Scale (HADS)	Arnetz 2014 LeMaster 2018	Anxiety, Depression	CHW	Arabic
25	Hassles Scale	LeMaster 2018	OTHER	CHW	unspecified
26	Home, Education/Eating, Activities, Drugs, Sexuality, Suicide/mental health (HEADSS) Questionnaire	Hirani 2016	OTHER	unspecified	English
27	Health Leaflet (HL)	Sondergaard 2003	PTSD	Self-assessment	unspecified
28	Kennedy et al. author-developed tool	Kennedy 1999	Depression, Anxiety, PTSD	Self-assessment	unspecified
29	Clinician-rated Health of the Nation Outcome Scores (HoNOS)	Young 2016	Depression, Substance Use Disorders, Disruptive Behaviour Disorders	MHS, PCP	unspecified
30	Clinician-rated Health of the Nation Child and Adolescent Outcome Scores (HoNOSCA)	Young 2016	Depression, Substance Use Disorders, Disruptive Behaviour Disorders	MHS, PCP	unspecified
31	Hopkins Symptom Checklist-25 (HSCL-25)	Jakobsen 2017 Javanbakht 2019 Kleijn 2001 Ovitt 2003 Schweitzer 2011 Sondergaard 2003 Tay 2013 Van Dijk 1999	Anxiety, Depression	MHS, PCP, CHW	Arabic, Farsi, Russian, Bosnian-Serbo-Croatian
32	Harvard Trauma Questionnaire (HTQ)	Arnetz 2014 Bertelsen 2018 Churbaji 2020 Geltman 2005 Jakobsen 2017 Kleijn 2001 LeMaster 2018 Rasmussen 2015 Schweitzer 2011 Sondergaard 2003 Tay 2013 Young 2016 Van Dijk 1999	PTSD	MHS, PCP, CHW	Arabic, Cambodian, Dutch, English, Farsi, French, Laotian, Russian, Serbo-Croatian, Vietnamese
33	Impact of Event Scale (IES-22)	Sondergaard 2003	Trauma	Self-rating	unspecified
34	Interpersonal Support Evaluation Checklist (ISEL)	LeMaster 2018	OTHER	CHW	unspecified
35	ICD-11 International Trauma Questionnaire (ITQ)	Barbieri 2019	PTSD	MHS, PCP, CHW	Arabic, English, French
36	Kaltenbach et al. author-developed questionnaire	Kaltenbach 2017	Daily Functioning	Clinical psychologists	unspecified
37	Karen Mental Health Screener	Brink 2016	PTSD, Depression	PCP	Karenic
38	Self-rated Kessler 10 (K-10)	Lillee 2015 Young 2016	OTHER	Self-administered (SA)	English, Kurdish, Pashto
39	Life Events Checklist (LEC-5)	Kaltenbach 2017	OTHER	unspecified	Arabic, Albanian, Farsi, Kurdish, Russian, Serbian, Somali

Table 3. *Cont.*

	Screening Tool	Studies	Mental Health Conditions Assessed	Administrator	Languages
39	Loutan et al. author-developed questionnaire	Loutan 1999	Anxiety, Depression, PTSD, and Traumatic Events	Nurse	French, English, Italian, Spanish and German
40	Multi-Adaptive Psychological Screening Software (MAPSS)	Morina 2017	Depression, PTSD	MHS, PCP	Arabic, Farsi, Tamil, Turkish
41	Mini International Neuropsychiatric Interview (MINI)	Churbaji 2020 Durieux-Paillard 2006 El Ghaziri 2019 Eytan 2007 Kaltenbach 2017 Richter 2015	Depression, Anxiety, Substance Use Disorders, Disruptive Behaviour Disorders, PTSD, Somatoform Disorders	MHS, PCP	70+ languages
42	Mini International Neuropsychiatric Interview for Children and Adolescents (MINI-KID)	El Ghaziri 2019	Depression, Anxiety, Substance Use Disorders, Disruptive Behaviour Disorders, PTSD, Somatoform Disorders	MHS, PCP	70+ languages
43	Monash Health Psychosocial Needs Assessment (Psychosocial Screening Tool)	Boyle 2019 Willey 2020	OTHER	MHS, PCP, CHW, LAY, Self-administered	unspecified
44	Montgomery-Asberg Depression Scale (MADRS)	Richter 2015	Depression	MHS, PCP	unspecified
45	Multidimensional Scale of Perceived Social Support (MSPSS)	El Ghaziri 2019	OTHER	MHS, PCP, CHW	unspecified
46	Nikendei et al. author-developed interviews	Nikendei 2019	Substance Use	Research personnel	English, German, French, Persian, Arabic, Turkish, Kurmanji (Northern Kurdish), Urdu, Hausa, Russian, Serbian, Albanian, Macedonian, Georgian, Mandinka, Tigrinya
47	Ovitt et al. author-developed client questionnaire	Ovitt 2003	OTHER		
48	Primary Care PTSD-4 (PC-PTSD-4)	Bjarta 2018	PTSD	MHS, PCP, CHW, LAY, SA	Arabic, Dari
49	PC-PTSD-5	Nikendei 2019	PTSD	Trained research assistants	English, German, French, Persian, Arabic, Turkish, Kurmanji (Northern Kurdish), Urdu, Hausa, Russian, Serbian, Albanian, Macedonian, Georgian, Mandinka, Tigrinya
50	PTSD Checklist for DSM-5 (PCL-5)	Barbieri 2019 Kaltenbach 2017	PTSD	MHS, PCP	Arabic, Albanian, Farsi, Kurdish, Russian, Serbian, Somali
51	Civilian version of the PTSD Checklist (PCL-C)	Arnetz 2014 Javanbakht 2019 LeMaster 2018	PTSD	CHW	Arabic
52	Posttraumatic Diagnostic Scale (PDS)	Kroger 2016 Mewes 2018 Wulfes 2019	PTSD	MHS, Self-assessment	German, Arabic, Persian, Kurdish, Turkish, English
53	Patient Health Questionnaire (PHQ-2)	Kroger 2016 Nikendei 2019 Poole 2020	Depression	Trained research assistants	English, German, French, Persian, Arabic, Turkish, Kurmanji (Northern Kurdish), Urdu, Hausa, Russian, Serbian, Albanian, Macedonian, Georgian, Mandinka, Tigrinya

Table 3. *Cont.*

	Screening Tool	Studies	Mental Health Conditions Assessed	Administrator	Languages
54	Patient Health Questionnaire (PHQ-8)	Poole 2020	Depression	Research personnel	
55	Patient Health Questionnaire (PHQ-9)	Bertelsen 2018 Bjarta 2018 Churbaji 2020 Mewes 2018 Wulfes 2019	Depression	MHS, PCP, Self-assessment	Arabic, Dari, Farsi, English, Kurdish
56	Patient Health Questionnaire—Panic Disorders (PHQ-PD)	Nikendei 2019	Panic Symptoms	Trained research assistants	English, German, French, Persian, Arabic, Turkish, Kurmanji (Northern Kurdish), Urdu, Hausa, Russian, Serbian, Albanian, Macedonian, Georgian, Mandinka, Tigrinya
57	Parentification Inventory (PI)	El Ghaziri 2019	OTHER	MHS, PCP, CHW	unspecified
58	Post-Migration Living Difficulties Checklist (PMLDC)	Schweitzer 2011	OTHER	CHW	unspecified
59	Process of Recognition and Orientation of Torture Victims in European Countries to Facilitate Care and Treatment (PROTECT) Questionnaire	Mewes 2018 Wulfes 2019	PTSD, Depression	MHS, PCP, LAY	English, German, Farsi, French, Persian, Arabic, Turkish, Kurdish, Kurmanji (Northern Kurdish), Urdu, Hausa, Russian, Serbian, Albanian, Macedonian, Georgian, Mandinka, Tigrinya
60	Present State Examination (PSE)	Hauff 1995	PTSD, psychiatric disorders	The first author	unspecified
61	Providing Online Resource and Trauma Assessment' (PORTA)	Sukale 2017	Trauma, Depression, Anxiety, Behavioural Problems, Self-Harm/Suicidality	Self-administered	German, English, French, Arabic, Dari/Farsi, Pashto, Tigrinja, Somali
62	PTSD Symptoms Scale (PSS)	Weine 1998	PTSD	MHS, CHW, LAY	Croatian
63	Posttraumatic Symptom Scale (PTSS-10-70)	Thulesius 1999	PTSD	unspecified	English, Serbo-Croatian
64	Reactions of Adolescents on Traumatic Stress (RATS)	van Os 2018	PTSD	unspecified	Arabic, Dari, Farsi, Somali
65	Resilience Scale	LeMaster 2018	OTHER	CHW	unspecified
66	Refugee Health Screener-13 (RHS-13)	Bjarta 2018 Kaltenbach 2017	Depression, Anxiety, SOM, PTSD, OTHER	MHS	Amharic, Arabic, Albanian, Burmese, Cuban Spanish, Farsi, French, Haitian Creole, Karen, Kurdish, Mexican Spanish, Nepali, Russian, Spanish, Serbian, Somali, Swahili, Tigrinya
67	Refugee Health Screener-15 (RHS-15)	Al-Obaidi 2015 Baird 2020 Hollifield 2013 Hollifield 2016 Johnson-Agbakwu 2014 Kaltenbach 2017 Polcher 2016 Stingl 2019 Yalim 2020	Depression, Anxiety, Somatoform Disorders, PTSD, OTHER	MHS, PCP, CHW	Amharic, Arabic, Albanian, Burmese, Cuban, English, Farsi, French, Haitian Creole, Karen, Kurdish, Mexican Spanish, Nepali, Russian, Spanish, Serbian, Somali, Swahili, Tigrinya
68	Refugee Trauma History Checklist (RTHC)	Sigvardsdotter 2017	OTHER	MHS, PCP	English, Arabic

Table 3. *Cont.*

	Screening Tool	Studies	Mental Health Conditions Assessed	Administrator	Languages
69	Savin et al. author-developed checklist derived from the DSM-IV	Savin 2005	Depression, Anxiety, PTSD	PCP, MHS	English
70	S-DAS	El Ghaziri 2019	Disruptive Behaviour Disorders, OTHER	MHS, PCP, CHW	unspecified
71	Structured Clinical Interview for DSM-IV (SCID)	Brink 2016 Tay 2013 Wulfes 2019	Depression, Anxiety, PTSD, Substance Use Disorders, Disruptive Behaviour Disorders, Somatoform Disorders	MHS, PCP	Danish, French, German, Greek, Hebrew, Karen, Italian, Portuguese, Spanish, Swedish, Turkish, Zulu
72	SCL-90-R	Hauff 1995 Weine 1998	Depression, Anxiety, Somatoform Disorders, Disruptive Behaviour Disorders, OTHER	MHS, PCP, CHW	Croatian
73	Strength and Difficulty Questionnaire (SDQ)	Green 2021 Hanes 2017 van Os 2018	OTHER	CHW, LAY	75+ languages
74	SF-10	El Ghaziri 2019	Depression, Anxiety, Disruptive Behaviour Disorders	MHS, PCP, CHW	unspecified
75	SF-12	El Ghaziri 2019	Depression, Anxiety, Disruptive Behaviour Disorders	MHW, PCP, CHW	unspecified
76	Shannon et al. author-developed questionnaire	Shannon 2015	Depression, PTSD, OTHER	Master's-level and doctoral-level research assistant, professional Karen interpreters	English and Karen
77	Stressful Life Events (SLE)	van Os 2018	OTHER	unspecified	Arabic, Dari, Farsi, Somali
78	Sondergaard et al. (2001) author-developed questionnaire	Sondergaard 2001	PTSD, Anxiety, Depression, OTHER	Professionals working with refugees	Arabic and Sorani
79	STAR-MH	Hocking 2018	Depression, PTSD	CHW	English
80	Trauma Exposure Questionnaire by Nickerson et al.	Barbieri 2019	PTSD	PCP	Arabic, English, French
81	Vietnamese Depression Scale (VDS)	Buchwald 1995	Depression	PCP	Vietnamese
82	WHO-5	Nikendei 2019 Richter 2015	Social Well-Being	LAY, MHS, PCP	English, German, French, Persian, Arabic, Turkish, Kurmanji (Northern Kurdish), Urdu, Hausa, Russian, Serbian, Albanian, Macedonian, Georgian, Mandinka, Tigrinya
83	WHO General Health Questionnaire	Masmas 2008	Psychological Health Status	PCP, MHS	unspecified
84	World Health Organization Quality of Life Brief Version (WHOQOL-Bref)	Bjarta 2018	OTHER	MHS, PCP, CHW, LAY, SA	28 languages (who.int)
85	World Health Organization PTSD screener	Lillee 2015	PTSD	unspecified	English, Kurdish, Pashto

Legend: PCP: Primary care provider. MHS: Mental health specialist. CHW: Community health worker. LAY: Layperson. SA: Self-administration.

12. Pre-Departure Mental Health Screening

The International Organization for Migration (IOM) conducts several pre-migration health activities at the request of receiving country governments to identify health conditions of public health importance and to provide continuity of care linking the pre-departure, travel, and post-arrival phases. These assessments include radiology services, laboratory services, treatment of communicable diseases, vaccinations, and detection of non-communicable diseases, including mental health assessments. We identified two grey literature reports which evaluated pre-departure screening programs for refugees [4,39].

In 2019, IOM conducted a total of 110,992 pre-departure health assessments for refugees [4]. Most assessments among refugees were conducted in Lebanon (11.7%), Turkey (11.1%), and Jordan (8.8%). The top destination countries were the United States (39.7%), Canada (27.9%), and Australia (14.6%). In total, 48.8 percent of assessments were conducted among females and 51.2 percent among males. The majority of health assessments were among refugees younger than 30 (67.1%), with the highest number in the under-10 age group. During 2019, mental health conditions were identified in 2249 pre-departure health assessments conducted among refugees (2.0%). Where indicated, refugees were referred to a specialist for further evaluation (1%). The report does not provide any further details on the specific conditions assessed or other administration details [4].

In 2016–2017, IOM collaborated with Public Health England (UK) to evaluate the pre-departure administration of the Global Mental Health Assessment Tool (GMHAT) among 200 Syrian refugees in a refugee camp in Lebanon [39]. These refugees had already been accepted for resettlement to the UK. This clinically validated, computerized assessment tool was administered by a range of healthcare staff and was designed to detect common psychiatric disorders and serious mental health conditions within the time span of 15–20 min [39].

Findings suggested that a pre-departure mental health assessment could be a useful tool to assist in the preparation for refugee arrivals to overseas resettlement facilities and serve as a valuable resource for general practitioners. Other potential benefits included overcoming barriers such as trust and language, expediting referral and treatment, increasing awareness of mental health issues, and improving support and integration of refugees by proactively addressing concerns [39].

Several considerations were identified to improve the impact and roll out of pre-departure mental health assessments [39]. Firstly, the GMHAT identified 9% of participants with a likely diagnosis of mental illness and an additional 1.5% of participants were referred post-arrival based on clinical judgment; as such, it was noted that the pre-arrival assessment should not be used in isolation or as a replacement for routine psychological assessments post-arrival, and that practitioners should use their clinical expertise to pick up on any missed diagnoses. Secondly, the use of the tool was deemed appropriate, but it was noted that participants' cases took longer to process than those who had not undergone an assessment. Though it was not possible to distinguish whether the GMHAT was the cause of the delay, this is an important consideration. An evaluation of the program indicated that additional information is needed to estimate the impacts on costs and case processing times. Further, the authors concluded it is important to ensure that the information obtained from the pre-assessment will not lead to the rejection of vulnerable refugees based on their mental health status nor based on the resettlement country's service availability. Clear parameters should be defined to determine the flow of information sharing, and usage should be defined a priori, as it was noted that some healthcare workers in this pilot study were unsure on how the information was intended to be used and whom it could be shared with, ultimately devaluing the purpose of this tool. Lastly, it is important to ensure adequate post-arrival mental health service delivery, since pre-departure assessments can also pose a risk of raising expectations of the care that refugees hope to receive upon resettlement. Although not unique to pre-departure screening procedures, several other concerns were raised including the risk of re-traumatization during assessments, the increased need for mental health services upon arrival, additional guidance and training for healthcare workers, and an increase in the provision of culturally appropriate services. This pilot study acknowledges concerns regarding the acceptability of screening for refugees but recommends that the GHMAT tool requires further modifications to be appropriate for use in the resettlement context [39].

13. Mental Health Screening for Survivors of Torture

We identified four studies which described screening approaches and tools for survivors of torture [45,78,80,105]. Masmas and colleagues identified a high prevalence of torture survivors among an unselected population of asylum seekers using the WHO's General Health Questionnaire and a clinical interview conducted by physicians [78]. Mewes and colleagues conducted a validation study among adult asylum seekers in Germany. They used the Process of Recognition and Orientation of Torture Victims in European Countries to Facilitate Care and Treatment (PROTECT) Questionnaire, which identifies symptoms of PTSD and depression and categorizes asylum seekers into risk categories, supporting a two-stage approach to mental health screening [80]. The questionnaire was specially developed to be administered by nonmedical/psychological staff for the early identification of asylum seekers who suffered traumatic experiences (e.g., experiences of torture). The tool was administered directly in refugee reception centres and refugee accommodations. The validity of the PROTECT Questionnaire was confirmed by Wulfes and colleagues, who concluded that the use of the PROTECT Questionnaire could be more efficient than other brief screening tools (eight-item short-form Posttraumatic Diagnostic Scale (PDS-8) and the Patient Health Questionnaire (PHQ-9)) because it detects two conditions at once [105].

Among included studies, most community-based programs were not offered specifically for victims of torture. In New York, USA, a hospital-based Program for Survivors of Torture (PSOT) exists to offer services to clients who experienced torture [45]. Referrals to this program typically came from asylum lawyers, other health care professionals when they learned about these clients' trauma histories, and word-of-mouth in the communities. At PSOT, asylum seekers were screened for PTSD with the Harvard Trauma Questionnaire (HTQ) and Major Depressive Disorder (MDD) screening was conducted with the Patient Health Questionnaire-9 (PHQ-9). If a client screened positive for MDD or PTSD at intake, they were referred for a mental health evaluation and management through PSOT. Severe cases were evaluated urgently by a PSOT psychologist or psychiatrist. Of those clients diagnosed with depression and PTSD, 94% received follow-up, defined as either referral to a psychiatrist, psychologist, or support group, or pharmacologic management by a primary care provider [45]. The high follow-up rate was attributed to the unique multidisciplinary medical home structure of the program, which has significantly more allied health professionals, live interpreters, and support staff than an average primary care clinic in the area [45].

14. Mental Health Screening Approaches for Refugee Women

Three publications described two mental health screening programs specifically for refugee women of reproductive age [47,69,104]. The report by Boyle and colleagues is a protocol for a screening program [47] whose acceptability and feasibility has been evaluated [104], but whose effectiveness (outcome) data are not yet available. Boyle et al. conducted their study in a Refugee Antenatal Clinic in Australia [47], while Johnson-Agbakwu et al. conducted their study in a Refugee Women's Health Clinic in the United States [69]. Both studies screened for mental health conditions post-arrival in a clinic specifically aimed at assessing and treating refugee women. Boyle et al. screened pregnant women in the perinatal and postnatal period at their first appointment, with screening repeated in the third trimester [47]. Johnson-Agbakwu et al. recruited women seeking obstetric and/or gynaecological care, not differentiating between pregnant and non-pregnant women [69]. The purpose of the screening programs was to improve resettlement and integration outcomes [69], and to identify the urgent needs of refugee women for referral to ensure continuity of care [47].

In the USA, Johnson-Agbakwu et al. administered the Refugee Health Screener-15 (RHS-15) with a cultural health navigator to screen women for PTSD, depression, and anxiety [69]. The aim was for women to complete the screening independently and confidentially without the presence of spouses, family members, or friends, as this may influence patient responses. However, this was difficult to enforce. In contrast, Boyle et al. have planned to use the Edinburgh Postnatal Depression Scale to assess depression and anxiety in the perinatal period [47]. In addition, Boyle et al. will use the Monash Health psychosocial needs assessment tool to assess perinatal mental health disorders, such as past birthing experiences, violence and safety, and social factors (finances and housing). Women will complete both assessments on a tablet in their chosen language and interpreters or bicultural workers are available to assist.

The Refugee Women's Health Clinic where Johnson-Agbakwi et al. conducted their study employed multilingual cultural health navigators; program managers skilled in social work who reflected the ethnic and cultural diversity of the patient population and helped with the administration of the screening tool [69]. They were all female, which helped to build strong rapport and trusting relationships for refugee women to feel more comfortable discussing sensitive concerns in their native language. The implementation of their program was dependent on a community-partnered approach and a sustainable interdisciplinary model of care, which was necessary to build trust, empower refugees towards greater receptivity to mental health services, and provide bi-directional learning. Johnson-Agbakwu et al. reported that interdisciplinary models of care, gender-matched multi-disciplinary health care providers, and patient health navigators and interpreters are necessary for integrated approaches and community empowerment [69].

Prior to the implementation of a screening program in Australia, little support was offered to refugee women as midwives were unsure of what services were available [104]. Following the implementation, midwives expressed they were now making more referrals using a co-designed referral pathway than before the screening program, and more information was available at the point of referral because of screening [104]. Finally, it was reported in the USA that while screening for mental health disorders amongst refugee women provides greater awareness and identifies those who need treatment, many women still do not enroll in mental health care [69]. This was either due to women declining care or a lack of health insurance [69]. It was speculated that one reason women may decline care is due to the social stigma of mental health which could be introduced via social desirability bias and may be heightened through the verbal administration of questionnaires [69].

15. Mental Health Screening Approaches for Refugee Children and Adolescents

Eleven studies were identified that investigated mental health screening approaches specific to refugee children and adolescents [52,57–59,61,62,67,82,89,97,100]. Children and adolescents between the ages of 6 months to 18 years old were included and all identified screening programs were completed post-arrival to the resettlement country. All studies included adolescent populations (ages 10–18) and fewer studies included children below the age of 10 [58,59,82,89,100]. The programs reported that there is variability in the timing of presentations of mental health disorders; thus, an early assessment of the psychological needs of children and families allows for timely targeted support [58,59].

Children and adolescent screening programs focused on a wider range of conditions which consider critical developmental stages. The psychological factors screened for included: emotional problems, conduct problems, hyperactivity, peer problems and prosocial behavior, stressful life events, PTSD [82,100], anxiety, depression [58,59,67,97], and somatization disorder [58]. Health risk behaviours, health-related quality of life, and physical and psychosocial well-being, including physical functioning, body pain, emotional problems, self-esteem, and family cohesion were also screened for [57,62]. The most common mental health condition screened for was PTSD, as 10/11 identified studies included a questionnaire which screened for it.

Various "child-centered" approaches were described. Two studies, consistent with trauma-informed care guidelines, offered children the possibility to be accompanied by a person they trusted as support [82,100]. In contrast, another study recommended seeing adolescents alone during consultations [62]. Children, regardless of their age, were offered help to read the items on the questionnaire, to clarify and ensure understanding of the concepts being screened for in the questionnaire [89]. When administering questionnaires to children, investigators noted that it is important to not overload them with various instruments as it may cause confusion and a decrease in completion rates [57]. Furthermore, children can experience difficulties with Likert scales and question formats, despite surveys being constructed with attention to literacy, linguistic, and culture issues [57]. The approaches emphasized the importance of interdisciplinary collaboration and discussions regarding confidentiality [59]. Children and adolescents often require diverse services; thus, multidisciplinary healthcare was recommended to manage health risk behaviours (e.g., medical, sexual, reproductive, mental, social services) [59,62].

Only two publications reported on the digital administration of mental health screening with adolescents. Of note, Jakobsen et al. utilized a computer-based system (laptops and touch-screen function) to administer their screening questionnaires to unaccompanied adolescents with limited school backgrounds [67]. Similarly, Sukale et al. administered a computer-based tool named 'Providing Online Resource and Trauma Assessment' (PORTA), which combines disorder-specific questionnaires on the topics of trauma (CATS), depression and anxiety (RHS + PHQ-9), behavioural problems (SDQ), and self-harm and suicidality (SITBI) [97]. Investigators found that regardless of how they rated their own reading and writing abilities, or how many years of formal schooling they had, they were able to complete the computer-based assessments independently, and there was a minimal need for interpreters [67].

Several studies included pediatric populations in addition to adults, but these studies were not exclusive to children or adolescents [60,65,66,70,92,107]. These studies represent community and primary care settings that do not separate out the children, adolescents, women, and men, but rather provide services to families and any individual patient.

16. Mental Health Screening Tool Validation Studies

A total of 25 studies evaluated the validity of mental health screening tools among a cumulative sample of N = 4341 refugees and asylum seekers [42,44,46,48,50,52,55,64–67,70, 72,80,82,86,87,89,95,99–101,105,106]. All of the included studies followed a cross-sectional study design. Screening took place post-arrival or in transit to the host country, which varied between studies and included the United States (n = 6), Sweden (n = 4), Germany (n = 5), Italy (n = 2), The Netherlands (n = 3), Australia (n = 1), Norway (n = 2), Greece (n = 1), and Switzerland (n = 1). Sixteen studies screened for mental health conditions among refugees, seven among asylum seekers, and one among unaccompanied migrant minors regardless of their legal migration status.

Screening targeted refugees and asylum seekers regardless of their age in nineteen studies [42,44,46,48,50,55,64–66,70,72,80,86,87,95,99,101,105,106], whereas it targeted adolescents and children (also referred to as minors) in five [52,67,82,89,100]. Studies seldom screened for just one mental health condition and most commonly screened for multiple; trauma-spectrum disorders, such as posttraumatic stress disorder (PTSD) and complex posttraumatic stress disorder (CPTSD), as well as traumatic events and experiences, were the most commonly screened conditions across studies (n = 21/25), followed by major depression (n = 12/25), anxiety (n = 8/25), somatization (n = 1/25), general psychological needs (n = 1/25), and environment safety (n = 1/25). Four screening tools emerged as the most commonly used among the identified validation studies:

The Harvard Trauma Questionnaire (HTQ) screened for posttraumatic stress disorder and traumatic events and was validated in six studies [42,67,72,87,95,101]. Translation of the tool to non-English languages was reported in four studies and the use of interpreters to facilitate its administration was reported in three. Sondergaard and colleagues discussed the superiority of the HTQ in screening PTSD compared to other screening tools [95]. Another study reported its higher sensitivity but warned of lower specificity [67]. Further, two studies reported the high validity of HTQ but discussed how certain items carry some threat to its validity when adapted across cultures [72,87]. Finally, Arnetz and colleagues discussed the importance of distinguishing two trauma subtypes when screening for PTSD using the HTQ: physical trauma and lack of necessities [42].

The Refugee Health Screener (RHS), both the 13- and 15-item versions, screened for depression, anxiety, and posttraumatic stress disorder and was validated in five studies [46,65,66,70,106]. The tool was translated in all studies and the use of interpreters to facilitate its administration was reported in four of five. All studies reported the adequate validity of the RHS tool in screening depression, anxiety, and posttraumatic stress disorder [46,65,66,70,106].

The Hopkins Symptom Checklist (HSCL-25) screened for depression and anxiety and was validated in two studies that translated the tool to the language of screened refugees and asylum seekers, and used interpretation services to facilitate its administration [67,72]. Jakobsen and colleagues reported the higher sensitivity but lower specificity of the tool when using a cut-off value of 2 [67]. Similarly, Kleijn and colleagues reported the high validity of the tool in screening depression and anxiety, but commented on the different meanings some items may carry across cultures [72].

The Mini International Neuropsychiatric Interview (MINI) was adapted and validated in two studies. The first study translated the instrument into Arabic and tested its validity in screening major depressive episodes, PTSD, panic disorders, generalized anxiety disorder, and agoraphobia among Syrian, Iraqi, and Palestinian refugees [50]. When compared to the PHQ-9, authors reported the high validity of the MINI instrument in screening for depression, anxiety, and PTSD [50]. The second study validated the major depression and PTSD sections of the French version of the MINI among asylum seekers from Europe, Asia, and Africa [55]. The authors of this study concluded that the tool could be used to systematically screen for depression and PTSD among refugees from different origins [55].

Other screening tools were sporadically tested for validity among refugees and asylum seekers and are described in Table 3 [44,48,64,80,82,89,99,105].

17. Discussion

Early screening and care programs for common mental health disorders in refugees and asylum seekers are emerging in many resettlement countries. Our scoping review aimed to characterize these approaches to inform a country-level resettlement policy and practice. We reported on two evaluations of pre-departure screening programs [4,39], 43 post-arrival screening programs, and 25 validation studies of screening tools/instruments. Our results characterized mental health assessment approaches, described approaches for special populations, such as women and children, and highlighted which screening tools are available, which have been validated among refugee populations, and where and how they have been used. Further, we summarized lessons learned and implementation considerations (see Box 2). Our results offered an overview of the international literature in this rapidly expanding area of refugee mental health research [108] and highlighted ongoing challenges and areas of uncertainty.

Box 2. Lessons learned and implementation considerations

Who administers mental health screening? Most mental health assessments are administered by a trained health professional with various levels of mental health expertise. This includes general practitioners, nurses, psychiatrists, psychologists, and community health workers. However, some tools can be self-administered (for example, the Refugee Health Screener) and completed on paper or using digital technology such as a tablet or computer. We identified a few mental health screening tools (PROTECT Questionnaire; STAR-MH; Refugee Health Screener) administered by staff without medical or psychological health training. Regardless of who administers the mental health assessment, numerous studies highlighted the importance of a trained interpreter or translator to assist in the assessment and prevent misinterpretations and miscommunications. Authors suggest the presence of trained interpreters improved the quality of communication and also served as cultural mediators [56].

Which mental health screening tool should be administered? There is no international consensus regarding the most effective mental health screening tool to be applied in the context of resettlement. While several tools are gaining popularity (for example, the Harvard Trauma Questionnaire or the Refugee Health Screener), there is currently insufficient effective research to guide the selection of mental health screening tools for national level programs. Currently, tools are chosen to reflect the cultural sensitivity and geographical diversity of refugee groups, but as migration patterns change rapidly, it is difficult to specify a singular set of tools that can be applicable to a large array of refugee populations [53]. It is well recognized that Western diagnostic classifications of mental health conditions have significant limitations with refugee populations because of variations in causality, sociocultural context, and symptom manifestation [6,66]. Authors agree that there is a need for culturally appropriate validated tools to detect mental health problems in refugees [48]. According to Poole et al. screening tools should be (1) self-reported or administered by trained non-medical health workers; (2) responsive to change; with (3) a demonstrated acceptable response rate, reliability, and validity in displaced populations; and (4) a minimal response burden [86].

When should mental health screening take place? Despite the existence of country-level guidance for pre-migration mental health screening (for example, from the USA [109], Australia [61], or New Zealand [110]), there are very few published reports evaluating these processes. The published literature shows that most assessments occur post-arrival to the resettlement state. Post-arrival programs can leverage community partnerships (e.g., [69]) and medical home models (e.g., [45]) to ensure efficient and appropriate linkages to care. Some studies noted the difficulty of following up with refugees as they often get transferred from one location to another in the first few months post-arrival [89,94]. Further, one Australian study reported challenges with the information transfer between and within pre-migration and post-arrival health systems, causing duplication of avoidable tests, increased costs, inefficiencies, and possible clinical consequences [61]. Evidence from the UK also identified critical operational issues with the information flow and supports the notion that further evaluation of pre-departure screening is warranted prior to widespread implementation [39]. To date, there is neither consensus nor sufficient program research to identify the optimal time to screen and assess the mental health needs of refugees and asylum seekers.

Where does mental health screening take place? The majority of mental health screening takes place in a primary care community setting, including refugee specific clinics or services where professionals were trained and familiar with the caseload. Buchwald et al. proposed that individuals presenting to primary care have come for help and accepted the "patient" role; therefore, psychiatric case finding and offering treatment may be less intrusive than it would be in other settings [49]. Furthermore, because this setting is not defined as "psychiatric," the stigma associated with mental health treatment may be more easily minimized [6,49]. One study reported a high rate of refusal during a clinic-based post-arrival health assessment and found that mental health screening was more effective when conducted during a home visit [40].

Do screening programs facilitate linkages to care? Post-arrival screening programs usually include a linkage to care, either on-site or through referrals to community organizations or further specialized care. Programs which operate a medical home model can offer direct multidisciplinary care with allied health professionals and interpreters [45]. The evidence on pre-departure screening is less conclusive: while this information could function as an "early warning" to help local authorities prepare for individuals needing additional support, the impact of the screening is likely to be limited by resource availability and access to specialist mental health services [39]. Existing community resources may not be appropriate for the specific mental health needs of refugees who have fled conflict or experienced violence, torture, or trauma. However, as these pre-departure reports provide valuable information which is usually not available on arrival or takes time and trust to elicit from a patient, pre-departure mental health screening may help primary care providers save time and take appropriate action more proactively, thereby expediting the referral and provision of care [39].

Box 2. *Cont.*

> **How can mental health screening be implemented?** Several studies highlighted that funding for mental health screening and care programs is essential [41,45,102]. Although many factors affect program success, the loss of program funds has been identified as the primary factor contributing to staff reductions and implementation failure [49]. Further, basic training about the context and important health issues of resettled refugees and administration procedures is necessary for all clinical and non-clinical staff [43]. Processes should be streamlined to reduce the time required to complete the assessment [39,43]. National training programs can provide technical assistance and support culturally relevant behaviours, attitudes, and policies in clinical practice [41,106], and help address mental health stigma [66]. Finally, the results from two studies suggest that sequential screening (i.e., categorizing refugees by level of risk to inform linkage to care) is a pragmatic strategy that can reduce the response burden and facilitate the detection of mental health conditions in settings with a scarcity of mental health specialists [80,86].

Among our identified studies, mental health screening programs were most common for adult refugee populations and most commonly delivered in primary care settings. We did identify studies on programs tailored to survivors of torture, women of reproductive age, and children and adolescents. We failed to identify studies on other vulnerable refugee subgroups, such as refugees who identify as LGBTQ+ and people living with disabilities. Cowen suggests that research on these vulnerable refugee populations is in its infancy [111]. For example, a 2019 report identified only six published studies on the mental health of sexual and gender minority refugees and asylum seekers [112]. These subgroups of refugees may be understudied due, in part, to complex intersecting identities and experiences which are not captured by immigration systems or other institutions. Concepts of "impairment", "disability", and "gender" can differ enormously among different cultures and societies, and these identities are often excluded from refugee registration and assistance programs [113]. Despite this, our findings noted that refugee mental health screening programs were often tailored to the refugee population by applying the principles of trauma-informed and person-centered care [114,115], including linguistically and culturally appropriate approaches and the evolution of gender- and age-specific programs.

Four studies focused on asylum seekers with an interest to identify and care for survivors of torture or violence [45,78,80,105]. Early health assessments and follow-ups for survivors of torture and violence are considered important to ensure the safety of these people [9]. Among survivors of torture, unmet mental health care needs are pervasive [116] and they are more likely to have PTSD and major depressive disorder in response to the trauma they had experienced [117]. Advocacy organizations, such as the Canadian Centre of Victims of Torture, can contribute to the resettlement of these populations by organizing networks of psychiatrists and refugee health practitioners, supporting mental health training, and providing medical-legal resources and general advocacy.

An overwhelming majority of studies (90%) reported on post-arrival mental health assessments. We only identified two reports on pre-departure mental health screening [4,39]. Pre-departure health assessments are an important established approach for individual and public health promotion, disease prevention, and facilitation of refugee integration in the resettlement country [19]. Due to the limited availability of and access to mental health services for refugees, countries such as the UK have identified a need for more pre-departure mental health screening to enable effective planning for resettlement [118]. However, the inclusion of mental health assessments within these pre-departure assessments is contentious given the lack of acceptability among refugee populations, lack of immediate and culturally appropriate interventions, and the challenges in information flow, suggesting that pre-departure mental health assessments are not ready to replace assessments on arrival [39,118,119].

Mental health screening was primarily administered by health professionals such as primary care providers (i.e., nurses, physicians) and mental health specialists (e.g., psychologists, psychiatrists). In some cases, a community health worker or research professional (often of the same cultural or linguistic group as the refugees themselves) conducted the assessments. We identified several studies where the assessment was made by a lay or administrative person [46,64,80,105]. Several studies also supported self-assessments, and demonstrated the potential value of digital approaches (e.g., laptops, tablets) when literacy levels allow [46,47,67,80,81,97]. Recent advances in automating screening with technologies such as mobile phones or tablets may facilitate the use of sequential screening in such settings [80,86]. Evidence that instrument performance is similar, regardless of the mode of administration (e.g., patient self-report, interviewer-administered either in-person or electronically) for self-reported depression supports the adoption of adaptive screening processes [81,86]. Mobile applications could offer youth, who otherwise lack independence, to access an assessment and information on their own [97,120]. Multidisciplinary programs for refugee children and their families have also suggested the merits and risks of including family members in the screening process [54].

A screening tool is assessed for sensitivity and specificity, but these are not constant or absolute performance measures. The performance of a tool will depend on the prevalence of the disorder within a population. The performance could also vary based on other characteristics of populations such as age, language, and culture. For this reason, a tool is often taken through a cross-cultural validation process to determine if it provides accurate and consistent measures across cultures. These tool characteristics are only the first part in the pathway to determining actual screening and care effectiveness (see Figure 1). A systematic review would be necessary to provide meaningful commentary on the effectiveness of tools along this care cascade (for e.g., [121]).

When selecting the most appropriate mental health screening tool, program developers must consider the specific refugee population, the estimated prevalence of mental health disorders, cultural idioms of distress, and the complex environmental stressors and traumatic events that may provoke mental health issues [21]. A comprehensive biopsychosocial assessment and meaningful intervention may need to occur over time with trusting, supportive therapeutic relationships and sometimes with specialized mental health care teams [21]. Literacy levels also play a role in determining the use of digital, self-administered, lay, or primary care provider assessment tools. Finally, women of a reproductive age often encounter their own unique challenges, and assessments should also factor in refugee lived experiences of pregnancy, childbirth, and raising children [21]. A recent review of mobile applications for women during pregnancy showed that technology-assisted approaches may improve timely access to mental health support and facilitate successful mental health care across different ethnicities [122]. Assessment tools for children may also need to include a broader spectrum of conditions and assess social determinants of health, developmental delays, family separation, and trauma [123].

18. Implications for Policy

The integration of refugees into society has significant health equity implications [124]. Policymakers need to ensure that new programs and policies are beneficial and not harmful for refugees prior to their implementation. While the benefit of the treatment of symptomatic mental illness among refugees is well-recognized [6], several factors influence the timing and feasibility of these assessments and subsequent treatment interventions. Ensuring refugee communities understand the goal and privacy of mental health screening, and ensuring access to care after screening, are essential factors for program success. Community-based screening with links to a holistic health settlement process is the most common and feasible approach. This may include formal routes of intersectoral collaboration between various services to provide multidisciplinary health care (e.g., medical, sexual, and reproductive health, mental health, allied health, educational agencies, social services, governmental bodies) [62]. Pre-departure overseas screening may provide some benefits, but more evaluation and refugee community support is required. Immigration policy should also be aware of mental health stigma and racism in the general population. Values of pluralism, equity, diversity, and inclusion within the receiving country's society may also play a role in the mental health of refugees [13].

19. Implications for Practice

Most refugee mental health assessments were held in refugee-specific clinics or services with interdisciplinary primary care, primary care clinics, and hospital services. As cultural idioms of distress and the presentation of mental health symptoms vary across cultures, it is essential that health care workers are supported and equipped with the training and tools to adequately assess the mental health of refugees and asylum seekers in a sensitive and culturally appropriate manner [6,13,21]. Mental health care is often specialized, but most refugees and asylum seekers will initially present to primary care clinics [21]. It is important to remember that mental health disorders are most often experienced as social, cultural, spiritual, and medical issues, and these can lead to a range of first presentations, often to family, friends, and religious leaders. Primary care clinics need interdisciplinary programs with co-located physical and mental health services [90], and these programs need screening and monitoring tools to help engage team members in identifying illness, monitoring care, and detecting the severity of symptoms. In addition to primary care support, there will also be a need for more specialized clinicians and experts in cultural psychiatry who can meet the serious or severe mental health needs of patients.

20. Implications for Research

Our review highlights an array of programs and screening and diagnostic assessment tools in various languages across several ethnic groups of varied ages and experiences. Nonetheless, there still remains a gap in understanding which tools may be the most useful in each context, including increasing screening capacity, addressing acceptability concerns, and building trust in team-based interdisciplinary care. It also remains unknown what type of services and supports must be in place in order to safely and effectively implement pre-departure screening programs. Future realist-informed research may reveal contextual factors that influence program success, such as community outreach programs, rapid screening tools, community leaders, and primary care clinics [29,125]. Additionally, there were only two reports that assessed pre-departure mental health assessments [4,39]. It is important to understand if there are evidence-based benefits to performing the assessment of mental health at different time points (i.e., pre-departure, during their transition, or post-arrival) in order to determine how the timing of the assessment can impact immigration, referral to care, access to support, and overall health outcomes. Further, we identified few studies conducted among asylum seekers in detention, and this population warrants further research. Future research could include how information from these screening tools serves to empower screening and care programs, as well as to support physicians in diagnosis, care, and monitoring of patients. Further, evaluations should consider the impact of mental health screening on long-term resettlement outcomes.

21. Strengths and Limitations

This comprehensive review captures a large number of studies on refugee mental health screening tools and programs. We searched multiple databases, sought grey literature, and followed rigorous scoping review methods as suggested by the Joanna Briggs Institute according to a published protocol [34]. As a scoping review, our methods were not geared to synthesize the benefits and harms of screening programs but instead focused on characterizing existing mental health screening approaches. Within our results, there are examples of innovative community programs, a rich array of validated tools for screening and monitoring, and years of primary care screening experience. With additional research, the tools could guide the development of frameworks for mobile applications to improve access and allow anonymous use.

We, nonetheless, recognize several limitations of this work. Our focus was the screening components of programs and not cultural psychiatric consultation, psychotherapy services, and cultural navigation. Additionally, we excluded qualitative publications that focused on patient experiences rather than characteristics of early screening approaches. We restricted the "resettlement" period to 12 months post-arrival. We recognize that many asylum seekers may not have received a decision or official refugee status within this time (i.e., they may spend several years as "asylum seekers" as in Australia and Europe). We focused only on refugees and asylum seekers during resettlement, and excluded studies among general immigrant populations, refugee camp populations, and internally displaced populations, as these groups may each have unique levels of needs and complex pathways to mental health care.

Displacement and resettlement are often experienced at a collective level [6,54], and mental health includes a dynamic interplay of family and community. However, screening tends to occur at the individual level. Understanding the relationship between the patient, family, community, and provider is an important concept to consider. This level of complexity was outside the scope of this review but has significant implications for designing screening programs.

22. Deviations from Protocol

Due to time constraints, our grey literature was limited to searching government websites and reaching out to migration health experts in the field. We did not complete a grey literature search using Google search engines for NGOs and IGOs. We did not conduct a grey literature search focused on Europe. In the protocol we had stated: "We will search OpenGrey for grey literature originating from Europe. We will also use a Google Custom Search Engine to search the websites of over 1500 non-governmental organizations (NGOs) and over 400 international governmental organizations (IGOs)" [34].

23. Conclusions

Many refugees and asylum seekers face protracted migration status uncertainty, isolation, trauma, and additional delays in resettlement. Our review suggests early refugee mental health screening and care are feasible and often linked to established post-arrival medical screening programs in primary care. Vulnerable population programs for women, children, and survivors of torture are also emerging. More programmatic and realist evaluation research is needed to help programs select the most appropriate tools and processes for mental health screening and care programs in their context. Pre-departure screening exists but needs more evaluation.

Supplementary Materials: The following supporting information can be downloaded at: https://www.mdpi.com/article/10.3390/ijerph19063549/s1, Supplementary File S1: List of resettlement states; Supplementary File S2: PRISMA-ScR; Supplementary File S3: PRISMA-S; Supplementary File S4: Search strategies; Supplementary File S5: Excluded studies with reasons.

Author Contributions: O.M. (Olivia Magwood), K.P., A.S. contributed to conceptualization and funding acquisition; O.M. (Olivia Magwood), K.P., A.K. contributed to methodology; A.K., A.S., D.M., O.M. (Olivia Magwood), O.M. (Oreen Mendonca), H.H., M.M., Y.T., D.R. contributed to data curation and abstraction. All authors contributed to writing and editing the manuscript. All authors have read and agreed to the published version of the manuscript.

Funding: This work was supported by Immigration, Refugees and Citizenship Canada, Government of Canada. The funders of the study had no direct role in data collection, data analysis, data interpretation, or writing of the report. The analysis is the responsibility of the authors and does not represent the views of the Government of Canada.

Institutional Review Board Statement: Not applicable.

Informed Consent Statement: Not applicable.

Data Availability Statement: Not applicable.

Acknowledgments: The authors would like to thank Lindsay Sikora, University of Ottawa, for her expert librarian support and review of the search strategy. The authors would like to thank Eric Agbata, Brianna Abboud, Zinnia Al-Najjar, Dana Ghanem, Rinila Haridas, and Jeremie Alexander for their assistance in study selection and data extraction.

Conflicts of Interest: K.P. led the Canadian evidence-based clinical guidelines for immigrants and refugees (2011) and the European Centre for Disease Prevention and Control public health guidance on screening and vaccination for infectious diseases in newly arrived migrants within the EU/EEA (2018). O.M. (Olivia Magwood) participated in the development of the European Centre for Disease Prevention and Control public health guidance on screening and vaccination for infectious diseases in newly arrived migrants within the EU/EEA (2018). The authors declare no other competing interests.

References

1. United Nations High Commissioner for Refugees (UNHCR). *Projected Global Resettlement Needs 2020*; UNHCR: Geneva, Switzerland, 2019.
2. Brickhill-Atkinson, M.; Hauck, F.R. Impact of COVID-19 on Resettled Refugees. *Prim. Care* **2021**, *48*, 57–66. [CrossRef] [PubMed]
3. UNHCR. *Projected Global Resettlement Needs 2022*; 27th Annual Tripartite Consultations on Resettlement; UNHCR: Geneva, Switzerland, 2021.
4. International Organization for Migration (IOM). *Migration Health Assessments and Travel Health Assistance: 2019 Overview of Pre-Migration Health Activities*; IOM: Geneva, Switzerland, 2020.
5. United Nations High Commissioner for Refugees The Global Report 2005. Available online: https://www.unhcr.org/publications/fundraising/4a0c04f96/global-report-2005.html (accessed on 27 February 2022).
6. Kirmayer, L.J.; Narasiah, L.; Munoz, M.; Rashid, M.; Ryder, A.G.; Guzder, J.; Hassan, G.; Rousseau, C.; Pottie, K. Common mental health problems in immigrants and refugees: General approach in primary care. *Can. Med. Assoc. J.* **2011**, *183*, E959–E967. [CrossRef] [PubMed]
7. Benjamen, J.; Girard, V.; Jamani, S.; Magwood, O.; Holland, T.; Sharfuddin, N.; Pottie, K. Access to Refugee and Migrant Mental Health Care Services during the First Six Months of the COVID-19 Pandemic: A Canadian Refugee Clinician Survey. *Int. J. Environ. Res. Public Health* **2021**, *18*, 5266. [CrossRef] [PubMed]
8. Beiser, M. The Health of Immigrants and Refugees in Canada. *Can. J. Public Health* **2005**, *96*, S30–S44. [CrossRef]
9. Sveaass, N.; Lie, B. *Early Assessment of Mental Health and Options for Documentation of Torture in Newly Arrived Asylum Seekers*; Oxford University Press: Oxford, UK, 2021; pp. 387–394. ISBN 978-0-19-883374-1.
10. Kronick, R. Mental Health of Refugees and Asylum Seekers: Assessment and Intervention. *Can. J. Psychiatry* **2018**, *63*, 290–296. [CrossRef]
11. Andermann, L.; Kanagaratnam, P.; Wondimagegn, D.; Pain, C. *Post-Traumatic Stress Disorder in Refugee and Migrant Mental Health*; Oxford University Press: Oxford, UK, 2021; ISBN 978-0-19-187215-0.
12. World Health Organization. *Health of Refugees and Migrants*; WHO: Geneva, Switzerland, 2018; p. 37.
13. Kassam, A.; Magwood, O.; Pottie, K. Fostering Refugee and Other Migrant Resilience through Empowerment, Pluralism, and Collaboration in Mental Health. *Int. J. Environ. Res. Public Health* **2020**, *17*, 9557. [CrossRef]
14. Kirmayer, L.J.; Pedersen, D. Toward a new architecture for global mental health. *Transcult. Psychiatry* **2014**, *51*, 759–776. [CrossRef]
15. Steel, Z.; Chey, T.; Silove, D.; Marnane, C.; Bryant, R.A.; van Ommeren, M. Association of Torture and other Potentially Traumatic Events with Mental Health Outcomes among Populations Exposed to Mass Conflict and Displacement: A Systematic Review and Meta-analysis. *JAMA* **2009**, *302*, 537–549. [CrossRef]
16. Charlson, F.J.; Flaxman, A.; Ferrari, A.J.; Vos, T.; Steel, Z.; Whiteford, H.A. Post-traumatic stress disorder and major depression in conflict-affected populations: An epidemiological model and predictor analysis. *Glob. Ment. Health* **2016**, *3*, e4. [CrossRef]
17. World Health Organization. *Depression and other Common Mental Disorders: Global Health Estimates*; World Health Organization: Geneva, Switzerland, 2017.
18. Stein, D.J.; McLaughlin, K.A.; Koenen, K.C.; Atwoli, L.; Friedman, M.J.; Hill, E.D.; Maercker, A.; Petukhova, M.; Shahly, V.; van Ommeren, M.; et al. DSM-5 and ICD-11 definitions of posttraumatic stress disorder: Investigating "narrow" and "broad" approaches. *Depress. Anxiety* **2014**, *31*, 494–505. [CrossRef]
19. Wickramage, K.; Mosca, D. Can Migration Health Assessments Become a Mechanism for Global Public Health Good? *Int. J. Environ. Res. Public Health* **2014**, *11*, 9954–9963. [CrossRef]
20. Mitchell, T.; Weinberg, M.; Posey, D.L.; Cetron, M. Immigrant and Refugee Health: A Centers for Disease Control and Prevention Perspective on Protecting the Health and Health Security of Individuals and Communities During Planned Migrations. *Pediatr. Clin. North. Am.* **2019**, *66*, 549–560. [CrossRef]
21. Pottie, K.; Greenaway, C.; Feightner, J.; Welch, V.; Swinkels, H.; Rashid, M.; Narasiah, L.; Kirmayer, L.J.; Ueffing, E.; MacDonald, N.E.; et al. Evidence-based clinical guidelines for immigrants and refugees. *Can. Med. Assoc. J.* **2011**, *183*, E824–E925. [CrossRef]
22. Ali, G.-C.; Ryan, G.; De Silva, M.J. Validated Screening Tools for Common Mental Disorders in Low and Middle Income Countries: A Systematic Review. *PLoS ONE* **2016**, *11*, e0156939. [CrossRef]
23. Amiri, S. Prevalence of Suicide in Immigrants/Refugees: A Systematic Review and Meta-Analysis. *Arch. Suicide Res.* **2020**, 1–36. [CrossRef]
24. Morina, N.; Akhtar, A.; Barth, J.; Schnyder, U. Psychiatric Disorders in Refugees and Internally Displaced Persons After Forced Displacement: A Systematic Review. *Front. Psychiatry* **2018**, *9*, 433. [CrossRef]
25. Blackmore, R.; Boyle, J.A.; Fazel, M.; Ranasinha, S.; Gray, K.M.; Fitzgerald, G.; Misso, M.; Gibson-Helm, M. The prevalence of mental illness in refugees and asylum seekers: A systematic review and meta-analysis. *PLoS Med.* **2020**, *17*, e1003337. [CrossRef]

26. Due, C.; Green, E.; Ziersch, A. Psychological trauma and access to primary healthcare for people from refugee and asylum-seeker backgrounds: A mixed methods systematic review. *Int. J. Ment. Health Syst.* **2020**, *14*, 71. [CrossRef]

27. Satinsky, E.; Fuhr, D.; Woodward, A.; Sondorp, E.; Roberts, B. Mental health care utilisation and access among refugees and asylum seekers in Europe: A systematic review. *Health Policy* **2019**, *123*, 851–863. [CrossRef]

28. Hassan, A.; Sharif, K. Efficacy of Telepsychiatry in Refugee Populations: A Systematic Review of the Evidence. *Cureus* **2019**, *11*, e3984. [CrossRef]

29. Gruner, D.; Magwood, O.; Bair, L.; Duff, L.; Adel, S.; Pottie, K. Understanding Supporting and Hindering Factors in Community-Based Psychotherapy for Refugees: A Realist-Informed Systematic Review. *Int. J. Environ. Res. Public Health* **2020**, *17*, 4618. [CrossRef]

30. Lu, J.; Jamani, S.; Benjamen, J.; Agbata, E.; Magwood, O.; Pottie, K. Global Mental Health and Services for Migrants in Primary Care Settings in High-Income Countries: A Scoping Review. *Int. J. Environ. Res. Public Health* **2020**, *17*, 8627. [CrossRef] [PubMed]

31. Gadeberg, A.K.; Montgomery, E.; Frederiksen, H.W.; Norredam, M. Assessing trauma and mental health in refugee children and youth: A systematic review of validated screening and measurement tools. *Eur. J. Public Health* **2017**, *27*, 439–446. [CrossRef]

32. Hollifield, M.; Warner, T.D.; Lian, N.; Krakow, B.; Jenkins, J.H.; Kesler, J.; Stevenson, J.; Westermeyer, J. Measuring Trauma and Health Status in RefugeesA Critical Review. *JAMA* **2002**, *288*, 611–621. [CrossRef] [PubMed]

33. Davidson, G.R.; Murray, K.E.; Schweitzer, R.D. Review of Refugee Mental Health Assessment: Best Practices and Recommendations. *J. Pac. Rim Psychol.* **2010**, *4*, 72–85. [CrossRef]

34. Magwood, O.; Muharram, H.; Saad, A.; Mavedatnia, D.; Madana, M.; Agbata, E.; Pottie, K. *Mental Health Screening Approaches for Refugees and Asylum Seekers: A Protocol for a Scoping Review*; Bruyère Research Institute: Ottawa, ON, Canada, 2021; p. 10.

35. Tricco, A.C.; Lillie, E.; Zarin, W.; O'Brien, K.K.; Colquhoun, H.; Levac, D.; Moher, D.; Peters, M.D.J.; Horsley, T.; Weeks, L.; et al. PRISMA Extension for Scoping Reviews (PRISMA-ScR): Checklist and Explanation. *Ann. Intern. Med.* **2018**, *169*, 467–473. [CrossRef]

36. Rethlefsen, M.L.; Kirtley, S.; Waffenschmidt, S.; Ayala, A.P.; Moher, D.; Page, M.J.; Koffel, J.B.; Blunt, H.; Brigham, T.; Chang, S.; et al. PRISMA-S: An extension to the PRISMA Statement for Reporting Literature Searches in Systematic Reviews. *Syst. Rev.* **2021**, *10*, 39. [CrossRef]

37. United Nations High Commissioner for Refugees UNHCR Resettlement Handbook and Country Chapters. Available online: https://www.unhcr.org/protection/resettlement/4a2ccf4c6/unhcr-resettlement-handbook-country-chapters.html (accessed on 27 February 2022).

38. Veritas Health Innovation. Covidence Systematic Review Software. Available online: https://www.covidence.org/ (accessed on 7 March 2022).

39. Hough, C.; O'Neill, E.; Dyer, F.; Beaney, K.; Crawshaw, A. *The Global Mental Health Assessment Tool (GMHAT) Pilot Evaluation: Final Report*; Public Health England: London, UK, 2019; p. 80.

40. Barnes, D.M. Mental Health Screening in a Refugee Population: A Program Report. *J. Immigr. Health* **2001**, *3*, 141–149. [CrossRef]

41. Al-Obaidi, A.; West, B.; Fox, A.; Savin, D. Incorporating Preliminary Mental Health Assessment in the Initial Healthcare for Refugees in New Jersey. *Community Ment. Health J.* **2015**, *51*, 567–574. [CrossRef] [PubMed]

42. Arnetz, B.B.; Broadbridge, C.L.; Jamil, H.; Lumley, M.A.; Pole, N.; Barkho, E.; Fakhouri, M.; Talia, Y.R.; Arnetz, J.E. Specific Trauma Subtypes Improve the Predictive Validity of the Harvard Trauma Questionnaire in Iraqi Refugees. *J. Immigr. Minority Health* **2014**, *16*, 1055–1061. [CrossRef]

43. Baird, M.B.; Cates, R.; Bott, M.J.; Buller, C. Assessing the Mental Health of Refugees Using the Refugee Health Screener-15. *West J. Nurs. Res.* **2020**, *42*, 910–917. [CrossRef]

44. Barbieri, A.; Visco-Comandini, F.; Alunni Fegatelli, D.; Schepisi, C.; Russo, V.; Calò, F.; Dessì, A.; Cannella, G.; Stellacci, A. Complex trauma, PTSD and complex PTSD in African refugees. *Eur. J. Psychotraumatol.* **2019**, *10*, 1700621. [CrossRef]

45. Bertelsen, N.S.; Selden, E.; Krass, P.; Keatley, E.S.; Keller, A. Primary Care Screening Methods and Outcomes for Asylum Seekers in New York City. *J. Immigr. Minority Health* **2018**, *20*, 171–177. [CrossRef]

46. Bjarta, A.; Leiler, A.; Ekdahl, J.; Wasteson, E. Assessing Severity of Psychological Distress Among Refugees With the Refugee Health Screener, 13-Item Version. *J. Nerv. Ment. Dis.* **2018**, *206*, 834–839. [CrossRef]

47. Boyle, J.A.; Willey, S.; Blackmore, R.; East, C.; McBride, J.; Gray, K.; Melvin, G.; Fradkin, R.; Ball, N.; Highet, N.; et al. Improving Mental Health in Pregnancy for Refugee Women: Protocol for the Implementation and Evaluation of a Screening Program in Melbourne, Australia. *JMIR Res Protoc.* **2019**, *8*, e13271. [CrossRef]

48. Brink, D.R.; Shannon, P.J.; Vinson, G.A. Validation of a brief mental health screener for Karen refugees in primary care. *Fam. Pract.* **2016**, *33*, 107–111. [CrossRef]

49. Buchwald, D.; Manson, S.M.; Brenneman, D.L.; Dinges, N.G.; Keane, E.M.; Beals, J.; Kinzie, J.D. Screening for Depression among Newly Arrived Vietnamese Refugees in Primary Care Settings. *West J. Med.* **1995**, *163*, 341–345.

50. Churbaji, D.; Lindheimer, N.; Schilz, L.; Böge, K.; Abdelmagid, S.; Rayes, D.; Hahn, E.; Bajbouj, M.; Karnouk, C. Development of a Culturally Sensitive Version of the MiniInternational Neuropsychiatric Interview (MINI) in Standard Arabic. *Fortschr. Neurol. Psychiatr.* **2020**, *88*, 95–104. [CrossRef]

51. Cook, T.L.; Shannon, P.J.; Vinson, G.A.; Letts, J.P.; Dwee, E. War trauma and torture experiences reported during public health screening of newly resettled Karen refugees: A qualitative study. *BMC Int. Health Hum. Rights* **2015**, *15*, 8. [CrossRef]

52. Di Pietro, M.L.; Zaçe, D.; Sisti, L.G.; Frisicale, E.M.; Corsaro, A.; Gentili, A.; Giraldi, L.; Bruno, S.; Boccia, S. Development and validation of a questionnaire to assess Unaccompanied Migrant Minors' needs (AEGIS-Q). *Eur. J. Public Health* **2021**, *31*, 313–320. [CrossRef]
53. Durieux-Paillard, S.; Whitaker-Clinch, B.; Bovier, P.A.; Eytan, A. Screening for major depression and posttraumatic stress disorder among asylum seekers: Adapting a standardized instrument to the social and cultural context. *Can. J. Psychiatry* **2006**, *51*, 587–597. [CrossRef] [PubMed]
54. El Ghaziri, N.; Blaser, J.; Darwiche, J.; Suris, J.-C.; Sanchis Zozaya, J.; Marion-Veyron, R.; Spini, D.; Bodenmann, P. Protocol of a longitudinal study on the specific needs of Syrian refugee families in Switzerland. *BMC Int. Health Hum. Rights* **2019**, *19*, 32. [CrossRef] [PubMed]
55. Eytan, A.; Durieux-Paillard, S.; Whitaker-Clinch, B.; Loutan, L.; Bovier, P.A. Transcultural Validity of a Structured Diagnostic Interview to Screen for Major Depression and Posttraumatic Stress Disorder among Refugees. *J. Nerv. Ment. Dis.* **2007**, *195*, 723–728. [CrossRef] [PubMed]
56. Eytan, A.; Bischoff, A.; Rrustemi, I.; Durieux, S.; Loutan, L.; Gilbert, M.; Bovier, P.A. Screening of Mental Disorders in Asylum-Seekers from Kosovo. *Aust. N. Z. J. Psychiatry* **2002**, *36*, 499–503. [CrossRef] [PubMed]
57. Geltman, P.L.; Grant-Knight, W.; Mehta, S.D.; Lloyd-Travaglini, C.; Lustig, S.; Landgraf, J.M.; Wise, P.H. The "Lost Boys of Sudan": Functional and Behavioral Health of Unaccompanied Refugee Minors Resettled in the United States. *Arch. Pediatr. Adolesc. Med.* **2005**, *159*, 585. [CrossRef] [PubMed]
58. Green, A.E.; Weinberger, S.J.; Harder, V.S. The Strengths and Difficulties Questionnaire as a Mental Health Screening Tool for Newly Arrived Pediatric Refugees. *J. Immigr. Minority Health* **2021**, *23*, 494–501. [CrossRef] [PubMed]
59. Hanes, G.; Sung, L.; Mutch, R.; Cherian, S. Adversity and resilience amongst resettling Western Australian paediatric refugees: Refugee resilience and adversity. *J. Paediatr. Child Health* **2017**, *53*, 882–888. [CrossRef]
60. Hauff, E.; Vaglum, P. Organised violence and the stress of exile. Predictors of mental health in a community cohort of Vietnamese refugees three years after resettlement. *Br. J. Psychiatry* **1995**, *166*, 360–367. [CrossRef]
61. Heenan, R.C.; Volkman, T.; Stokes, S.; Tosif, S.; Graham, H.; Smith, A.; Tran, D.; Paxton, G. I think we've had a health screen: New offshore screening, new refugee health guidelines, new Syrian and Iraqi cohorts: Recommendations, reality, results and review: 'I think we've had a health screen'. *J Paediatr. Child Health* **2019**, *55*, 95–103. [CrossRef]
62. Hirani, K.; Cherian, S.; Mutch, R.; Payne, D.N. Identification of health risk behaviours among adolescent refugees resettling in Western Australia. *Arch. Dis. Child* **2018**, *103*, 240–246. [CrossRef]
63. Hobbs, M.; Moor, C.; Wansbrough, T.; Calder, L. The health status of asylum seekers screened by Auckland Public Health in 1999 and 2000. *N. Z. Med. J.* **2002**, *115*, 1160.
64. Hocking, D.C.; Mancuso, S.G.; Sundram, S. Development and validation of a mental health screening tool for asylum-seekers and refugees: The STAR-MH. *BMC Psychiatry* **2018**, *18*, 69. [CrossRef] [PubMed]
65. Hollifield, M.; Verbillis-Kolp, S.; Farmer, B.; Toolson, E.C.; Woldehaimanot, T.; Yamazaki, J.; Holland, A.; St. Clair, J.; SooHoo, J. The Refugee Health Screener-15 (RHS-15): Development and validation of an instrument for anxiety, depression, and PTSD in refugees. *Gen. Hosp. Psychiatry* **2013**, *35*, 202–209. [CrossRef] [PubMed]
66. Hollifield, M.; Toolson, E.C.; Verbillis-Kolp, S.; Farmer, B.; Yamazaki, J.; Woldehaimanot, T.; Holland, A. Effective Screening for Emotional Distress in Refugees: The Refugee Health Screener. *J. Nerv. Ment. Dis.* **2016**, *204*, 247–253. [CrossRef]
67. Jakobsen, M.; Meyer DeMott, M.A.; Heir, T. Validity of screening for psychiatric disorders in unaccompanied minor asylum seekers: Use of computer-based assessment. *Transcult. Psychiatry* **2017**, *54*, 611–625. [CrossRef]
68. Javanbakht, A.; Amirsadri, A.; Abu Suhaiban, H.; Alsaud, M.I.; Alobaidi, Z.; Rawi, Z.; Arfken, C.L. Prevalence of Possible Mental Disorders in Syrian Refugees Resettling in the United States Screened at Primary Care. *J. Immigr. Minority Health* **2019**, *21*, 664–667. [CrossRef]
69. Johnson-Agbakwu, C.E.; Allen, J.; Nizigiyimana, J.F.; Ramirez, G.; Hollifield, M. Mental health screening among newly arrived refugees seeking routine obstetric and gynecologic care. *Psychol. Serv.* **2014**, *11*, 470–476. [CrossRef]
70. Kaltenbach, E.; Härdtner, E.; Hermenau, K.; Schauer, M.; Elbert, T. Efficient identification of mental health problems in refugees in Germany: The Refugee Health Screener. *Eur. J. Psychotraumatol.* **2017**, *8*, 1389205. [CrossRef]
71. Kennedy, J.; Seymour, D.J.; Hummel, B.J. A comprehensive refugee health screening program. *Public Health Rep.* **1999**, *114*, 469–477. [CrossRef]
72. Kleijn, W.C.; Hovens, J.E.; Rodenburg, J.J. Posttraumatic Stress Symptoms in Refugees: Assessments with the Harvard Trauma Questionnaire and the Hopkins Symptom Checklist–25 in Different Languages. *Psychol. Rep.* **2001**, *88*, 527–532. [CrossRef]
73. Kleinert, E.; Müller, F.; Furaijat, G.; Hillermann, N.; Jablonka, A.; Happle, C.; Simmenroth, A. Does refugee status matter? Medical needs of newly arrived asylum seekers and resettlement refugees—A retrospective observational study of diagnoses in a primary care setting. *Confl. Health* **2019**, *13*, 39. [CrossRef]
74. Kröger, C.; Frantz, I.; Friel, P.; Heinrichs, N. Posttraumatische und depressive Symptomatik bei Asylsuchenden. *Psychother Psychosom. Med. Psychol.* **2016**, *66*, 377–384. [CrossRef]
75. LeMaster, J.W.; Broadbridge, C.L.; Lumley, M.A.; Arnetz, J.E.; Arfken, C.; Fetters, M.D.; Jamil, H.; Pole, N.; Arnetz, B.B. Acculturation and post-migration psychological symptoms among Iraqi refugees: A path analysis. *Am. J. Orthopsychiatry* **2018**, *88*, 38–47. [CrossRef]

76. Lillee, A.; Thambiran, A.; Laugharne, J. Evaluating the mental health of recently arrived refugee adults in Western Australia. *J. Public Ment. Health* **2015**, *14*, 56–68. [CrossRef]
77. Loutan, L.; Bollini, P.; Pampallona, S.; Haan, D.B.D.; Gar, F. Impact of trauma and torture on asylum-seekers. *Eur. J. Public Health* **1999**, *9*, 93–96. [CrossRef]
78. Masmas, T.N.; Student, E.M.; Bunch, V.; Jensen, J.H.; Hansen, T.N.; Jørgensen, L.M.; Kj, C.; Oxholm, A.; Worm, L.; Ekstrøm, M. Asylum seekers in Denmark—A study of health status and grade of traumatization of newly arrived asylum seekers. *Torture Q. J. Rehabil. Torture Vict. Prev. Torture* **2008**, *18*, 10.
79. McLeod, A.; Reeve, M. The health status of quota refugees screened by New Zealand's Auckland Public Health Service between 1995 and 2000. *N. Z. Med. J.* **2005**, *118*, 1224.
80. Mewes, R.; Friele, B.; Bloemen, E. Validation of the Protect Questionnaire: A tool to detect mental health problems in asylum seekers by non-health professionals. *Torture J.* **2018**, *28*, 2. [CrossRef]
81. Morina, N.; Ewers, S.M.; Passardi, S.; Schnyder, U.; Knaevelsrud, C.; Müller, J.; Bryant, R.A.; Nickerson, A.; Schick, M. Mental health assessments in refugees and asylum seekers: Evaluation of a tablet-assisted screening software. *Confl. Health* **2017**, *11*, 18. [CrossRef]
82. Nehring, I.; Sattel, H.; Al-Hallak, M.; Sack, M.; Henningsen, P.; Mall, V.; Aberl, S. The Child Behavior Checklist as a Screening Instrument for PTSD in Refugee Children. *Children* **2021**, *8*, 521. [CrossRef]
83. Nikendei, C.; Kindermann, D.; Brandenburg-Ceynowa, H.; Derreza-Greeven, C.; Zeyher, V.; Junne, F.; Friederich, H.-C.; Bozorgmehr, K. Asylum seekers' mental health and treatment utilization in a three months follow-up study after transfer from a state registration-and reception-center in Germany. *Health Policy* **2019**, *123*, 864–872. [CrossRef]
84. Ovitt, N.; Larrison, C.R.; Nackerud, L. Refugees' Responses to Mental Health Screening: A Resettlement Initiative. *Int. Soc. Work* **2003**, *46*, 235–250. [CrossRef]
85. Polcher, K.; Calloway, S. Addressing the Need for Mental Health Screening of Newly Resettled Refugees: A Pilot Project. *J. Prim. Care Community Health* **2016**, *7*, 199–203. [CrossRef]
86. Poole, D.N.; Liao, S.; Larson, E.; Hedt-Gauthier, B.; Raymond, N.A.; Bärnighausen, T.; Smith Fawzi, M.C. Sequential screening for depression in humanitarian emergencies: A validation study of the Patient Health Questionnaire among Syrian refugees. *Ann. Gen. Psychiatry* **2020**, *19*, 5. [CrossRef]
87. Rasmussen, A.; Verkuilen, J.; Ho, E.; Fan, Y. Posttraumatic stress disorder among refugees: Measurement invariance of Harvard Trauma Questionnaire scores across global regions and response patterns. *Psychol. Assess.* **2015**, *27*, 1160–1170. [CrossRef]
88. Richter, K.; Lehfeld, H.; Niklewski, G. Waiting for Asylum: Psychiatric Diagnoses in the central reception facility in Bavaria. *Gesundheitswesen* **2015**, *77*, 834–838. [CrossRef]
89. Salari, R.; Malekian, C.; Linck, L.; Kristiansson, R.; Sarkadi, A. Screening for PTSD symptoms in unaccompanied refugee minors: A test of the CRIES-8 questionnaire in routine care. *Scand. J. Public Health* **2017**, *45*, 605–611. [CrossRef]
90. Savin, D.; Seymour, D.J.; Littleford, L.N.; Bettridge, J.; Giese, A. Findings from Mental Health Screening of Newly Arrived Refugees in Colorado. *Public Health Rep.* **2005**, *120*, 224–229. [CrossRef]
91. Schweitzer, R.D.; Brough, M.; Vromans, L.; Asic-Kobe, M. Mental Health of Newly Arrived Burmese Refugees in Australia: Contributions of Pre-Migration and Post-Migration Experience. *Aust. N. Z. J. Psychiatry* **2011**, *45*, 299–307. [CrossRef]
92. Seagle, E.E.; Vargas, M. Prevalence of Mental Health Screening and Associated Factors among Refugees and other Resettled Populations ≥ 14 Years of Age in Georgia, 2014–2017. *J. Immigrant Minority Health* **2019**, *21*, 1191–1199. [CrossRef]
93. Shannon, P.J.; Vinson, G.A.; Wieling, E.; Cook, T.; Letts, J. Torture, War Trauma, and Mental Health Symptoms of Newly Arrived Karen Refugees. *J. Loss Trauma* **2015**, *20*, 577–590. [CrossRef]
94. Söndergaard, H.P.; Ekblad, S.; Theorell, T. Self-reported life event patterns and their relation to health among recently resettled Iraqi and Kurdish refugees in Sweden. *J. Nerv. Ment. Dis.* **2001**, *189*, 838–845. [CrossRef] [PubMed]
95. Sondergaard, H.P.; Ekblad, S.; Theorell, T. Screening for post-traumatic stress disorder among refugees in Stockholm. *Nord. J. Psychiatry* **2003**, *57*, 185–189. [CrossRef] [PubMed]
96. Stingl, M.; Knipper, M.; Hetzger, B.; Richards, J.; Yazgan, B.; Gallhofer, B.; Hanewald, B. Assessing the special need for protection of vulnerable refugees: Testing the applicability of a screening method (RHS-15) to detect traumatic disorders in a refugee sample in Germany. *Ethn. Health* **2019**, *24*, 897–908. [CrossRef] [PubMed]
97. Sukale, T.; Hertel, C.; Möhler, E.; Joas, J.; Müller, M.; Banaschewski, T.; Schepker, R.; Kölch, M.G.; Fegert, J.M.; Plener, P.L. Diagnostics and initial assessment in the case of underage refugees. *Nervenarzt* **2017**, *88*, 3–9. [CrossRef]
98. Tay, K.; Frommer, N.; Hunter, J.; Silove, D.; Pearson, L.; San Roque, M.; Redman, R.; Bryant, R.A.; Manicavasagar, V.; Steel, Z. A mixed method study of expert psychological evidence submitted for a cohort of asylum seekers undergoing refugee status determination in Australia. *Soc. Sci. Med.* **2013**, *98*, 106–115. [CrossRef]
99. Thulesius, H.; Håkansson, A. Screening for posttraumatic stress disorder symptoms among Bosnian refugees. *J. Traum. Stress* **1999**, *12*, 167–174. [CrossRef]
100. Van Os, E.C.C.; Zijlstra, A.E.; Knorth, E.J.; Post, W.J.; Kalverboer, M.E. Recently arrived refugee children: The quality and outcomes of Best Interests of the Child assessments. *Int. J. Law Psychiatry* **2018**, *59*, 20–30. [CrossRef]
101. Van Dijk, D.G.L.; Kortmann, F.A.M.; Kooyman, M.; Bot, J. The Harvard Trauma Questionnaire. A cross-cultural instrument for screening posttraumatic stress disorder in hospitalized refugees. *Tijdschr. Psychiatr.* **1999**, *41*, 45–49.

102. Vergara, A.E.; Miller, J.M.; Martin, D.R.; Cookson, S.T. A Survey of Refugee Health Assessments in the United States. *J. Immigr. Health* **2003**, *7*, 67–73. [CrossRef]
103. Weine, S.M.; Vojvoda, D.; Becker, D.F.; McGlashan, T.H.; Hodzic, E.; Laub, D.; Hyman, L.; Sawyer, M.; Lazrove, S. PTSD Symptoms in Bosnian Refugees 1 Year after Resettlement in the United States. *Am. J. Psychiatry* **1998**, *155*, 562–564. [CrossRef]
104. Willey, S.M.; Gibson-Helm, M.E.; Finch, T.L.; East, C.E.; Khan, N.N.; Boyd, L.M.; Boyle, J.A. Implementing innovative evidence-based perinatal mental health screening for women of refugee background. *Women Birth* **2020**, *33*, e245–e255. [CrossRef]
105. Wulfes, N.; del Pozo, M.A.; Buhr-Riehm, B.; Heinrichs, N.; Kröger, C. Screening for Posttraumatic Stress Disorder in Refugees: Comparison of the Diagnostic Efficiency of Two Self-Rating Measures of Posttraumatic Stress Disorder: Screening for PTSD in Refugees. *J. Trauma. Stress* **2019**, *32*, 148–155. [CrossRef]
106. Yalim, A.C.; Zubaroglu-Ioannides, P.; Sacco, S. Implementation of an Initial Mental Health Assessment for Newly Arrived Refugees. *J. Soc. Serv. Res.* **2021**, *47*, 199–206. [CrossRef]
107. Young, P.; Gordon, M.S. Mental health screening in immigration detention: A fresh look at Australian government data. *Australas Psychiatry* **2016**, *24*, 19–22. [CrossRef]
108. Sweileh, W.M.; Wickramage, K.; Pottie, K.; Hui, C.; Roberts, B.; Sawalha, A.F.; Zyoud, S.H. Bibliometric analysis of global migration health research in peer-reviewed literature (2000–2016). *BMC Public Health* **2018**, *18*, 777. [CrossRef]
109. CDC. Mental Health Technical Instructions for Panel Physicians. Available online: https://www.cdc.gov/immigrantrefugeehealth/panel-physicians/mental-health.html (accessed on 16 December 2021).
110. Immigration New Zealand (INZ). Refugee Settlement Health Assessments. Available online: https://www.immigration.govt.nz/assist-migrants-and-students/other-industry-partners/panel-physician-network/refugee-settlement-health-assessments (accessed on 16 December 2021).
111. Cowen, T.; Stella, F.; Magahy, K.; Strauss, K.; Morton, J. *Sanctuary, Safety and Solidarity: Lesbian, Gay, Bisexual, Transgender Asylum Seekers and Refugees in Scotland*; University of Glasgow: Glasgow, UK, 2011.
112. White, L.C.; Cooper, M.; Lawrence, D. Mental illness and resilience among sexual and gender minority refugees and asylum seekers. *Br. J. Gen. Pract* **2019**, *69*, 10–11. [CrossRef]
113. Women's Refugee Commission. *Disabilities Among Refugees and Conflict-Affected Populations*; Women's Refugee Commission: New York, NY, USA, 2010; ISBN 978-1-58030-072-8.
114. Purkey, E.; Patel, R.; Phillips, S.P. Trauma-informed care. *Can. Fam. Physician* **2018**, *64*, 170–172.
115. Crocker, E.; Webster, P.D. *Developing Patient- and FamilyCentered Vision, Mission, and Philosophy of Care Statements*, 2nd ed.; Institute for Patient- and Family-Centered Care: Bethesda, MD, USA, 2012.
116. Griswold, K.S.; Vest, B.M.; Lynch-Jiles, A.; Sawch, D.; Kolesnikova, K.; Byimana, L.; Kefi, P. "I just need to be with my family": Resettlement experiences of asylum seeker and refugee survivors of torture. *Glob. Health* **2021**, *17*, 27. [CrossRef]
117. Member Centers of the National Consortium of Torture Treatment Programs (NCTTP). Descriptive, inferential, functional outcome data on 9025 torture survivors over six years in the United States. *Torture* **2015**, *25*, 34–60.
118. Dunn, T.J.; Browne, A.; Haworth, S.; Wurie, F.; Campos-Matos, I. Service Evaluation of the English Refugee Health Information System: Considerations and Recommendations for Effective Resettlement. *Int. J. Environ. Res. Public Health* **2021**, *18*, 10331. [CrossRef]
119. Regmi, P.R.; Aryal, N.; van Teijlingen, E.; Simkhada, P.; Adhikary, P. Nepali Migrant Workers and the Need for Pre-departure Training on Mental Health: A Qualitative Study. *J. Immigr Minor. Health* **2020**, *22*, 973–981. [CrossRef]
120. Grist, R.; Porter, J.; Stallard, P. Mental Health Mobile Apps for Preadolescents and Adolescents: A Systematic Review. *J. Med. Internet Res.* **2017**, *19*, e176. [CrossRef]
121. Magwood, O.; Bellai Dusseault, K.; Fox, G.; McCutcheon, C.; Adams, O.; Saad, A.; Kassam, A. *Diagnostic Test Accuracy of Screening Tools for Post-Traumatic Stress Disorder Among Refugees and Asylum Seekers: A Protocol for a Systematic Review of Diagnostic Test Accuracy Studies*; Cochrane Equity Methods: Ottawa, ON, Canada, 2021.
122. Saad, A.; Magwood, O.; Aubry, T.; Alkhateeb, Q.; Hashmi, S.S.; Hakim, J.; Ford, L.; Kassam, A.; Tugwell, P.; Pottie, K. Mobile interventions targeting common mental disorders among pregnant and postpartum women: An equity-focused systematic review. *PLoS ONE* **2021**, *16*, e0259474. [CrossRef] [PubMed]
123. Cleveland, J.; Rousseau, C.; Guzder, J. Cultural Consultation for Refugees. In *Encountering the Other in Mental Health Care*; Springer: Amsterdam, The Neatherlands, 2014; pp. 245–268. ISBN 978-1-4614-7614-6.
124. Ng, E.; Pottie, K.; Spitzer, D. Official language proficiency and self-reported health among immigrants to Canada. *Health Rep.* **2011**, *22*, 15–23. [PubMed]
125. Pottie, K.; Hadi, A.; Chen, J.; Welch, V.; Hawthorne, K. Realist review to understand the efficacy of culturally appropriate diabetes education programmes. *Diabet. Med.* **2013**, *30*, 1017–1025. [CrossRef] [PubMed]

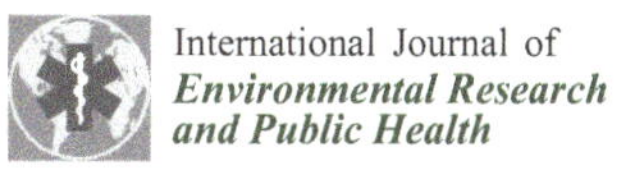

International Journal of
Environmental Research and Public Health

MDPI

Article

Mental Health in the Transit Context: Evidence from 10 Countries

Maria Caterina Gargano [1], Dean Ajduković [2] and Maša Vukčević Marković [3,4,*]

1. Department of Psychology, Kroc Institute for International Peace Studies, University of Notre Dame, 390 Corbett Family Hall, Notre Dame, IN 46556, USA; mcgargano@nd.edu
2. Department of Psychology, University of Zagreb, Ivana Lucica 3, 10000 Zagreb, Croatia; dean.ajdukovic@ffzg.hr
3. Department of Psychology, Faculty of Philosophy, University of Belgrade, 11000 Belgrade, Serbia
4. Psychosocial Innovation Network, 11000 Belgrade, Serbia
* Correspondence: masa.vukcevic@f.bg.ac.rs; Tel.: +381-63-723-4658

Abstract: Most interventions for mental health and psychosocial support (MHPSS) have been developed in contexts and with populations that differ significantly from the realities of migration. There is an urgent need for MHPSS in transit; however, transit-specific aspects of MHPSS provision are often neglected due to the inherent challenges transit poses to traditional conceptualizations of practice. The Delphi method, which consisted of three iterative rounds of surveys, was applied with the goal of identifying challenges to and adaptations of MHPSS in the transit context. Twenty-six MHPSS providers working with refugees in 10 European transit countries participated; 69% of participants completed all three survey rounds. There was consensus that a flexible model of MHPSS, which can balance low intensity interventions and specialized care, is needed. Agreement was high for practice-related and sociopolitical factors impacting MHPSS in transit; however, the mandate of MHPSS providers working in the transit context achieved the lowest consensus and is yet to be defined. There is a need to rethink MHPSS in the refugee transit context. Providing MHPSS to refugees on the move has specificities, most of which are related to the instability and uncertainty of the context. Future directions for improving mental health protection for refugees, asylum seekers, and migrants in transit are highlighted.

Keywords: migration; mental health promotion; refugees; transit; MHPSS; Delphi method

Citation: Gargano, M.C.; Ajduković, D.; Vukčević Marković, M. Mental Health in the Transit Context: Evidence from 10 Countries. *Int. J. Environ. Res. Public Health* **2022**, *19*, 3476. https://doi.org/10.3390/ijerph19063476

Academic Editors: Greg Armstrong and Shameran Slewa-Younan

Received: 30 December 2021
Accepted: 9 March 2022
Published: 15 March 2022

Publisher's Note: MDPI stays neutral with regard to jurisdictional claims in published maps and institutional affiliations.

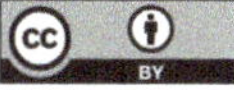

1. Introduction

According to UNHCR reports, by the end of 2020, the number of people who were forced to leave their home countries in order to escape war, persecution, and human rights violations and to search for safety reached 82.4 million [1]. The current refugee crisis in Europe has lasted for years now, and recent events indicate that new challenges are to be expected [2]. As noted at the 20th Berlin Conference on Refugee Rights in 2020 [3], this crisis has long been exacerbated by inadequate investment in sustainable asylum systems. As a result, states increasingly seek to avoid their human rights obligations to asylum seekers and to place human rights at odds with border management. This rhetoric and the policy choices stemming from it have increased the time spent in transit, leading to substantial consequences for the daily lives and wellbeing of refugees, migrants, and asylum seekers.

It is important to note that, while crisis language is often used to frame refugee movements, for refugees, each decision to move is part of a much longer journey [4]. After leaving their home countries, refugees, asylum seekers, and migrants (For better readability and simplicity, the term refugee will be used throughout the text regardless of individuals' legal status) often try to reach destination countries in Western Europe, where they seek international protection and can start rebuilding their lives. One of the main land transit routes refugees are using, with over 150,000 crossings in 2019 [5], is the Western Balkan route, which includes Turkey, Greece, Bulgaria, North Macedonia, Montenegro, Albania,

Croatia, Bosnia and Herzegovina, and Kosovo (This designation is without prejudice to positions on status and is in line with UNSCR 1244/1999 and the ICJ Opinion on the Kosovo declaration of independence [5]. After EU migration governance policies sought to close the Balkan route following the spring of 2016, refugees are increasingly pushed to try "The Game", informal travel into Western Europe [6]. For the majority, transit from their homes to the destination countries does not represent a journey but rather the advent of transit as a new reality of living on the move. It has been documented that transit can last from several months to several years [7]. Transit usually includes a long and risky route across the sea and land where refugees are exposed to detention or extended stays in camps [8] and illegal pushbacks [9], as well as physical and psychological violence [7,10,11], human trafficking [12], and other life-threatening situations [13]. In addition, prolonged periods of time in transit usually entail poor housing, limited access to essential services such as healthcare [14,15], discrimination by the local community, and separation from family and friends, which can lead to a lack of social support, isolation, and loneliness [13,16]. The urgency of improving conditions in transit is evidenced by the conclusions of the Second Berlin Conference on Libya in 2021, which called for increased respect for human rights, addressing human trafficking and the use of detention, and the development of a comprehensive approach to migration in the Libyan transit context [17].

The situation of protracted transit, in addition to bringing numerous risks for refugees, also leads to various challenges for countries along transit routes who are obliged to provide protection and care to people currently residing in their territories. These responsibilities include ensuring protection of rights, access to adequate shelter, food, and other basic living necessities, and access to healthcare and social services, as well as to the asylum procedure for those seeking international protection. The provision of these protections and services is even more difficult for countries that are already struggling with limited resources, particularly when it comes to health and social protection systems, which is often the case in countries along transit routes. For many state systems, the current refugee crisis has highlighted preexisting gaps in social services and infrastructure as well as the need to rethink existing practices and policies. This is not only due to limited resources, but also stems from specific characteristics that are inherent in the transit context and the population of concern, which may call into question if and how some traditionally conceptualized services respond to the needs of refugees on the move.

1.1. Implications of the Transit Context for Existing Mental Health and Psychosocial Support Practices and Policies

Most interventions for mental health and psychosocial support (MHPSS) have been developed and tested in contexts that differ significantly from the realities of refugee life on the move. Namely, the unpredictability of circumstances in the transit context presents challenges for informed treatment planning and, accordingly, deciding which interventions should be applied. In addition, health care systems in most transit countries are often under-resourced and provide limited access to MHPSS services, while services funded by international agencies and civil society usually lack continuity and sustainability. Therefore, the standard frequency and duration of treatment may not be achievable. Typically, there is a shortage of trained interpreters and cultural mediators, as well as MHPSS practitioners sensitized for work in the context of migration. Furthermore, refugees' short duration of stay in one country and the lack of cross-country cooperation mean that it is not possible to ensure continuity of care. All of these factors pose challenges to the way MHPSS practice has traditionally been conceptualized in the stable and well-resourced contexts of European and North American destination countries.

Additional challenges to traditional MHPSS practice stem from other characteristics of the transit context and the population in question, including the high prevalence of mental health difficulties that have been identified in refugee populations [18–22] due to continuous exposure to stressful and traumatic experiences [7,23–26], the role of interpreters and cultural mediators in providing care [27,28], ethical dilemmas in conducting research [29], and a deficit of cultural understanding in MHPSS treatments [30]. Finally, it is important to investigate to what extent existential threats, including numerous legal and socio-economic issues refugees are facing [16], may limit the overall effectiveness of MHPSS interventions [31]. Under these circumstances, the role of MHPSS practitioners can hardly be limited to traditional norms when defining roles and boundaries. It can be assumed that MHPSS practitioners in the transit context are more involved in advocacy work, as well as cooperation with multidisciplinary teams that are jointly providing protection and support to refugees.

1.2. The Present Study

The aim of the current study was to identify challenges and areas requiring adaptation within MHPSS in the refugee transit context. Additionally, the study aimed to provide essential evidence to inform the adaptation of MHPSS guidance to the transit context in order to improve future research and practice.

2. Materials and Methods

2.1. Delphi Process

The Delphi method [32] is commonly used to harness the value of experts' opinions and experiences in order to identify areas of consensus or lack thereof, which can inform future research, practice, and decision-making. It is particularly useful in situations where there is insufficient evidence or in new areas of research. In the field of psychology, the Delphi method has been used to create guidelines for post-disaster psychosocial care [33], to develop training programs [34], and to identify research priorities [35]. The present study adopts this method with the goal of using experts' opinions to identify obstacles and therefore areas that need to be addressed in future research and practice in the provision of evidence-based MHPSS services to refugees.

2.2. Statement Development

For the purpose of the present study, a group of experts convened to develop the initial statements. This group consisted of members of the Research Working Group of the Consortium on Refugees' and Migrants' Mental Health (CoReMH). The Consortium on Refugees' and Migrants' Mental Health was established in 2020 with the goal of facilitating international cooperation between mental health experts and practitioners working on the ground with refugees in the transit context. The CoReMH is devoted to identifying and addressing prominent issues in mental health protection for refugees, asylum seekers, and migrants, through evidence-based practice, research, and advocacy work. The authors are members of the CoReMH. In total, eleven experts from Serbia, Croatia, Turkey, Italy, Bulgaria, and Kosovo, 91% of whom were female, participated in the statement development process. Initially, open-ended questions and general topics were developed during the first online meeting. Subsequently, the initial set of statements was collaboratively produced, and the subsections of the survey as well as methodological details such as the inclusion criteria and sampling method were discussed and defined. The resulting initial survey draft was sent to all experts who participated in statement development as a Google form. They were asked to provide their opinion on the inclusion and wording of each statement by choosing between "include as is", "remove completely", or "reword/change". If they chose the third option, they were asked to include their reasoning or suggested changes. Further, space for additional comments, questions, ideas, or concerns was provided at the end of each section, as well as at the end of the survey to allow the experts to express their opinions and provide suggestions. The resulting data were used to inform a new draft of the survey and a second experts' meeting was convened. At this meeting, the final version of the Initial Survey was completed.

Ultimately, the Initial Survey consisted of 12 sections. At the beginning of the survey, key terms were defined, and demographic questions were asked. Section 1 of the Initial Survey focused on understanding the mandate of mental health practitioners in the transit context and how they define their job. Sections 2–4 asked participants to consider the impact of the transit context on MHPSS interventions, identify contextual challenges to MHPSS, and consider what does and does not work in this context. Section 5 explored how the professional roles, settings, and boundaries in transit are similar to or different from those in a standard context. Sections 6–8 delved into evidence-based practice in the transit context, as well as ethical and methodological challenges that are inherent when working with refugees, and realistic measures of assessing effectiveness. Sections 9–11 focused on the mental health of practitioners themselves; specifically, they examined the impact this work has on them, the way that they perceive the value and efficacy of their interventions, and their cooperation with other providers. Section 12 consisted of two open-ended general conclusion questions regarding what else people should know about MHPSS provision in the transit context and why rethinking MHPSS of that context may be plausible.

The surveys were administered using Google Forms.

2.3. Participants

The inclusion criterion for participants was defined as having a minimum of one year of experience working in the provision of MHPSS services to refugees in the transit context. Participants were recruited through the CoReMH, as well as other providers in members' networks, using a snowballing sampling strategy. During Round 1, 26 participants completed the survey of which 3 self-identified as male (11.5%) and 23 identified as female (88.5%). Participants' ages ranged from 24 to 70 years (mean = 36.5, median = 32.5, sd = 12.7) and they were from 10 countries (Albania, Bosnia and Herzegovina, Bulgaria, Croatia, Greece, Hungary, Italy, Kosovo, Serbia, and Turkey). Years of experience ranged from 1 to 29 (mean = 6.8, median = 4.5, sd = 7.9). The vast majority of the participants ($n = 22$) described their professional and educational background as related to psychology, including clinical psychology, psychological rehabilitation, psychological counseling, psychiatry, psychotherapy, and having a master's degree in psychology. Other professions included workshop management, social work, child protection, academia, and nonprofit leadership. During Round 2, 24 of the original participants completed the survey with an acceptable attrition rate of 7.69%. Eighteen of the original participants completed the Round 3 (Final) Survey with an overall attrition rate of 30.77% from Round 1.

2.4. Procedure

The study included three rounds of data collection. During the first round, the participants were asked to rate their level of agreement with each statement using a 10-point Likert scale where 1 indicated strong disagreement and 10 indicated strong agreement. In addition, they were asked to explain their rationale, leave comments, or suggest the addition or removal of statements. The statements that reached high consensus after the first round were not included in the following survey rounds, meaning that the number of statements being assessed decreased in each round. The statements that had not reached sufficient consensus were reviewed and adapted to be clearer and to better capture the concept in question or deleted, based on statistics and qualitative data obtained in the first round.

Panelists were then asked to complete Round 2 of the survey and assess 87 statements. This time they were provided with contextual data: each item was accompanied by the average agreement score and the level of consensus from Round 1. Each participant was also able to see the score they had assigned to items in the previous round. They could choose to keep their previous score or change it based on the contextual information provided and were asked to justify their reasoning for this decision. The same process was repeated in Round 3 when 30 statements were assessed with a final survey.

2.5. Data Analysis

Agreement levels for each statement were based on the mean of the assessment the panelists chose on the 10-point scale. This agreement level is a measure of the importance attributed to each particular statement related to MHPSS in the transit context.

The consensus level reached for each statement was derived from the coefficient of variation (CV), a measure that takes into account both mean and standard deviation [36]. The CV is inversely related to the level of consensus such that a smaller CV indicates less variation in individual scores for a given statement and is evidence of a higher level of consensus. Statements were considered high or low consensus if they had a CV of less than 0.2 or above 0.2, respectively. Only statements that fell into the high consensus category (CV < 0.2) were retained in the final list of statements that reached consensus (Appendix A (Table A1).

RStudio Cloud (Version 4.0.3, RStudio Team, Boston, MA, USA) [37–41] and Google Sheets (Google LLC, Mountain View, CA, USA), were used for all statistical and data visualization purposes.

3. Results

3.1. Round 1

The first round of the Delphi study indicated a fairly high overall level of agreement with the contents of the initial 92 statements: the average rating across all participants and statements was 7.71 points on the 10-point scale. A high level of consensus was achieved for 27 statements.

Out of the remaining statements, based on statistics and suggestions from the participants, 34 were reformulated, 16 were deleted, and 13 were kept in their original form. Based on the qualitative data collected in the survey, one new section (Section 13) consisting of 28 statements was introduced, entitled "Impact of Sociopolitical Context on MHPSS in the Transit Context," which focused on policies and other structural characteristics of the transit context.

3.2. Round 2

As in the first round, there was a high overall level of agreement with the contents of the statements included in the second-round survey. Of the 87 statements panelists were asked to rate, 46 met requirements for high consensus.

Of the remaining statements, 5 were reformulated, 12 were dropped, and 26 were kept in their original form.

3.3. Round 3

In Round 3, high consensus was reached for 20 statements. Ten statements failed to achieve a high level of consensus.

3.4. Emerging Themes

In total, 93 statements reached consensus. These statements are listed by theme in Appendix A (Table A1) To the right of each statement, the average score is provided as a metric of how strongly participants agreed with the statements that reached consensus.

The highest overall average score was observed for the importance for close cooperation between MHPSS practitioners from different countries on the route (M = 9.39). Of all the statements that reached consensus, only two had average scores below 7, indicating an attribution of lower importance to these particular aspects of MHPSS. The first focused on whether the ethical, practical, and methodological concerns limit possibilities for conducting research in transit (M = 5.89); the second addressed whether the transit context decreases clients' motivation to engage with MHPSS services (M = 6.61).

Three main themes emerged from our findings. First, the failure to reach consensus on certain statements related to the mandate of MHPSS providers working in the transit context revealed that this professional role and identity remain unclear and require further definition. For example, when considering which types of interventions make sense in the transit context, panelists showed the highest support for occupational workshops and activities being an important part of MHPSS for people on the move (M = 9.31) but failed to agree upon two typically central tenets of MHPSS providers' jobs: providing specialized services for diagnosed mental health disorders (CV = 0.34) and helping people process potentially ongoing traumatic and stressful experiences (CV = 0.30). Despite the lack of consensus on these two statements, study results show that there is considerable agreement on certain aspects of providers' mandate. The most strongly agreed upon aspects were raising awareness of the importance of MHPSS for people on the move (M = 9.00), recognizing and validating clients' existing capacities and strengths (M = 9.13), and connecting clients with other resources (M = 9.19). These high-agreement statements can provide insights into how practitioners think about their role in transit and can serve as a starting point for future discussions on the mandate of MHPSS providers in transit that seek to explore and address the identified areas of disagreement.

Second, a trend in the data across several sections was that many features inherent in the transit context present challenges to the ways in which both practice and research are usually carried out. Of the statements in Section 2, which focused on the impact of transit on MHPSS interventions, the importance of a flexible model of care that could meet clients' needs wherever they are reached the highest level of agreement (M = 8.83). When considering challenges to MHPSS in transit, participants most strongly agreed that MHPSS interventions should be adapted to consider the impact of circumstantial factors in transit (M = 8.96). This complicates and presents both ethical and practical challenges for the application of methods for treatment and data collection in transit that were originally developed for use in contexts with different resources and were likely tested on populations with different needs and backgrounds. Nevertheless, there was a high level of agreement regarding the need for more evidence on the effectiveness of MHPSS intervention implementation in transit (M = 8.42), which highlights that, despite the numerous challenges identified, providers agree that more transit-specific research, which could enable evidence-based practice, is urgently needed.

Third, a high level of agreement was exhibited for most statements from Section 13 on the impact of the sociopolitical context on MHPSS in transit. Specifically, border-related violence (M = 8.78), the high level of uncertainty (M = 8.70), the undesired extension of time spent in transit (M = 8.70), stress surrounding the asylum procedure and the low likelihood of obtaining asylum (M = 8.39), and the present political context (M = 8.22) were all identified by providers as stressors, which negatively impact the mental health of people on the move. These findings highlight the importance of considering social determinants of mental health, including environmental conditions created or reinforced by migration governance policies, in the design and provision of MHPSS services in transit.

4. Discussion

The main aim of the current study was to identify challenges to and areas for adaptation within MHPSS services in the refugee transit context as well as to provide the evidence needed to guide that adaptation. The study findings fall into three broad themes.

4.1. Identity of MHPSS Providers

This study showed there is a common understanding of the importance of some aspects of MHPSS providers' mandate. Namely, the panelists overwhelmingly assessed as important and agreed that their mandate involves maintaining clients' mental health and wellbeing, helping people survive and cope in healthy ways, raising awareness of the importance of MHPSS, and bolstering extant resilience capacities. Interestingly, the highest level of agreement in the mandate section corresponded to connecting people on the move to other resources, highlighting the multiplicity of roles that MHPSS providers are expected to play in the transit context.

Surprisingly, the experts did not agree that the job of MHPSS practitioners working with refugees in transit should include treating diagnosed mental health disorders. Upon reviewing the qualitative data linked to this topic, it was found that those who agreed with the statement mainly argued that this was a central part of their work, as it is essential to prevent deterioration of mental health, especially for those presenting with severe symptoms (e.g., "It is a necessary part of our job. Of course it will be done in a team (e.g., in collaboration with the psychiatrists), but if this is not the job of MHPSS practitioners providing MHPSS support to people on the move, I do not understand whose it should be"). Conversely, those who did not agree with the statement expressed concern about limited resources, potentially inadequate training and competencies, ethical issues in medicalizing symptoms, and the lack of continuity of care. It is important to highlight that these factors have also been identified as legitimate concerns by past research, which has found harmful effects linked to these factors for both providers and clients. Low resources are often linked to increased caseloads for providers, which has been shown to be associated with emotional exhaustion and burnout in community mental health care providers [42]. Inadequate cultural competency training and treatment adaptation has been shown to cause harm, and the dominance of the biomedical model of mental health has been challenged, especially in work with refugee populations [43].

In addition, there was a lack of consensus around the importance of helping refugees to process potentially ongoing trauma. As with the previous statement, those who agreed expressed that this was a large part of their job and that it was their responsibility to provide such support ("This is probably the primary job and it's the job that takes up the most time in this kind of setting."). Those who were opposed argued that it is more appropriate to help the refugees process trauma when people have settled in a destination country and achieved a basic state of safety and stability ("Besides the basic interventions, it is best to start treatment once the person reaches a destination country and other preconditions for continuous therapeutic work and life circumstances are stabilized"). Whether providers considered this an important aspect of their mandate or not in the transit context, they emphasized the need to acknowledge individual preferences across clients and the beneficiary's perspective ("Processing of traumatic experiences in my opinion should not be instigated by the MHPSS practitioner if it is not on the agenda of the beneficiary." "If they want to, there are many clients who do not wish to go through trauma with MHPSS professionals, and that has to be respected"). The unanticipated contentiousness of these statements demonstrates how, in the transit context, even the most basic functions of mental health care provision are called into question.

There are several potential causes for these findings. It is possible that the lack of universal standards on required qualifications for MHPSS care providers poses a concern regarding the expertise needed to ensure the required quality of care for refugees who have experienced several traumatic events. This could explain why some providers are hesitant when it comes to the more sensitive aspects of MHPSS work, such as providing treatment to persons with mental health disorders or processing traumatic experiences. In addition, it seems there are dilemmas among care providers about whether certain types of MHPSS interventions, primarily specialized care, should be applied before refugees arrive at their destination and achieve some form of life stability. However, the importance of providing an opportunity to process ongoing trauma whenever it is introduced by the client was highlighted ("It is not ours to decide when the need for support in processing traumatic and stressful experiences will appear, but to be ready to provide support whenever that happens. And experience says it might happen while people are still in transit"). Interestingly, there is agreement, both within and outside of our study, on the provision of mental health services in the post-migration context. Healthcare professionals have stressed the importance of mental health care provision for newly arriving refugees as well as strengthening continuity of care [44]. A qualitative study conducted with refugees who had recently arrived in seven European countries also identified psychological distress as a main health problem, as well as a need to address the deficit in continuity of care for this population [45]. Both provision and continuity of mental health care are equally important in transit, yet they may be even more challenging to achieve in this context due to time and resource limitations.

The short time refugees tend to spend in transit countries could also account for the avoidance of the aforementioned interventions. However, previous studies have shown that time spent in transit varies from several months to several years [7], so it is hard to justify the sustained lack of specialized care observed in this context. Finally, a potential explanation may be the recent paradigm shift from more substantial specialized treatment to low intensity peer-support models of MHPSS [46], which may have impacted the way care providers' understand the expectations and goals of their work.

Furthermore, the methods that are currently promoted by most international bodies and donors supporting MHPSS services, particularly in low- and middle-income countries, mainly include basic psychosocial support. Individual specialized care is rarely funded by international donors and is consequently rarely part of project-based MHPSS care providers' mandates. This, in the long run, may influence the way MHPSS care providers conceptualize their professional identity and, accordingly, the way they orient their practice towards or away from treating mental health disorders and trauma ("I think that while trying not to stigmatize people with mental health difficulties we slip into the opposite extreme and have started stigmatizing mental health disorders as such. They might be disorders, but they can also be treatable, and people should be encouraged to address them, and MHPSS care providers should provide support along this process"). Overall, this study showed polarization among care providers, which highlights the urgent importance of rethinking core aspects of MHPSS care providers' identity and their understanding of their mandate.

When it comes to other aspects of MHPSS practitioners' mandate, including setting, roles, and boundaries, there was agreement that the transit context differs from that of standard work in several ways. These include lack of proper premises for delivering MHPSS services, working with interpreters, and MHPSS practitioners balancing multiple roles in relation to their clients, all of which make maintaining boundaries more difficult than in the standard context. Furthermore, this study revealed that advocacy work is conceptualized as one of the core aspects of MHPSS work in the transit context. This includes working in multidisciplinary teams, advocating for clients' rights, informing policy development, and striving to achieve a political impact that will be protective for the mental health of refugees. Thus, MHPSS providers' responsibility for education on human rights violations and for supporting clients in knowing their rights and reporting any violations in order to avoid perpetuating an inhumane system was highlighted ("These systemic stressors are exactly the reason why MHPSS providers should engage with and actively contribute to organized advocacy efforts and politically engaged consultancy, campaigning, publishing, etc., which is needed for an influential impact on political decision making"). Therefore, the study revealed an evolving aspect of MHPSS providers' mandate, which emerged as a response to job requirements in such precarious and dynamic circumstances and confirmed the need to rethink and adjust definitions of the role of MHPSS providers in the transit context.

4.2. Specifics of MHPSS in the Transit Context

The study revealed a need to define suitable MHPSS interventions for the transit context. There was support for developing a more flexible model of care ranging from community-based to specialized care, in accordance with past research on meeting mental health needs in the transit context [47]. This model should be adjusted to the needs of people on the move, which could be enabled by continuously assessing needs and by including refugees themselves in the design and provision of MHPSS services in the transit context. Furthermore, this model should be adjusted to transit-specific systemic factors, such as unpredictability, lack of control over time, and major life events that refugees might experience during transit, all of which are related to mental health and, consequently, impact the types of MHPSS interventions that should be applied in the transit context. These findings align with those of past research, which has underscored the importance of incorporating an understanding of environmental factors into MHPSS service provision [48]. The transit-specific contextual factors our study identified could add to the cumulative load of environmental stress a person of refugee background experiences as posited by Kashyap and colleagues' (2021) "Psychological Interaction with Environment (PIE) Matrix Model" of refugee mental health and should be investigated further in the future [48]. Additionally, several other material factors limiting the efficacy of practice in the transit context, such as lack of funding and referrals for people in remote locations where support is not available, were considered important. This echoes findings from other researchers who have emphasized the need to increase accessibility to care in transit [47].

It was also pointed out that trust, which is foundational for successful MHPSS interventions, is much more difficult to establish in the transit context given the uncertainty created by sociopolitical factors. Our qualitative data offers an example of how some providers conceptualize the impact of transit-related factors on the establishment of trust ("Re-traumatization, exacerbation of symptoms, and impaired functionality impacted trust in MHPSS experts and services. [There could be] serious deterioration of mental health due to interventions which shouldn't be implemented before basic preconditions (such as safety/stability/basic needs) are met").

Other researchers have highlighted the importance of strengths, values, and action-based intervention approaches in the transit context [49], an approach that was also supported by our qualitative data ("In my opinion [processing traumatic and stressful experiences] should mean focusing on survival, successful coping, strengths and resources"). The variance in ideas about which types of interventions are and are not appropriate in transit reflects an ongoing debate in the field regarding how best to adapt MHPSS care provision to the specific contextual factors of life on the move.

These contextual factors were also seen as impacting care providers' mental health and creating feelings of hopelessness, guilt, and anger ("It was often the case to have questions on migration policies within psychological sessions. It caused and triggered my feelings of shame and helplessness, and the awareness that I am also part of that system which failed to provide protection and abandoned people, as well as the fact that I did not do enough to change it.").

Furthermore, the need to conduct more research within the transit context to inform practice as well as for additional training for MHPSS practitioners on research methodology, in order to support future evidence-based practice in transit, was recognized. Moreover, the panelists agreed that there is a need to define what can be considered "evidence" when discussing evidence-based practice in the transit context.

However, despite the numerous contextual limitations, there was a high level of agreement on the perceived value and effectiveness of MHPSS in the transit context, which can be attributed to a belief that MHPSS in the transit context can make a difference, regardless of the myriad obstacles inherent in transit.

4.3. Sociopolitical Factors

Another insight from this study is the importance of considering the impact of the sociopolitical context on MHPSS in the transit context. Sociopolitical context and European migration and border governance policies were recognized as risk factors that impact refugees' mental health and the effectiveness of MHPSS interventions. Moreover, numerous factors introduced by the sociopolitical context represent under-researched areas and are typically not accounted for in MHPSS. These include, but are not limited to, border-related violence, pushbacks, the undesired extension of time spent in transit, high level of uncertainty, lack of legal and safe pathways for refugees, unpredictability and unfairness of migration procedures, police violence and exposure to violence from criminal groups, and stress surrounding the asylum procedure, including potential retraumatization [50] and the low likelihood of obtaining asylum. These findings largely align with past work on social determinants of health, which has demonstrated that the environmental conditions in which people live, shaped by systemic inequities and structural violence, can impact health between and within societies [51]. The concept of social determinants has also been applied to mental health, highlighting the relationship between social inequalities and exposure to risk factors for many mental health disorders [52]. Qualitative data from many participants in our study highlight providers' agreement regarding how foundational social determinants, including sociopolitical factors, are in both shaping refugees' daily lived experiences and MHPSS care provision. ("For any disadvantaged population, socio-economic and political factors that lead to and maintain discrimination and racism play a role in mental health and wellbeing, particularly if disadvantages and inequalities are trans-generational").

This study also highlighted that the stressful and traumatic experiences refugees go through during transit constitute another round of trauma, sometimes consisting of more traumatic events than were experienced in the country of origin, whose negative effects on refugees' mental health have been demonstrated in previous studies [7]. In addition, the study provided insights into how the wider sociopolitical context is represented in refugees' narratives and shared during psychological support sessions as well as how this can consequently trigger additional stress for refugees ("I also would like to emphasize that potential retraumatization, low likelihood of obtaining asylum, bureaucracy of seeking asylum, limited access to basic needs, health, education and high level of uncertainty, inconsistent policies have a greater effect on the mental health of this vulnerable group"). While, to our knowledge, social determinants of mental health specific to transit have not been studied, researchers have investigated social determinants of mental health in the post-migration and resettlement contexts. Chen and colleagues found evidence to suggest that the social environment in the post-migration context is essential for humanitarian migrants' mental health [53]. Others have concluded that interventions should incorporate elements designed to address broader social, political, economic, and material conditions of post-migration life, a conclusion also reached in our study [54]. Similarly, Li, Liddell, and Nickerson discussed how sociopolitical factors can impact refugees' psychosocial functioning in the post-migration context [55]. Unfortunately, there is evidence that, as a result of the COVID-19 pandemic, the existing inequalities driving social determinants of mental health for refugees, as well as challenges to accessing MHPSS services, have been exacerbated in the post-migration context [56].

Our study findings on the asylum process as a stressor are supported by past research, which has both found that the asylum procedure is a source of stress and recognized policies related to migration as having shaped many social determinants of health for migrant populations [54,55,57]. Participants in our study repeatedly focused on the potential impacts of the asylum process and related stressors on refugees' wellbeing. This is evidenced by both survey data, for instance the high agreement with statement 81 in Appendix A (Table A1), as well as qualitative data ("While waiting for asylum approval and going through interviews and new procedures, people often experience stress that affects their memory, sleep and relationships with people"). While several social determinants overlap between transit and post-migration contexts, there is a need for further research that could identify and evaluate ways to address transit-specific social determinants of mental health, such as border-related violence.

The study points out that mental health protection for refugees on the move cannot be ensured by interventions at the individual level alone, without addressing wider systemic and sociopolitical factors, as it would be hard to speak about the long-term effectiveness of MHPSS interventions ("[The] global political situation, asylum policies and rules, and closing borders often cause additional distress and disrupt wellbeing and progress that has been made").

4.4. Study Limitations and Future Directions

The Delphi method included 26 panelists, of which 18 assessed the statements in all three rounds. The retention rate of 69.23% of the initial pool of panelists throughout the three iterations and over a two-month data collection period probably reflects more dedicated and perhaps more experienced providers. The uneven representation of female and male panelists, although a possible source of bias, in fact broadly corresponds to the situation in the MHPSS field in countries on the refugee route to Western European destination countries, where most often the providers are female. The panelists had a variety of professional backgrounds and many of them had an activist history. This may have impacted the lack of consensus on statements regarding specialized care provision, given that some panelists did not have competencies in this area. The uneven number of statements across sections of the Delphi survey reflects the possible bias of the group of experts who identified the initial areas of MHPSS provision in the transit context to be assessed and their concern with the vague definition of the mandate and job of providers under these circumstances. However, during the three Delphi iterations, the panelists had the opportunity to influence the formulation of statements, their rejection, and even the inclusion of new sections.

5. Conclusions

Ultimately, this study reinforces the importance of recognizing how the transit context impacts the standard view of MHPSS that is typically provided in much more stable and well-resourced conditions.

The study highlights several important aspects of the current state of the field that need to be reconsidered. First, there is a need for a clearer understanding of the versatile and multidimensional mandate of MHPSS practitioners in the refugee transit context. Second, the importance of considering specificities of the transit context when designing and implementing MHPSS services is highlighted. To this end, providers advocated for a more flexible model of MHPSS that can adapt to the changing needs of refugees on the move and meet them where they are at. This model should be neither so 'zoomed-in' on specialized care that it loses sight of the vast number of people needing other kinds of support, nor so 'zoomed-out' that it loses sight of the individual needs of each person within the range of MHPSS possibilities. Third, the study reveals the importance of addressing both individual and systemic risk factors for mental health in order to ensure sustainable and comprehensive mental health protection for people on the move. Finally, the study pointed to several key future directions for improving MHPSS in the transit context. These include a need for closer cooperation between MHPSS practitioners from different countries along the route to enable continuity of care, as well as to exchange knowledge, experiences, and lessons learned. The need for collaboration is also evidenced by calls for the production of guiding documents, which could inform research, practice, and advocacy work in the transit context, thus enabling appropriate mental health protection and care for refugees on the move.

Author Contributions: Conceptualization: M.V.M. and M.C.G.; methodology: D.A.; validation: M.V.M.; formal analysis: M.C.G., M.V.M. and D.A.; investigation: M.C.G., M.V.M. and D.A.; resources: M.V.M.; data curation: M.C.G.; writing—first draft: M.C.G.; writing—review & editing: M.V.M. and D.A.; supervision: M.V.M. and D.A.; project administration: M.V.M.; funding acquisition: M.V.M. All authors have read and agreed to the published version of the manuscript.

Funding: This research was funded by PIN (Psychosocial Innovation Network) and the Open Society Foundation. MVM receives institutional support from the Ministry of Education, Science and Technological Development of the Republic of Serbia.

Institutional Review Board Statement: The study was conducted in accordance with the Declaration of Helsinki and was approved by the Institutional Review Board of the Department of Psychology, Faculty of Philosophy, University of Belgrade, Serbia, under protocol number #2021-104.

Informed Consent Statement: Informed consent was obtained from all subjects involved in the study.

Data Availability Statement: The data and R code for the study are available upon request from the corresponding author.

Acknowledgments: This study is part of the work of the Consortium on Refugees' and Migrants' Mental health (CoReMH), and the authors would like to thank all the providers and members of the CoReMH who participated in the study.

Conflicts of Interest: The authors declare no conflict of interest. The funders had no role in the design of the study; in the collection, analyses, or interpretation of data; in the writing of the manuscript; or in the decision to publish the results.

Appendix A

Table A1. Statements that reached consensus and average score for each of the 93 statements.

Section 1: Mandate of MHPSS Practitioners in the Transit Context	Average
1. The job/mandate of MHPSS practitioners working with people on the move in the transit context is to connect people with other resources (legal, medical, practical, etc.).	9.19
2. The job/mandate of MHPSS practitioners working with people on the move in the transit context is to recognize and validate internal capacities, strengths, and successes.	9.13
3. The job/mandate of MHPSS practitioners working with people on the move in the transit context is to raise awareness of the importance of MHPSS for people on the move.	9.00
4. The job/mandate of MHPSS practitioners working with people on the move in the transit context is to encourage positive coping mechanisms.	8.89
5. The job/mandate of MHPSS practitioners working with people on the move in the transit context is to maintain/stabilize the mental health and well-being of the client.	8.89
6. The job/mandate of MHPSS practitioners working with people on the move in the transit context is to provide a space of safety and interpersonal trust.	8.83
7. The job/mandate of MHPSS practitioners working with people on the move in the transit context is to help people on the move to cope with their psychological trauma.	8.78
8. The job/mandate of MHPSS practitioners working with people on the move in the transit context is to help people develop a toolbox for their well-being that they can take with them on the route.	8.69
9. The job/mandate of MHPSS practitioners working with people on the move in the transit context is to prevent deterioration of the client's psychological condition.	8.65
10. The job/mandate of MHPSS practitioners working with people on the move in the transit context is to help the client survive and make sense of the situation.	8.54
11. The job/mandate of MHPSS practitioners working with people on the move in the transit context is to triage in order to stretch the available resources to address the most urgent needs.	8.31
12. The job/mandate of MHPSS practitioners working with people on the move in the transit context is to mitigate destructive coping mechanisms such as substance abuse.	8.28
13. The job/mandate of MHPSS practitioners working with people on the move in the transit context is to strive for improvement of their psychological condition.	8.22
14. The job of MHPSS practitioners working within the transit context differs from standard work.	8.15
15. The job/mandate of MHPSS practitioners working with people on the move in the transit context is to screen for mental health disorders and refer clients to the appropriate specialized services.	8.13
16. Advocacy is an important part of the job/mandate of MHPSS providers working in the transit context.	7.87
Section 2: Impact of the Transit Context on MHPSS Interventions	
17. In the transit context, it is important to have a flexible model of care, including a range of specialized and peer/community-based services that can meet individual clients where they are at.	8.83
18. It is important to assess the risk of retraumatization to the people on the move providing translation, interpretation, and cultural mediation services with other people on the move.	8.74
19. Positive effects of MHPSS cannot be expected to be at the same level in situations where basic safety and survival needs have not yet been met, which is sometimes the case in the transit context.	8.65
20. Care should be provided even if the MHPSS interventions cannot be completed due to clients leaving the country.	8.61

Table A1. *Cont.*

Section 2: Impact of the Transit Context on MHPSS Interventions	
21. It is important to assess the risk of retraumatization and other harm for people on the move providing and receiving peer support services.	8.57
22. Psychiatric care adjusted to the transit context is an important component of MHPSS in the transit context.	8.52
23. Expected results and overall reach of MHPSS interventions should be adjusted to the limitations and characteristics of the transit context.	8.48
24. There is a need to define suitable interventions for the transit context.	8.48
25. MHPSS should be adapted as the needs of people on the move change.	8.35
26. Peer based support is an important component of MHPSS in the transit context.	8.22
27. Even though there is likely a strong impact of circumstances, it is possible to successfully implement MHPSS interventions in the transit context.	8.17
28. MHPSS services in the transit context require unexpected adaptations.	7.96
29. Standard MHPSS interventions applied in the transit context cannot be as effective as they are in the standard context.	7.78
30. MHPSS interventions based on evidence from other populations and in other contexts can only be successfully applied in the transit context if they are properly adapted for that purpose.	7.78
31. There is a risk of doing harm by applying trauma-related interventions that cannot be completed due to the lack of available time in the transit context.	7.56
32. The transit context decreases clients' motivation to engage in MHPSS services.	6.61
Section 3: Challenges to MHPSS in the Transit Context	
33. MHPSS interventions in the transit context should be adapted taking into consideration the impact of circumstances which may include major life events, stressors, and losses.	8.96
34. MHPSS interventions in the transit context should be adapted taking into consideration the impact of the lack of continuity of care.	8.77
35. Unpredictability of the transit context has an impact on the types of MHPSS which should be applied.	8.31
36. Unpredictability of the transit context has an impact on the overall effectiveness of MHPSS interventions.	8.04
Section 4: What makes sense in the transit context?	
37. Occupational workshops and activities (sports, arts, language classes) are an important component of MHPSS in the transit context.	9.31
38. Psychoeducational workshops and activities are an important component of MHPSS in the transit context.	8.81
39. Community based support is an important component of MHPSS in the transit context.	8.81
40. Psychotherapeutic interventions adjusted to the transit context are an important component of MHPSS in the transit context.	8.73
Section 5: Setting, Roles, and Boundaries	
41. When you are providing MHPSS in the transit context you are usually more than just a MHPSS practitioner to your client.	8.30
42. The setting in which interventions take place in the transit context differs from that of standard work.	7.83
43. The numerous systemic risk factors for mental health associated with transit, which are beyond the control of MHPSS practitioners (such as difficulty meeting basic needs and violation of social and economic rights), decrease MHPSS practitioners' motivation for provision of MHPSS services.	7.65
44. Maintaining boundaries with clients is more difficult in the transit context than in standard work.	7.35
45. Limitations of the transit context and the numerous risk factors for mental health that it brings increase feelings of helplessness among MHPSS practitioners.	7.22

Table A1. *Cont.*

Section 6: Evidence-Based Practice in the Transit Context	
46. We need more evidence on the effectiveness of MHPSS services implemented in the transit context.	8.391
47. There is a need to define what can be considered "evidence" when discussing evidence-based practice in the transit context.	8.087
48. It is important to follow evidence-based treatment protocols as much as possible, taking into account the transit circumstances.	7.611
Section 7: Ethical and Methodological Concerns of Research in Transit	
49. It is important to include people on the move in the design and provision of MHPSS services in the transit context.	8.42
50. We should conduct research in the transit context despite the challenges it presents to standard research practices.	8.39
51. There is a need to conduct more research within the transit context in order to inform practice.	8.17
52. There is a need for additional training for MHPSS practitioners on research methodology and implementation in order to support future evidence-based practice in the transit context.	8.04
53. The typical methodological requirements from standard contexts are harder to meet in the transit context.	7.96
54. It is problematic to define treatment as usual (TAU) in the transit context due to lack of continuity of care, universal standards, and equal distribution of services on the route.	7.94
55. The ethical, practical, and methodological concerns of conducting research within the uncertainty of transit limit the possibilities for research in the transit context.	5.89
Section 8: Realistic Measurements of Effectiveness	
56. Well-recognized and commonly used measures and outcome variables should be included in assessing the effectiveness of MHPSS interventions in the transit context (e.g., well-being, symptoms of psychological difficulties, quality of life, etc.)	7.72
57. The level of evidence in evaluating the effectiveness of MHPSS interventions in the transit contexts should not be expected to be the same as in the standard context.	7.70
58. There is a need to introduce new, transit-informed outcome measures for assessing the effectiveness of MHPSS services in the transit context.	7.61
Section 9: Impact on MHPSS on Practitioners	
59. Awareness of the possibility that we are the first point where a person has the opportunity to receive care increases the motivation and responsibility for providing MHPSS services.	8.19
Section 10: Perceived Value & Effectiveness of Interventions	
60. MHPSS has the potential to be beneficial not only for mental health but also for overall quality of life of the people on the move.	8.885
61. MHPSS interventions are of particular importance in the transit context, due to numerous risk factors for mental health people in these circumstances are exposed to.	8.731
62. Experience of safety and responsiveness during MHPSS interventions can be of crucial importance for long-term wellbeing of people on the move.	8.692
63. Experience and insights from MHPSS may help people make informed and constructive decisions, which is of particular importance in the risky circumstances of the transit context.	8.462
64. Experience from MHPSS services/interventions can impact major life decisions of people in the transit context.	8.038
Section 11: Cooperation with Other Actors and Experts	
65. There is a need for closer cooperation between MHPSS practitioners from the different countries along the route in order to exchange knowledge, experience and lessons learned.	9.39
66. There is a need for closer cooperation between MHPSS practitioners from different countries along the route, in order to enable continuity of care.	8.92
67. The purpose and the importance of MHPSS in the transit context is adequately recognized by MHPSS professionals.	8.08

Table A1. *Cont.*

Section 12: General Conclusions	
68. The specific knowledge and experience of MHPSS practitioners working in the transit context should be consulted in migration policy development.	8.52
69. There is a need to integrate an understanding of how systemic factors can negatively impact the psychosocial wellbeing of people on the move, when conducting MHPSS interventions in the transit context.	8.30
70. There is a need for best practices and guiding principles for MHPSS provision in the transit context.	8.17
71. There is a need to rethink MHPSS in the transit context.	8.11
72. There is a need to rethink the role of MHPSS providers in the transit context.	7.83
Section 13: Impact of the Sociopolitical Context on MHPSS in the Transit Context	
73. MHPSS providers are not in a vacuum, they are part of local and international systems, and as such their jobs are interrelated with these systems.	8.78
74. Stress surrounding the asylum procedure (potential retraumatization, low likelihood of obtaining asylum, bureaucracy of seeking asylum) limits the effectiveness of MHPSS services provided to people on the move in transit.	8.78
75. Border-related violence (such as pushbacks) is a stressor, which can negatively impact the wellbeing and mental health of people on the move.	8.78
76. Unresolved existential threats (such as threats to basic safety) people on the move face have an impact on the effectiveness of MHPSS interventions.	8.72
77. MHPSS interventions in the transit context should be adapted taking into consideration the impact of unpredictability (especially of time/length of potential interaction of MHPSS providers with the clients).	8.72
78. The high level of uncertainty in the transit context is a stressor, which can negatively impact the wellbeing and mental health of people on the move.	8.70
79. The undesired extension of time spent in the transit context is a stressor, which can negatively impact the wellbeing and mental health of people on the move.	8.70
80. Migration policies that are informed by the experience of MHPSS experts in the transit context would be protective for the mental health and wellbeing of people on the move.	8.44
81. Stress surrounding the asylum procedure (potential retraumatization, low likelihood of obtaining asylum, bureaucracy of seeking asylum) is a stressor, which negatively impacts the wellbeing and mental health of people on the move.	8.39
82. In the transit context, existing inequalities and vulnerabilities are reinforced, potentially making certain groups more vulnerable for experiencing new traumatic events.	8.33
83. Evidence on the impact of migration-related stressors on mental health and wellbeing in the transit context should be used to shape migration policies in order to mitigate these stressors.	8.22
84. The present political context is a stressor, which can negatively impact the wellbeing and mental health of people on the move.	8.22
85. Unresolved existential threats (such as threats to basic safety) people on the move face have an impact on the types of MHPSS which should be applied.	8.13
86. Unpredictability of the transit context has an impact on the delivery of MHPSS interventions.	8.13
87. Major life events (leaving one's country, separation from or death of family members), which often happen to the people in the transit context, have an impact on the types of MHPSS which should be applied.	8.04
88. When treating a person on the move, there is a concern related to what will happen and who will take over the provision of the MHPSS intervention after the person leaves the country.	8.00
89. European migration and border governance policies are a stressor, which can negatively impact the wellbeing and mental health of people on the move.	7.96
90. The impact of mental health on people on the move's memory, decision-making, and ability to adapt to a new environment is not adequately taken into consideration in the creation of migration policies.	7.96

Table A1. *Cont.*

Section 13: Impact of the Sociopolitical Context on MHPSS in the Transit Context	
91. Major life events (leaving one's country, separation from or death of family or friends), which often happen to the people in the transit context, have an impact on the effectiveness of MHPSS interventions.	7.94
92. The undesired extension of the time spent in the transit context limits the effectiveness of MHPSS services provided to people on the move in transit.	7.87
93. The high level of uncertainty limits the effectiveness of MHPSS services provided to people on the move in transit.	7.87

References

1. United Nations High Commissioner for Refugees. Global Trends in Forced Displacement—2020. Available online: https://www.unhcr.org/statistics/unhcrstats/60b638e37/global-trends-forced-displacement-2020.html (accessed on 29 December 2021).
2. Siegfried, K. The Refugee Brief—27 August 2021. UNHCR The Refugee Brief. 2021. Available online: https://www.unhcr.org/refugeebrief/the-refugee-brief-27-august-2021/ (accessed on 27 December 2021).
3. Mijatović, D. *Protecting Refugees in Europe: The ECHR and Beyond*; Council of Europe Commissioner for Human Rights: Strasbourg, France, 2020. Available online: https://www.coe.int/en/web/commissioner/-/protecting-refugees-in-europe-the-echr-and-beyond (accessed on 24 February 2022).
4. El-Shaarawi, N.; Razsa, M. Movements upon Movements: Refugee and Activist Struggles to Open the Balkan Route to Europe. *Hist. Anthropol.* **2019**, *30*, 91–112. [CrossRef]
5. Frontex European Border and Coast Guard Agency. *Risk Analysis for 2020*; Frontex European Border and Coast Guard Agency: Warsaw, Poland, 2020.
6. Minca, C.; Collins, J. The Game: Or, 'the Making of Migration' along the Balkan Route. *Political Geogr.* **2021**, *91*, 102490. [CrossRef]
7. Purić, D.; Vukčević Marković, M. Development and Validation of the Stressful Experiences in Transit Questionnaire (SET-Q) and Its Short Form (SET-SF). *Eur. J. Psychotraumatol.* **2019**, *10*, 1611091. [CrossRef] [PubMed]
8. Van de Wiel, W.; Castillo-Laborde, C.; Francisco Urzúa, I.; Fish, M.; Scholte, W.F. Mental Health Consequences of Long-Term Stays in Refugee Camps: Preliminary Evidence from Moria. *BMC Public Health* **2021**, *21*, 1290. [CrossRef] [PubMed]
9. Aulsebrook, G.; Gruber, N.; Pawson, M. Pushbacks on the Balkan Route: A Hallmark of EU Border Externalisation. *Forced Migr. Rev.* **2021**, *68*, 13–15.
10. Vukčević, M.; Dobrić, J.; Purić, D. *Study of the Mental Health of Asylum Seekers in Serbia*; UNHCR Serbia: Belgrade, Serbia, 2014.
11. Guarch-Rubio, M.; Byrne, S.; Manzanero, A.L. Violence and Torture against Migrants and Refugees Attempting to Reach the European Union through Western Balkans. *Torture J.* **2020**, *30*, 67–83. [CrossRef]
12. Hebebrand, J.; Anagnostopoulos, D.; Eliez, S.; Linse, H.; Pejovic-Milovancevic, M.; Klasen, H. A First Assessment of the Needs of Young Refugees Arriving in Europe: What Mental Health Professionals Need to Know. *Eur. Child Adolesc. Psychiatry* **2016**, *25*, 1–6. [CrossRef] [PubMed]
13. Ben Farhat, J.; Blanchet, K.; Juul Bjertrup, P.; Veizis, A.; Perrin, C.; Coulborn, R.M.; Mayaud, P.; Cohuet, S. Syrian Refugees in Greece: Experience with Violence, Mental Health Status, and Access to Information during the Journey and While in Greece. *BMC Med.* **2018**, *16*, 40. [CrossRef] [PubMed]
14. Pottie, K.; Martin, J.P.; Cornish, S.; Biorklund, L.M.; Gayton, I.; Doerner, F.; Schneider, F. Access to Healthcare for the Most Vulnerable Migrants: A Humanitarian Crisis. *Confl. Health* **2015**, *9*, 16. [CrossRef] [PubMed]
15. Orcutt, M.; Spiegel, P.; Kumar, B.; Abubakar, I.; Clark, J.; Horton, R. Lancet Migration: Global Collaboration to Advance Migration Health. *Lancet* **2020**, *395*, 317–319. [CrossRef]
16. Vukčević Marković, M.; Živanović, M.; Bjekić, J. Post-Migration Living Difficulties and Mental Health in Refugees and Asylum Seekers in Serbia. *Polit. Psychol.* **2019**, *1*, 32–45.
17. Federal Foreign Office of Germany. The Second Berlin Conference on Libya. Available online: https://www.auswaertiges-amt.de/en/newsroom/news/berlin-2-conclusions/2467750 (accessed on 26 February 2022).
18. Fazel, M.; Wheeler, J.; Danesh, J. Prevalence of Serious Mental Disorder in 7000 Refugees Resettled in Western Countries: A Systematic Review. *Lancet* **2005**, *365*, 1309–1314. [CrossRef]
19. Giacco, D.; Laxhman, N.; Priebe, S. Prevalence of and Risk Factors for Mental Disorders in Refugees. *Semin. Cell Dev. Biol.* **2018**, *77*, 144–152. [CrossRef] [PubMed]
20. Henkelmann, J.-R.; de Best, S.; Deckers, C.; Jensen, K.; Shahab, M.; Elzinga, B.; Molendijk, M. Anxiety, Depression and Post-Traumatic Stress Disorder in Refugees Resettling in High-Income Countries: Systematic Review and Meta-Analysis. *BJPsych Open* **2020**, *6*, e68. [CrossRef] [PubMed]
21. Vukčević, M.; Dobrić, J.; Purić, D. Psychological Characteristics of Asylum Seekers from Syria. In *Survey of the Mental Health of Asylum Seekers in Serbia*; UNHCR Serbia: Belgrade, Serbia, 2014; pp. 73–85.
22. Vukčević Marković, M.; Gašić, J.; Bjekić, J. *Refugees' Mental Health*; Psychosocial Innovation Network: Belgrade, Serbia, 2017.

23. Cantekin, D.; Gençöz, T. Mental Health of Syrian Asylum Seekers in Turkey: The Role of Pre-Migration and Post-Migration Risk Factors. *J. Soc. Clin. Psychol.* **2017**, *36*, 835–859. [CrossRef]
24. Carswell, K.; Blackburn, P.; Barker, C. The Relationship between Trauma, Post-Migration Problems and the Psychological Well-Being of Refugees and Asylum Seekers. *Int. J. Soc. Psychiatry* **2011**, *57*, 107–119. [CrossRef] [PubMed]
25. Turrini, G.; Purgato, M.; Acarturk, C.; Anttila, M.; Au, T.; Ballette, F.; Bird, M.; Carswell, K.; Churchill, R.; Cuijpers, P.; et al. Efficacy and Acceptability of Psychosocial Interventions in Asylum Seekers and Refugees: Systematic Review and Meta-Analysis. *Epidemiol. Psychiatr. Sci.* **2019**, *28*, 376–388. [CrossRef] [PubMed]
26. Vukcevic, M.; Momirovic, J.; Puric, D. Adaptation of Harvard Trauma Questionnaire for Working with Refugees and Asylum Seekers in Serbia. *Psihologija* **2016**, *49*, 277–299. [CrossRef]
27. Björn, G.J. Ethics and Interpreting in Psychotherapy with Refugee Children and Families. *Nord. J. Psychiatry* **2005**, *59*, 516–521. [CrossRef] [PubMed]
28. Bolton, J. The Third Presence: A Psychiatrist's Experience of Working with Non-English Speaking Patients and Interpreters. *Transcult. Psychiatry* **2002**, *39*, 97–114. [CrossRef]
29. Vukčević Marković, M.; Bjekić, J. Methods and Ethics in Refugee Research. In *Forced Migration and Social Trauma*; Routledge: London, UK, 2018; pp. 126–135.
30. Im, H.; Rodriguez, C.; Grumbine, J. A Multitier Model of Refugee Mental Health and Psychosocial Support in Resettlement: Toward Trauma-Informed and Culture-Informed Systems of Care. *Psychol. Serv.* **2019**, *18*, 345–364. [CrossRef] [PubMed]
31. Djelantik, A.A.A.M.J.; de Heus, A.; Kuiper, D.; Kleber, R.J.; Boelen, P.A.; Smid, G.E. Post-Migration Stressors and Their Association With Symptom Reduction and Non-Completion During Treatment for Traumatic Grief in Refugees. *Front. Psychiatry* **2020**, *11*, 407. [CrossRef] [PubMed]
32. Dalkey, N.; Helmer, O. An Experimental Application of the Delphi Method to the Use of Experts. *Manag. Sci.* **1963**, *9*, 458–467. [CrossRef]
33. Bisson, J.I.; Tavakoly, B.; Witteveen, A.B.; Ajdukovic, D.; Jehel, L.; Johansen, V.J.; Nordanger, D.; Garcia, F.O.; Punamaki, R.-L.; Schnyder, U.; et al. TENTS Guidelines: Development of Post-Disaster Psychosocial Care Guidelines through a Delphi Process. *Br. J. Psychiatry* **2010**, *196*, 69–74. [CrossRef]
34. Graham, L.F.; Milne, D.L. Developing Basic Training Programmes: A Case Study Illustration Using the Delphi Method in Clinical Psychology. *Clin. Psychol. Psychother.* **2003**, *10*, 55–63. [CrossRef]
35. Davidson, P.; Merritt-Gray, M.; Buchanan, J.; Noel, J. Voices from Practice: Mental Health Nurses Identify Research Priorities. *Arch. Psychiatr. Nurs.* **1997**, *11*, 340–345. [CrossRef]
36. Lovie, P. Coefficient of Variation. In *Encyclopedia of Statistics in Behavioral Science*; John Wiley & Sons, Ltd.: Hoboken, NJ, USA, 2005. [CrossRef]
37. RStudio Team. *RStudio: Integrated Development Environment for R*; RStudio PBC: Boston, MA, USA, 2021.
38. Revelle, W. *Psych: Procedures for Personality and Psychological Research*; Northwestern University: Evanston, IL, USA, 2020.
39. Huntington-Klein, N. Vtable: Variable Table for Variable Documentation; CRAN Repository. 2021. Available online: https://cran.r-project.org/web/packages/vtable/vtable.pdf (accessed on 8 March 2022).
40. Ooms, J. Writexl: Export Data Frames to Excel "xlsx" Format; CRAN Repository. 2021. Available online: https://cran.r-project.org/web/packages/writexl/writexl.pdf (accessed on 8 March 2022).
41. Wickham, H. Tidyr: Tidy Messy Data; CRAN Repository. 2022. Available online: https://cran.r-project.org/web/packages/tidyr/tidyr.pdf (accessed on 8 March 2022).
42. Kim, J.J.; Brookman-Frazee, L.; Gellatly, R.; Stadnick, N.; Barnett, M.L.; Lau, A.S. Predictors of Burnout among Community Therapists in the Sustainment Phase of a System-Driven Implementation of Multiple Evidence-Based Practices in Children's Mental Health. *Prof. Psychol. Res. Pract.* **2018**, *49*, 131–142. [CrossRef] [PubMed]
43. Fennig, M.; Denov, M. Regime of Truth: Rethinking the Dominance of the Bio-Medical Model in Mental Health Social Work with Refugee Youth. *Br. J. Soc. Work* **2019**, *49*, 300–317. [CrossRef]
44. Mechili, E.-A.; Angelaki, A.; Petelos, E.; Sifaki-Pistolla, D.; Chatzea, V.-E.; Dowrick, C.; Hoffman, K.; Jirovsky, E.; Pavlic, D.R.; Dückers, M.; et al. Compassionate Care Provision: An Immense Need during the Refugee Crisis: Lessons Learned from a European Capacity-Building Project. *J. Compassionate Health Care* **2018**, *5*, 2. [CrossRef]
45. Van Loenen, T.; van den Muijsenbergh, M.; Hofmeester, M.; Dowrick, C.; van Ginneken, N.; Mechili, E.A.; Angelaki, A.; Ajdukovic, D.; Bakic, H.; Pavlic, D.R.; et al. Primary Care for Refugees and Newly Arrived Migrants in Europe: A Qualitative Study on Health Needs, Barriers and Wishes. *Eur. J. Public Health* **2018**, *28*, 82–87. [CrossRef] [PubMed]
46. Inter-Agency Standing Committee (IASC). IASC Guidelines on Mental Health and Psychosocial Support in Emergency Settings. 2008. Available online: https://doi.org/10.1037/e518422011-002 (accessed on 27 December 2021).
47. Topalovic, T.; Episkopou, M.; Schillberg, E.; Brcanski, J.; Jocic, M. Migrant Children in Transit: Health Profile and Social Needs of Unaccompanied and Accompanied Children Visiting the MSF Clinic in Belgrade, Serbia. *Confl. Health* **2021**, *15*, 32. [CrossRef] [PubMed]
48. Kashyap, S.; Keegan, D.; Liddell, B.J.; Thomson, T.; Nickerson, A. An Interaction Model of Environmental and Psychological Factors Influencing Refugee Mental Health. *J. Trauma Stress* **2021**, *34*, 257–266. [CrossRef] [PubMed]

49. Posselt, M.; Eaton, H.; Ferguson, M.; Keegan, D.; Procter, N. Enablers of Psychological Well-Being for Refugees and Asylum Seekers Living in Transitional Countries: A Systematic Review. *Health Soc. Care Community* **2019**, *27*, 808–823. [CrossRef] [PubMed]
50. Vukčević Marković, M.; Kovačević, N.; Bjekić, J. Refugee Status Determination Procedure and Mental Health of the Applicant: Dynamics and Reciprocal Effects. *Front. Psychiatry* **2021**, *11*, 1635. [CrossRef]
51. Commission on Social Determinants of Health. *Closing the Gap in a Generation: Health Equigy through Action on the Social Determinants of Health*; World Health Organization: Geneva, Switzerland, 2008.
52. Allen, J.; Balfour, R.; Bell, R.; Marmot, M. Social Determinants of Mental Health. *Int. Rev. Psychiatry* **2014**, *26*, 392–407. [CrossRef] [PubMed]
53. Chen, W.; Hall, B.J.; Ling, L.; Renzaho, A.M. Pre-Migration and Post-Migration Factors Associated with Mental Health in Humanitarian Migrants in Australia and the Moderation Effect of Post-Migration Stressors: Findings from the First Wave Data of the BNLA Cohort Study. *Lancet Psychiatry* **2017**, *4*, 218–229. [CrossRef]
54. The Social Determinants of Refugee Mental Health in the Post-Migration Context: A Critical Review—Michaela Hynie. 2018. Available online: https://journals.sagepub.com/doi/full/10.1177/0706743717746666 (accessed on 21 February 2022).
55. Li, S.S.Y.; Liddell, B.J.; Nickerson, A. The Relationship between Post-Migration Stress and Psychological Disorders in Refugees and Asylum Seekers. *Curr. Psychiatry Rep.* **2016**, *18*, 82. [CrossRef] [PubMed]
56. Benjamen, J.; Girard, V.; Jamani, S.; Magwood, O.; Holland, T.; Sharfuddin, N.; Pottie, K. Access to Refugee and Migrant Mental Health Care Services during the First Six Months of the COVID-19 Pandemic: A Canadian Refugee Clinician Survey. *Int. J. Environ. Res. Public. Health* **2021**, *18*, 5266. [CrossRef]
57. Silove, D.; Ventevogel, P.; Rees, S. The Contemporary Refugee Crisis: An Overview of Mental Health Challenges. *World Psychiatry* **2017**, *16*, 130–139. [CrossRef]

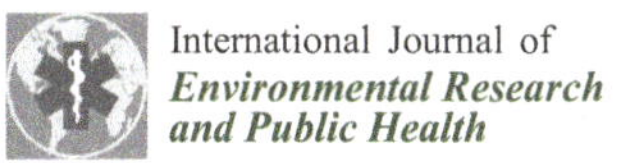

International Journal of
*Environmental Research
and Public Health*

MDPI

Article

Promoting Mental Health and Wellbeing in Multicultural Australia: A Collaborative Regional Approach

Ilse Blignault [1,*], Hend Saab [2,3], Lisa Woodland [4,5], Klara Giourgas [2] and Heba Baddah [2]

[1] Translational Health Research Institute, Western Sydney University, Penrith 2751, Australia
[2] South Eastern Sydney Local Health District, Multicultural Health Service, Darlinghurst 2010, Australia; hend.saab@health.nsw.gov.au (H.S.); klara.giourgas@health.nsw.gov.au (K.G.); heba.baddah@health.nsw.gov.au (H.B.)
[3] St George Community Mental Health, Kogarah 2172, Australia
[4] South Eastern Sydney Local Health District, Population and Community Health, Darlinghurst 2010, Australia; lisa.woodland@health.nsw.gov.au
[5] Centre for Primary Health Care and Equity, UNSW Sydney, Sydney 2052, Australia
* Correspondence: i.blignault@westernsydney.edu.au

Citation: Blignault, I.; Saab, H.; Woodland, L.; Giourgas, K.; Baddah, H. Promoting Mental Health and Wellbeing in Multicultural Australia: A Collaborative Regional Approach. *Int. J. Environ. Res. Public Health* **2022**, *19*, 2723. https://doi.org/10.3390/ijerph19052723

Academic Editors: Shameran Slewa-Younan and Greg Armstrong

Received: 31 January 2022
Accepted: 24 February 2022
Published: 26 February 2022

Publisher's Note: MDPI stays neutral with regard to jurisdictional claims in published maps and institutional affiliations.

Abstract: Migrant communities are often under-served by mental health services. Lack of community engagement results in missed opportunities for mental health promotion and early intervention, delayed care, and high rates of untreated psychological distress. Bilingual clinicians and others who work with these communities lack linguistically and culturally appropriate resources. This article reports on the implementation and evaluation of a community-based group mindfulness program delivered to Arabic and Bangla-speaking communities in Sydney, Australia, including modifications made to the content and format in response to the COVID-19 pandemic. The program was positioned within a stepped-care model for primary mental health care and adopted a collaborative regional approach. In addition to improved mental health outcomes for face-to-face and online program participants, we have documented numerous referrals to specialist services and extensive diffusion of mindfulness skills, mostly to family members, within each community. Community partnerships were critical to community engagement. Training workshops to build the skills of the bilingual health and community workforce increased the program's reach. In immigrant nations such as Australia, mainstream mental health promotion must be complemented by activities that target specific population groups. Scaled up, and with appropriate adaptation, the group mindfulness program offers a low-intensity in-language intervention for under-served communities.

Keywords: mindfulness-based intervention; stress management; mental health promotion; stepped care model; evaluation; migrant; Arabic speakers; Bangla speakers; Muslim; cultural adaptation

1. Introduction

The increasing number of international migrants and refugees worldwide presents a challenge for the delivery of health services and health promotion programs in destination countries. In 2020, there were 281 million international migrants [1], with refugees accounting for approximately 12 percent of the total [2]. Since WWII, Australia has been a major receiving country [3]. At the 2016 Census, 28% of Australia's population were born overseas [4], a level that is higher than most countries within the Organisation for Economic Co-operation and Development [5]. Another 21% of the population had one or both parents who were born overseas [4].

In 2016, multicultural Australia was home to people with more than 300 different ancestries and speaking over 300 different languages [4]. Such diversity is recognised as a national strength [6]. It is captured in the collective term 'culturally and linguistically diverse (CALD)' which refers to "the non-Indigenous cultural and linguistic groups represented in the Australian population who identify as having cultural or linguistic connections with their place of birth, ancestry or ethnic origin, religion, preferred language or language spoken at home" [7] (p. 3).

Mental health is a state of wellbeing whereby individuals recognise their abilities, are able to cope with normal stresses of life, work productively and fruitfully and contribute to their communities [8]. Migrants face numerous stressors that can affect their mental health and place them at heightened risk of developing mental disorders [9]. For example, the ability to find meaningful work may be compromised by difficulty gaining recognition for educational qualifications and employment credentials [10]. Other common stressors relate to changes to traditional gender roles and intergenerational conflicts within the family [10,11], and to discrimination and social exclusion on the part of the host society [10,12]. Refugees, fleeing war and conflict in their country of origin, have experienced violence and loss and the psychological impact of an often uncertain and prolonged journey [13]. Their distress is often exacerbated by social, economic, and legal circumstances in the new country [14].

Australia has long been a leader in mental health policy and service development, with a strategy of ongoing national reform [15]. The National Mental Health Policy 2008, which embedded a whole of government approach to mental health, also embedded mental health promotion and prevention into services [15]. As defined in the NMHP, "Mental health promotion aims to maximise the ability of [individuals] to realise their potential, cope with normal stresses of life, and participate meaningfully in their communities. It also seeks to increase awareness and understanding of mental health problems and mental illness, reduce stigma and discrimination, and encourage help-seeking behaviour where this is needed" [15] (p. 13). Mental health promotion works by strengthening individuals, strengthening communities, and reducing structural barriers to health [16]. Successful programs typically involve many different government agencies and community organisations and integrate the levels of action [15,16].

In the Fifth National Mental Health and Suicide Prevention Plan 2017-22, all Australian governments committed to working together to achieve integration in planning and service delivery at a regional level [17]. The Plan extended the role of the newly established Primary Health Networks (PHNs) to provide a regionally driven stepped care approach to mental health service delivery: from promotion and prevention to early intervention, treatment, and recovery [18,19]. As service commissioners and system integrators, an important aspect of the PHN role is mitigation of identified gaps and inequities for under-served groups, including people from CALD backgrounds [20].

The stepped care model for primary mental health care is summarised in Figure 1 [21]. In Step 1 the focus is promotion and prevention for the well population, mainly publicly available information, and self-help resources. In Step 2 the focus is early intervention for at-risk groups (people with early symptoms or previous illness), mainly self-help resources, including digital mental health (online and phone support). In Step 3 the focus is access to low intensity services for people with mild mental illness through a mix of self-help resources and low intensity face-to-face services, with psychological services for those who require them. Steps 4 and 5 focus on face-to-face clinical care for people with moderate and severe mental illness.

The CALD Mindfulness Program is an ongoing program of research involving the development, implementation, and evaluation of mindfulness-based interventions (MBIs) tailored for migrant and refugee communities. MBIs, such as mindfulness-based stress reduction, can significantly alleviate depression, anxiety and stress and improve physical and psychological functioning [22,23]. The program's genesis lies in the experience of a bilingual (Arabic/English speaking) psychologist employed at a Community Mental Health Service in the South Eastern Sydney Local Health District (SESLHD) who saw a need for an in-language mindfulness resource to use with Arabic-speaking clients.

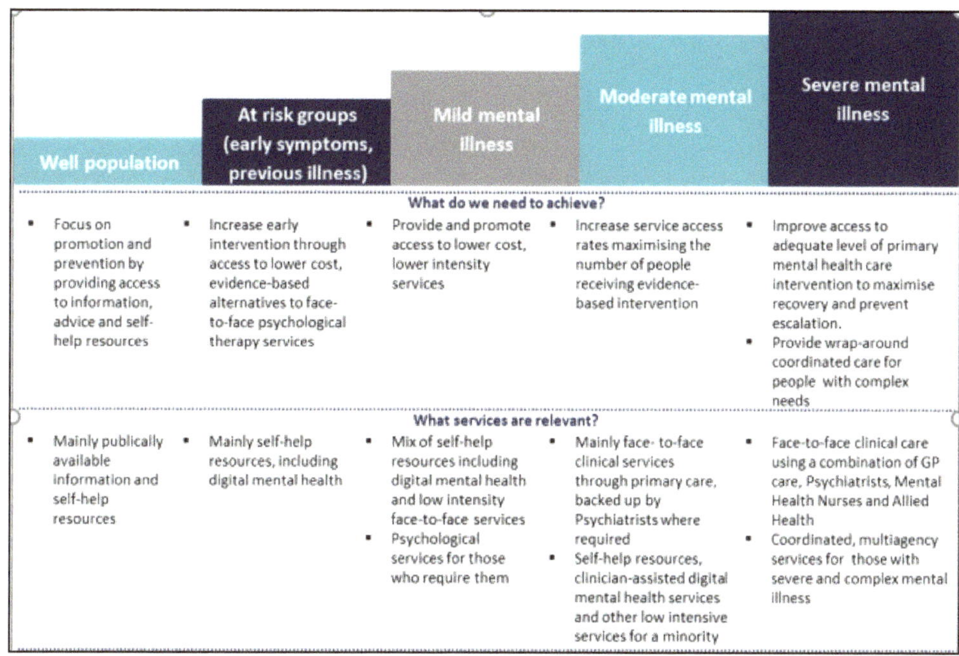

Figure 1. Stepped care model for primary mental health care service delivery [21].

The Arabic Mindfulness compact disc (CD) is a cultural adaptation of a resource produced by Dr Russ Harris, whose self-help books and CDs are very popular in Australia. The educational CD is 60 min in duration and contains five tracks [24]. During 2012–13, it was informally evaluated through interviews with Arabic-speaking clients who used the resource in conjunction with standard therapy. Positive feedback led to a series of formal evaluations focussing on mental health outcomes, cultural acceptability, and participant experience. The first two studies demonstrated that the Arabic Mindfulness CD was culturally and spiritually relevant and effective when used as a self-management tool in the home setting [24] and within a 5-week group program [25]. The MBI resulted in improved psychological wellbeing and was compatible with their cultural and religious practices [24,25]. The group program, which was promoted to newly arrived Arabic speaking women with refugee-like backgrounds, also provided opportunities for connecting with others and peer support [25].

Subsequently, the Central and Eastern Sydney Primary Health Network (CESPHN), commissioned the SESLHD Multicultural Health Service to deliver the group mindfulness program to CALD communities in their region. Within the stepped care model, the program corresponds to Step 3 (mix of self-help resources and low-intensity face-to-face services with psychological services as needed). The objectives were to deliver the program to Arabic speakers and Bangla speakers in the CESPHN region in order to reduce psychological distress, depression, anxiety, and stress; to provide in-language resources to support the program; and to train bilingual mental health clinicians and community workers in MBIs. The third study aimed to establish whether the group mindfulness program produced expected outcomes under normal operational conditions and to test its transferability to a second language group (Bangla) and scalability [26]. The program was shown to be culturally acceptable and effective, producing clinically and statistically significant improvements in mental health, facilitating access to mental health care and boosting mental health literacy for both language groups [26].

In March 2020, following the outbreak of COVID-19, health services ceased all face-to-face groups. Program resources were initially adapted to support the Arabic-speaking community through regular text messages that encouraged mindfulness practice at a time of changing and challenging circumstances. Additionally, the clinical lead (Hend Saab, HS) recorded a short video introducing mindfulness concepts and linking to the existing audio resources, which was disseminated through social media and community networks. The group program (Arabic and Bangla) was adapted for online delivery via videoconferencing (four sessions with a focus on stress management). It was also offered as a one-off refresher session for previous participants and as an open one-off session for new participants. Since December 2019, the mindfulness audio resources in Arabic, Bangla and English have been publicly available on the NSW Multicultural Health Communication Service website [27]. Resources for Mandarin and Nepali speakers have also been produced, with Spanish resources in development.

This article reports new findings from research with the two language groups that have been the focus of the CALD Mindfulness program to date (Arabic and Bangla), including online group outcomes, referrals to other mental health supports, diffusion through social networks, and in-language resource downloads. Additionally, it presents findings from a follow-up evaluation of the workforce capacity-building component of the broader project and interviews with community partners.

2. Materials and Methods

2.1. Regional Setting and Program Partners

Central and Eastern Sydney Primary Health Network (CESPHN) is the second largest of the 31 Primary Health Networks across Australia, with a resident population of approximately 1.6 million. The region is characterised by cultural diversity, with 40% of residents born overseas, 38% speaking a language other than English at home, and 6.9% not speaking English well or at all [28]. There is a focus on people experiencing socioeconomic disadvantage, including people from CALD backgrounds, as well as people experiencing complex health issues, poor health literacy and the impact of social isolation on health and wellbeing. Mental health is a priority [29]. Both local health districts within the CESPHN region were involved, SESLHD as the program lead and SLHD as a partner. The collaborative regional approach brought together key health services and fifteen community partners, including nine community organisations and six individuals (independent bilingual community workers or clinicians).

2.2. Target Groups

Arabic speakers have a significant cultural presence in Australia and in Central and south eastern Sydney where this work took place [3,29]. Bangla speakers are a new and emerging community in the region [30]. Nationally, Arabic is the third most spoken language after English and Mandarin [4]. The Arabic-speaking population is comprised of numerous cultural and ethnic communities and includes both Muslims and Christians. Members vary in country of origin, circumstances of arrival and length of residence in Australia, as well as age and education [3]. They form the majority of the refugee population [31]. Language maintenance is high [32]. The great majority of Australia's Bangla speakers come from Bangladesh and are Muslim. Most are relative newcomers under the skilled migration program [33].

2.3. Group Mindfulness Program (Face-to-Face and Online)

The 4-week online program, introduced in response to the COVID-19 pandemic, was a modification of the 5-week face-to-face group mindfulness program described elsewhere [25,26]. Box 1 provides an overview of the 4-week online program. Appendix A includes the (English-language) mnemonics developed to summarise the content of each session. Appendix B provides a brief comparison of the two programs.

Box 1. Overview of the Online CALD Mindfulness Stress Reduction Program.

> **Group session 1: Introduction and Debriefing**
> **Aim:** To discuss signs of stress and vulnerabilities experienced by participants, identify helpful and unhelpful stress responses and provide a set of motivating and practical stress management skills.
> **Video:** Mindfulness in Challenging Times.
> **Mindfulness practice:** Grounding exercise with sensory awareness.
> **Mnemonic:** HOPEFUL + L, a set of cognitive and practical tips to stay afloat during stressful times.
> **Group session 2: Stress Experiences and Responses, Mindfulness**
> **Aim:** To educate participants about stress from an evolutionary perspective, introduce mindfulness concepts and explore their cultural and spiritual applicability, and provide a set of mindfulness stress management skills.
> **Mindfulness practice:** Mindfulness breathing exercise.
> **Mnemonic:** Five 'A's of mindfulness—awareness, acknowledgement, actions, acceptance and appreciation.
> **Group session 3: Mindfulness Based Stress Reduction Strategies**
> **Aim:** To promote participants' awareness of the interconnectedness of thoughts, feelings and behaviours, differentiate themselves from their thoughts, introduce mindfulness-based stress management skills.
> **Mindfulness practice:** Leaves on a stream exercise, Body scan exercise.
> **Mnemonic:** BE PRESENT, a set of mindfulness-based stress management skills and practices to help reduce distress.
> **Group Session 4: Loving Kindness and Self-Compassion, Review**
> **Aim:** To define sense of self, emphasise self-care practices through loving kindness and self-compassion and review stress management skills learnt throughout the program. To reflect and recap topics and discussions from previous sessions.
> **Mindfulness practice:** Loving kindness and self-compassion exercise.
> **Mnemonic:** REFLECTION, a program summary.

Originally derived from Buddhist practices, mindfulness has become a popular evidence-based tool for managing mental health problems in Western countries. Mindfulness is often taught through a variety of meditation exercises and MBIs usually incorporate meditation practice together with various cognitive and/or behavioural techniques [24]. The group program content, which was organised around the mindfulness audio tracks, was informed by clinical experience and knowledge of the target groups [25,26]. It drew on a range of psychological concepts and methods that fall under the umbrella of the 'third wave' of cognitive behavioural therapy, including mindfulness-based stress reduction, mindfulness-based cognitive therapy and acceptance and commitment therapy [34], and incorporated a strong spiritual element [24].

The first of the four online sessions was primarily designed to create an emotionally safe space for group participants to share and normalise their experiences in the context of the COVID-19 pandemic. In particular, guided discussion in the online session assisted participants in recognising helpful and unhelpful strategies they had been applying in managing pandemic-related stressors (social restrictions, including lockdown). Both programs were facilitated by a bilingual mental health clinician (psychologist) with support from a bilingual community worker.

Community partners were responsible for taking registrations, keeping attendance lists and general organisation. For the online program, only women were recruited due to high demand and gender sensitivity. Referrals for further mental health care were managed in various ways. Linguistic and cultural needs and preferences and financial and personal circumstances were taken into consideration as well as clinical needs. All participants who scored 30 or above on the K10 (likely to have a severe mental disorder) or as 'severe' or 'extremely severe' on the DASS21 were contacted by the clinical lead [35,36]. If the psychologist facilitator noticed a participant was distressed they would reach out to them. In the face-to-face groups, participants were also able to approach the facilitator privately during breaks or after the session and request assistance with referral.

2.4. In-Language Resources

Since the Arabic Mindfulness CD [24], a suite of audio and video mindfulness resources has been developed. These can be streamed or downloaded from the NSW Health Multicultural Health Communication Service (MHCS) website at no cost (see Appendix B for details) [27].

Audio resources (CDs and USBs (Universal Serial Bus)) were provided to group participants to assist with their ongoing mindfulness practice and later uploaded to the MHCS website. Individuals are able to use them as a self-help resource by downloading the tracks and completing the mindfulness exercises in their own time. Short videos, 'Mindfulness in Challenging Times', were produced to support community members during the COVID-19 lockdown. They also introduce the CALD Mindfulness Program.

2.5. Workforce Capacity Building

Workforce capacity building was designed to increase the reach of the CALD Mindfulness Program, with free training offered to bilingual mental health professionals, community workers and others interested in facilitating future mindfulness groups. The full-day workshop was divided into four sections: introduction to mindfulness and background to the CALD Mindfulness Program; stress management and the observing self; loving kindness and self-compassion; and managing painful emotions. Training materials included a copy of the CALD Mindfulness Program Participant Handbook, handouts, and scripts for six mindfulness exercises (developed from various resources and designed to be culturally acceptable and easy to translate).

2.6. Evaluation

2.6.1. Group Mindfulness Program (Face-to-Face and Online)

Methods and tools used to evaluate the face-to-face group program have been published previously [25,26]. A similar approach was adopted for the online group program, with data collected by questionnaire at the first and final session. Sociodemographic items included age, gender, country of birth, years of residence in Australia, main language spoken at home, religion, education, and postcode. Participants were asked about health professionals, including mental health professionals, seen in the last four weeks. The final questionnaire assessed program experience using two questions ("What effect did the program have on your overall wellbeing?" and "Overall, how would you rate your experience of the program?"), with participants recording their responses on a 5-point Likert Scale ('poor' to 'excellent'). It also included a question on skills transfer: "Over the past four weeks, have you shared your mindfulness skills with anyone? If yes, who?"

While the face-to-face program utilised two translated and validated mental health outcome measures (DASS21 and K10+), the online program employed only the K10+ to reduce the evaluation burden on participants. In addition to a global measure of psychological distress (K10), the K10+ includes four questions asking about the individual's ability to work and carry out day-to-day activities, the number of times the person has seen a doctor or other health professional due to mental health issues, and how often physical health problems have been the main cause of these issues [37]. All other tools were translated into Arabic and Bangla by accredited translators and checked by other accredited translators and community members. The co-facilitators kept a record of group attendance and referrals made during and following the program. Participant feedback was noted verbatim if in English and translated if in Arabic or Bangla. Post program, community partners debriefed with the clinical lead, providing feedback on their experiences and observations for inclusion in the program summary and future program planning.

Analyses were conducted separately for Arabic and Bangla speakers. Sociodemographic and attendance data for the online groups were summarised using descriptive statistics. Pre- and post-measures of mental health were compared using the nonparametric sign test for paired samples (two-sided) as the data were not normally distributed, using SPSS v27 [38]. The null hypothesis was that the median difference in the pre- and post-measures would be zero.

Referrals were counted for all face-to-face and online group programs held between March 2017 and September 2021. We distinguished between referrals made for the participant themselves (if the person was referred to two separate services, this was counted as two referrals) and referrals made for a family member (e.g., a participant's children, grandchildren, or partner). Destination of referral was classified as 'private psychologist', 'General Practitioner (GP) for referral', 'family therapist' or 'other' (e.g., private psychiatrist, domestic violence service, pain clinic, or the NSW Service for the Treatment and Rehabilitation of Torture and Trauma Survivors). Destination percentages were calculated after excluding those already receiving mental health care. Referrals that involved reconnection with a previous service provider were noted. Specific needs for referral (beyond anxiety or depression symptoms) were noted also.

We counted the number of participants who reported sharing the mindfulness skills and examined both the pattern and extent of spread. We classified reported recipients/beneficiaries according to the following categories: 'any family', 'family unspecified', 'immediate family' (including 'spouse', 'child', 'parent', 'sibling'), 'extended family', 'friend' and 'other'. We also coded sharing with a 'person overseas' when it was reported. We then counted the number of participants who shared the skills across the various categories. We used the chi-square statistic to examine if language group (Arabic vs. Bangla), delivery format (face-to-face vs. online), gender (female vs. male) or age group (16–35 years vs. 36 years and over) were associated with skills transfer (not shared vs. shared); adopting a p value of 0.5. Further, we estimated extent of spread from the number of recipients/beneficiaries reported with each relationship category. To manage this, if a participant indicated a single person from a particular category (e.g., 'daughter' or 'friend') we counted one. If a participant indicated more than one person from a particular category (e.g., 'sons and daughter' or 'friends') we counted two, although in practice it could have been more. The resulting totals were, therefore, conservative.

2.6.2. In-Language Resources

Unfortunately, we did not keep a complete record of the number of Arabic Mindfulness CDs distributed to program participants and, more widely, on request and through community events (several hundred). USBs were produced in Arabic (60), Bangla (60) and English (20). We counted the number of downloads of the online audio resources from 1 July to 31 December 2021 and video views on the SESLHD YouTube website since June 2020.

2.6.3. Workforce Capacity Building

The training was evaluated through feedback forms distributed at the end of the workshops and an online follow-up survey. The feedback forms focussed on training content and delivery (process). The survey asked about key learnings and application of the learnings (outcomes and impact). Both were anonymous.

The feedback form contained 13 statements to which trainees were invited to show their level of agreement using a 5-point Likert Scale ('strongly disagree' to 'strongly agree'), followed by two open-ended questions asking what they like most and what could be improved. In October 2019, people who had attended any of the first six workshops (delivered between August 2017 and May 2018) were invited by email to complete a questionnaire created on Survey Monkey. The survey contained nine questions with a mix of pre-coded and open-ended responses. Questions 1–5 covered gender, language spoken, role, primary work setting and date of training. Questions 6–7 asked about key learnings and applying the learnings. Question 8 asked how much impact the training had on their practice using a 5-point Likert Scale ('no impact' to 'high impact'). Likert Scale responses and answers to the pre-coded questions were tabulated (frequencies and percentages) in

Microsoft Excel. Responses to the open-ended questions were systematically coded and tabulated by Ilse Blignault (IB).

2.6.4. Community Partnerships

We sought a better understanding of the role of community partners in supporting program rollout and reach through a series of interviews with facilitators, co-facilitators, and community workers. Individuals who had been involved in one or more face-to-face or online programs in the last two years were invited to take part in a 30-min semi-structured telephone interview conducted by a project officer recruited for this purpose. The interview guide contained 12 open-ended questions, two of which asked: "As an employee of [partner organisation], how do you think your contribution has supported the delivery and influenced the program outcomes?" "What were some of the challenges encountered as a partner organisation?" The interviews were not recorded; however, the project officer took extensive notes that informants were given the opportunity to review. Responses to the two questions were closely examined by HS to identify common experiences and issues, and the emergent findings reviewed at a research team meeting (IB, HS, HB (Heba Baddah) and project officer).

3. Results

3.1. Group Mindfulness Program

Between March 2017 and September 2021, 43 in-language group programs were facilitated across the region: 37 face-to-face and 5 online. They attracted a total of 489 participants, 397 of whom completed the program. Additionally, ten one-off online stress management sessions were conducted in Arabic and Bangla (results not reported here).

3.1.1. Online Groups

Forty-four Arabic and Bangla-speaking women aged 16 years and over enrolled in the online program and 35 (73% of Arabic speakers and 94% of Bangla speakers) completed it. The five groups ranged in size from 7 to 11 people.

Of the 26 Arabic-speaking women recruited, most were aged 26 to 55 years. All but two were born overseas, mostly in Lebanon, Syria, or Iraq, and all but three were Muslim. Thirteen had lived in Australia for under nine years. Seventeen spoke mainly Arabic at home, the rest Arabic and English. Eighteen possessed a post-school qualification, either trade or university. Pre-intervention, 20 scored as 'moderate' (25–29) or 'severe' (30–50) on the K10. All 19 women who completed the program attended at least three of the four sessions. Reasons for dropping out included health and family issues. Lack of access to technology and unreliable internet also affected participation.

Of the 18 Bangla-speaking women recruited, we have pre-program data for only 17. Most fell into the 26–35 age group. All but one were born in Bangladesh and all were Muslim; eleven had lived in Australia for under nine years. Twelve spoke mainly Bangla at home, the rest Bangla and English. All possessed a university qualification. Pre-intervention, 11 scored as 'moderate' or 'severe' on the K10. All 17 women who completed the program attended at least three sessions. One woman dropped out for work reasons.

For both language groups, post-program measures on the K10+ showed improvement. Post-program, fewer participants scored as 'moderate' and none as 'severe' (Table 1) and there was a statistically significant reduction in psychological distress ($p < 0.001$) (Table 2). For Arabic speakers, there was also a significant reduction in days of cutting down work due to mental health issues in the past four weeks ($p < 0.01$) (Table 2).

Table 1. Pre-post comparisons on the K10 category for program completers.

K10 Category	Arabic Speakers (*N* = 18)		Bangla Speakers (*N* = 17)	
	Pre-Program	Post-Program	Pre-Program	Post-Program
Well (10–19)	0	4	1	11
Mild (20–24)	4	10	5	5
Moderate (25–29)	6	4	8	1
Severe (30–50)	8	0	3	0

Table 2. Pre-post comparisons on K10+ scores for program completers.

Language Group Variable	Mean Score		Sign Test for Pre-Post Change	
	Pre-Program M (SD)	Post-Program M (SD)	z	1-Sided *p*
Arabic speakers (*N* = 18)				
K10 score	28.6 (4.8)	21.3 (3.1)	−4.24	<0.001
Q11. Days of inability to work due to mental health issues in past four weeks	0.9 (1.5)	0.7(1.4)	−1.34	0.180
Q12. Days of cutting down work due to mental health issues in past four weeks (apart from days in Q11)	5.8 (6.2)	4.7 (5.5)	−2.89	<0.01
Bangla speakers (*N* = 17)				
K10 score	26.1 (4.6)	18.5 (3.5)	−4.12	<0.001
Q11. Days of inability to work due to mental health issues in past four weeks	0.4 (1.2)	0.2 (0.5)	−0.58	0.564
Q12. Days of cutting down work due to mental health issues in past four weeks (apart from days in Q11)	4.9 (8.1)	3.3 (3.9)	0	1

All program completers reported that their experience of the program was positive. Across both language groups, 85% indicated that the effect on their overall wellbeing was 'very good' or 'excellent' and 97% rated their experience of the program as 'very good' or 'excellent'. Box 2 gives examples of the feedback received from participants at the end of the program.

Box 2. Participant feedback (translated from Arabic and Bangla as necessary).

Online group 3, Arabic
- "I am aware of my thoughts and able to let go."
- "My son is doing his [final exams] and I learnt to manage my anxiety so I don't impact him."

Online group 4, Arabic
- "I am very happy to have found this program in my language and culture. I am able to better understand and relate to the topics."

Online group 5, Bangla
- "I used to live in the past I now live in the moment and I enjoy it."
- "I have learnt a lot and I am applying them in my daily life."
- "This is very much needed in our community."

Online group 6, Arabic
- "I saw a psychologist but never benefitted like this, despite this is being virtual."

3.1.2. Referrals

Across the face-to-face and online programs combined, 302 Arabic and 187 Bangla speakers were recruited, including 444 women and 45 men. The Bangla participants tended to be younger than the Arabic speakers, most of whom were aged 36–55 years with a sizeable number aged 56–55 years. They had also spent less time in Australia on average (Bangla 8.6 years vs. Arabic 20.3 years).

At program commencement, 8.7% of face-to-face and 15.9% of online program participants were already receiving mental health care. In both delivery formats, Arabic speakers were more likely than Bangla speakers to be receiving such care (Table 3). The overall comparison by language was statistically significant: 9.6% Arabic vs. 4.3% Bangla, X^2 (1, N = 489 = 4.68, $p < 0.05$).

Table 3. Participants already receiving mental health care and referrals made.

Group Language and Format	Participants Recruited	Receiving Mental Health Care [a]	Referrals				
			Private Psychologist [b]	Family Therapist [b]	GP for Referral [b]	Other Service [b]	Total [b]
	N	n (%)	n (%)	n (%)	n (%)	n (%)	n (%)
Arabic							
Face-to-face	276	22 (8.0)	45 (17.8)	4 (1.6)	3 (1.2)	8 (3.1)	60 (23.6)
Online	26	7 (26.9)	4 (21.1)	0	0	3 (15.7)	7 (36.8)
Total	302	29 (9.6)	49 (17.9)	4 (1.5)	3 (1.1)	11 (4.0)	67 (24.5)
Bangla							
Face-to-face	169	8 (4.7)	22 (13.7)	2 (1.2)	1 (0.6)	5 (3.1)	30 (18.6)
Online	18	0	9 (50.0)	0	0	0	9 (50.0)
Total	187	8 (4.3)	31 (17.3)	2 (1.1)	1 (0.6)	5 (2.8)	39 (21.8)
Overall							
Face-to-face	445	30 (8.7)	67 (16.1)	6 (1.4)	4 (1.0)	13 (3.1)	90 (21.7)
Online	44	7 (15.9)	13 (35.1)	0	0	3 (8.1)	16 (43.2)
Total	489	37 (7.6)	83 (18.4)	6 (1.3)	4 (0.9)	16 (3.5)	106 (23.5)

[a] Percentage of all participants recruited. [b] Percentage of participants recruited who were not already receiving mental health care.

As a result of all group programs, an additional 106 referrals were made for specialist care (Table 3), including 11 referrals for a participant's family member. In the two Bangla online programs, half the participants were referred. Overall, referral was significantly more likely from the online groups than face-to-face groups—43.2% online vs. 21.7% face-to-face, X^2 (1, N = 452) = 8.79, $p < 0.01$). Over three-quarters (78.3%) of all referrals were to a private psychologist due to language needs. Four participants were reconnected with a service provider whom they had previously seen, usually a private psychologist. Six were referred to a family therapist (psychologist or mental health social worker) and four were referred to their GP to obtain a psychiatrist/psychologist referral. Sixteen were referred elsewhere: to a general health, social service, or community organisation (Table 3). Specific needs for referral included relationship issues, trauma, grief, and child specialist.

3.1.3. Skills Transfer

Overall, 95.2% of participants who completed the face-to-face or online program reported sharing the mindfulness skills they had learned with others in their social circle. We estimated that, collectively, the 397 participants shared the mindfulness skills with at least 922 other people, an average of 2.3 people each. Relatives were the most common recipients or beneficiaries. Over three-quarters (78.1%) of program completers reported sharing with a family member (Table 4). A minority (18.6%) simply indicated family without specifying the nature of the relationship. When this was stated, 75.8% indicated immediate family (usually spouse or child) and 6.8% indicated extended family. Just under half (45.8%) of participants reported sharing with a friend and 8.1% with another person (e.g., neighbour or colleague). Fourteen people shared with someone overseas.

Table 4. Sharing of skills by recipient for program completers.

Group Language and Format	Program Completers N	Recipient		
		Family n (%)	Friend n (%)	Other n (%)
Arabic				
Face-to-face	224	170 (75.9)	91 (40.6)	18 (7.4)
Online	18	13 (72.2)	9 (50.0)	0
Total	242	183 (75.6)	100 (41.3)	18 (7.4)
Bangla				
Face-to-face	138	117 (84.8)	72 (52.2)	13 (9.4)
Online	17	10 (58.8)	10 (58.8)	1 (5.9)
Total	155	127 (81.9)	82 (52.9)	14 (93.3)
Overall				
Face-to-face	362	287 (79.3)	163 (45.0)	31 (8.6)
Online	35	23 (65.7)	19 (54.3)	1 (2.9)
Total	397	310 (78.1)	182 (45.8)	32 (8.1)

The percentage of participants who reported sharing their new skills did not differ significantly by language (93.8% Arabic vs. 97.4% Bangla), group format (95.0% face-to-face vs. 97.1% online), gender (95.4% female vs. 93.1% male) or age group (96% 16–35 years vs. 94.7% 36+ years). However, Bangla speakers were significantly more likely than Arabic speakers to share with their spouse, 47.0% vs. 22.9%, X^2 (1, N = 378) = 24.02, $p < 0.001$); while Arabic speakers were more likely to share with their child, 37.0% vs. 15.9%, X^2 (1, N = 378) = 19.80, $p < 0.001$). Similarly, younger participants (16–35 years) were significantly more likely than older participants (36+ years) to share with their spouse, 44.4% vs. 25.2%, (1, N = 378) = 13.04, $p < 0.001$); while older participants were more likely to share with their child, 39.7% vs. 10.4%, X^2 (1, N = 378) = 37.57, $p < 0.001$).

3.2. In-Language Resources

The web-based in-language audio and video mindfulness resources expanded the CALD Mindfulness Program's reach within Australia and internationally. Table 5 shows how many times the different audio tracks were downloaded from 1 July to 31 December 2021.

Table 5. Mindfulness audio resources accessed from 1 July to 31 December 2021.

Track Title	Downloads		
	Arabic	Bangla	English
Introduction	36	10	20
Grounding Exercise with Sensory Awareness	54	5	52
Mindful Breathing	64	6	61
Leaves on a Stream	40	8	28
Body Scan	53	8	56
Practicing Loving Kindness and Self-Compassion	32	13	48
Sitting with Difficult Emotions	20	20	113

Since June 2020, the 'Mindfulness in Challenging Times' video in Arabic has received 2837 views and the English video 1275 views. Since October 2020, the Bangla video has received 1006 views.

3.3. Workforce Capacity Building

Between August 2017 and December 2019, seven full-day workshops were offered across the region, attracting a total of 83 participants, including a few from outside the region connected through professional networks. Another workshop was run in June 2021 with 15 participants (results not included below).

The great majority (88.0%) of trainees were women; 45.8% were bilingual community workers and 35.0% were bilingual mental health professionals, mostly psychologists and social workers. Arabic (49.4%) and Bangla (24.1%) were the most commonly spoken community languages. Other trainees spoke Cantonese, Greek, Hindi, Indonesian, Macedonian, Mandarin, Nepali, Russian, Sinhala, Spanish, Tamil, or Urdu. Eighty-two (99%) of the trainees provided post-workshop feedback, all of whom found the training engaging and the content both practical and relevant.

Seventy-one of the trainees from the first six workshops were emailed the follow-up survey, the others being uncontactable. Forty-five (63%) responded. Comparison on gender, role and language spoken suggested that the follow-up sample was reasonably representative of everyone trained. Key learnings related to core mindfulness concepts and techniques and how cultural and religious tailoring of MBIs enhances acceptability to CALD communities. Nearly three-quarters (73%) of respondents indicated that they had applied mindfulness skills for self-care. Both bilingual mental health professionals and bilingual community workers had facilitated mindfulness groups, with 19 (42%) facilitating at least two groups. They incorporated mindfulness into their clinical/counselling sessions and community wellbeing programs, and as an adjunct to mental health care and other interventions. All indicated at least 'moderate impact' on their practice and 60% 'significant impact' or 'high impact'.

3.4. Community Partnerships

We identified 17 people who met the eligibility criteria from the 15 community partners and were able to interview all but one: 10 from the Arabic speaking community, 4 from the Bangla speaking community, and 2 English-speakers who were employed by a community partner (Sydney Multicultural Community Services and the NSW Refugee Health Service). Twelve were community organisation staff while the other four, including two psychologists, worked independently. Thirteen of the informants had attended the 1-day training on MBIs for CALD communities.

All community partners reported that they were kept busy before, during and after the program, with completion of tasks often taking longer than expected. Being aligned with the organisation's operational plan and having committed and supportive management and dedicated staff (bilingual if available, paid or volunteer) and resources (venue, equipment, and refreshments) were important enablers of success. During the program, depending on their role, the community partners facilitated, co-facilitated, or provided support to the group by encouraging participants to ask questions, contributing to the group discussion, and helping to explain the presented concepts using culturally and religiously appropriate anecdotes. The presence of a familiar face also made participants feel comfortable. The bilingual community workers provided assistance with completing the evaluation measures in the first and final sessions when required, and technical support for the online groups.

Common recruitment challenges experienced by the partners included promoting and explaining mindfulness, which was a novel concept for most people, mental health stigma and geographic restrictions under the funding agreement. Recruiting homogeneous groups (similar age, gender, and level of education) presented an additional challenge. It took time to educate and reassure community members who were hesitant to discuss mental health-related issues outside their family by emphasising group confidentiality. Once the program was established, word-of-mouth proved to be the most effective means of promotion and limiting the number of participants in the group was sometimes a problem. Adhering to the program's geographical boundaries resulted in difficult conversations for community partners and led to feelings of abandonment and marginalisation among community members who lived outside the CESPHN region. All activities took time. Maintaining weekly contact between sessions to keep participants motivated and follow-up calls to gauge their experience with the program and its impact on their day-to-day lives could involve several phone calls. Helping participants to complete relevant paperwork and supporting online participants with technical issues added an extra burden on under-resourced and already stretched individuals and community organisations.

It was apparent that relationships were fundamental to successful community engagement and program outcomes. 'Trust' was mentioned repeatedly, e.g., "Having an established relationship with the community and having their trust [in] providing beneficial programs" and "Participants trusted the facilitator and felt more comfortable to seek support following the program". Community partners commented on the professionalism and expertise of the clinician facilitators from the same cultural and linguistic background and their skill in tailoring the program to make the content relevant and accessible, with consideration of each group's unique needs (often conveyed by partner organisation to facilitator).

4. Discussion

The population health framework underpinning Australian mental health policy and practice recognises that there are a complex range of determinants and consequences of mental health and illness across diverse population groups [15]. Mainstream or general population initiatives must be consolidated, expanded, and complemented by activities that target specific groups [15]. As in other immigrant nations [10,39], Australia's CALD communities are typically under-served by both primary and specialist mental health services [9,40,41]. The CALD Mindfulness Program seeks to address some of the barriers to mental health care (including self-care) through a suite of interventions designed to support de-stigmatisation, assist people to cope with negative experiences and stressful situations, and facilitate their access to professional mental health care when needed. Over the past 5.5 years, 302 Arabic-speaking and 187 Bangla speaking adults, mostly women, have participated in the 5-week face-to-face and 4-week online group programs. Both language groups, in both delivery formats, showed clinical and statistical improvements in mental health outcomes. Across all programs, 21.6% of those recruited were referred for further care.

Achieving high-levels of recruitment, retention, and adherence to protocol in community-based interventions is challenging for mainstream health services, particularly when dealing with marginalised populations [42]. Trauma-informed practices and an attitude of cultural humility can facilitate access to mental health care for minorities in a multicultural society [43]. Having a culturally competent research team and program staff who are embedded in the community and belong to the target community, who possess good interpersonal skills and are well trained is critical [42,44]. In the group programs, integration of spiritual or religious illustrations and anecdotes was pivotal to explaining mindfulness concepts to participants who were mostly of Islamic faith, facilitating their understanding and engagement. If presented appropriately, mindfulness-based approaches are very feasible and highly resonant with Islamic thought and practice [45].

Australia's multicultural health and community workforce is an important national resource. By training 98 bilingual mental health professionals and community workers in MBIs and cultural tailoring, the CALD Mindfulness Program has strengthened individual, organisational and community capacity to respond to mental health issues in CALD communities in the CESPHN region. In the follow-up survey, 63% of respondents indicated that the training had positively influenced their practice. The fact that 73% of respondents reported applying mindfulness skills for self-care provides further evidence of relevance and cultural acceptability. Over the course of the CALD Mindfulness Program, the bilingual (Arabic/English) clinical lead has supervised three bilingual (Arabic/English) psychology interns.

Community partners have played a major role in promoting the program, engaging individuals from the target communities, and encouraging weekly attendance and mindfulness practice. Interviews with 16 community partners reinforced the importance of weekly contact by a trusted person for retention. Shared culture and language convey cultural safety which has been defined by as "an environment that is spiritually, socially and emotionally safe for people, where there is no assault, challenge, or denial of their identity, of who they are and what they need" [46] (p. 213). Trust between community partners, community members and program providers formed the basis for the program and was reinforced through program processes and outcomes.

Culturally competent mental health promotion and care must address the social and cultural determinants of health [16,47]. Since 2020, the usual stressors associated with migration and settlement have been compounded by the COVID-19 pandemic. The impact of lockdown-related unemployment, school and business closure and social disconnection has disproportionately affected already vulnerable and marginalised populations, including CALD communities and people on low incomes [48]. An early Australian study found that overseas-born respondents were more likely to report clinically significant levels of anxiety [49]. Concurrently, the pandemic has accelerated the use of digital health interventions and telemedicine as a means of supporting mental health and wellbeing [50,51], including technology assisted MBIs [52,53].

Compared to face-to-face, more of the online participants possessed post-school qualifications (62.3% vs. 81.4%, respectively). It is likely that education and digital literacy account for some of the difference in retention between Arabic and Bangla speakers in the online program. While most are keen to return to the face-to-face format, it is clear that the online format, or possibly a blended format, has a place in responding to mental health needs, particularly for Bangla and other language groups who embrace this technology. Through sharing experiences of the pandemic, wellbeing was nurtured, and cultural identities and connections celebrated. A place (actual or virtual) that is respectful, engaging, and supportive is more likely than a mainstream service to be used by minority groups and those most in need [54].

Although online interventions typically have relatively high attrition [55], the online mindfulness group program had an overall retention rate of approximately 80%, comparable to the face-to-face program [26]. We attribute this exceptional result to the 'human element', i.e., the encouragement provided by the facilitators and community partners, as well as the supportive and culturally safe group format [54]. Support for this conclusion is provided by a randomised controlled trial of 4-week internet-based MBI with Chinese university students. Participants who received peer counsellor support demonstrated significantly less attrition and more course completion and reported significantly greater pre-post improvements in daily stress ratings and depression than those in the no support condition [55].

A minority of participants (8.7% face-to-face and 15.9% online) were already receiving mental health care. In both delivery formats, Arabic speakers were more likely than Bangla speakers to be receiving such care. The Arabic community in Sydney (and Australia generally) is much larger and longer established, so has greater knowledge of the health system and more resources and networks to draw upon, including a cohort of bicultural/bilingual health professionals who have been educated and trained in Australia. As a result of all group programs, an additional 106 referrals were made for specialist mental health care, the majority to bilingual psychologists in private practice: an indicator of previously unmet need.

In addition to program participants who benefited directly through a process of dissemination (i.e., active and planned efforts to encourage target groups to adopt an innovation), many other people benefited through a process of diffusion (i.e., passive spread through social networks) [56]. As participants experienced the benefits of mindfulness and other mental health self-help strategies for themselves, they were eager to share the skills and knowledge with others. Sharing of positive experiences resulted in increased demand for the program and likely reduced mental health stigma, although we did not measure this. The online resources, available in Arabic, Bangla and English and an increasing number of other community languages, are regularly downloaded.

Our research has demonstrated that the group mindfulness program provides an effective and culturally acceptable low-intensity mental health intervention for the target communities as is capable of integration into the wider health system [26]. Geographical restrictions associated with the current funding model present a predicament for implementation and further scaling up. Service boundaries defined by government departments do not necessarily align with community expectations. For many CALD communities, sense of identity and community is tied to shared experiences, practices, language, beliefs, and history, rather than geographical boundaries, and members will often travel to access programs and services aligned with their cultural values [3,9]. The mismatch between these understandings of community (a geographical place versus a group of people who depend on and interact with each other and with their environment [57]) is a barrier to identifying and responding to community needs in an effective, efficient, and meaningful way. The challenge ahead lies in extending this collaborative regional approach, which brings together health services and community partners, to other regions within the metropolitan Sydney and more broadly. This is currently hampered by a lack of mechanisms to scale up effective interventions for under-served populations at state and national levels.

This research has strengths and limitations. On the strengths side, the large multicomponent intervention, which was refined and extended over several years, had evaluation embedded across all aspects and employed mental health outcome measures translated and validated with Arabic and Bangla speakers. Referral numbers, based data collected over 43 group programs that attracted 489 participants, are likely to reflect population need. Retention and program adherence were high in both the face-to-face and online formats. We achieved a good response to the follow-up survey of trainees from the mindfulness workshops and the community partner interviews. Limitations include the small number of participants (all female) in the pre-post study of the online program. In the absence of a control group, it is impossible to conclusively demonstrate causality; however, the results are consistent with a pre-post study with a wait-list control group for the face-to-face program [24]. We did not assess understanding or application of mindfulness using a validated questionnaire and did not conduct a follow-up. Importantly, CALD communities are not homogeneous, and our results are from Arabic and Bangla speakers in the CESPHN region, mostly women. Further research is required to extend the group program to men and young people and to determine its suitability, with appropriate adaptation, for use with other language groups and in other settings.

5. Conclusions

The CALD Mindfulness Program, which was designed to address the mental health needs of under-served CALD communities in metropolitan Sydney, has proved very successful. This innovative community-based program, with its emphasis on promotion of mental health and wellbeing, sits well within Australia's stepped care model for primary mental health care. The in-language and culturally tailored mental health self-help resources, and low-intensity interventions delivered face-to-face and online through a collaborative regional approach, were readily adopted by participants from the target communities (Arabic and Bangla speakers) and shared with others in their family and community networks. The program provides a non-stigmatising soft-entry point to mental health services for the Arabic and Bangla communities who live in the CESPHN region. Future directions include extension of the CALD Mindfulness Program to other language groups, further exploration of technology mediated MBIs, and further integration of the program across the health system.

Author Contributions: Conceptualization, I.B., H.S. and L.W.; methodology, I.B., H.S. and L.W.; formal analysis, I.B., H.B. and H.S.; investigation, H.S., H.B. and K.G.; resources, L.W.; data curation, H.S. and K.G.; writing—original draft preparation, I.B.; writing—review and editing, H.S., L.W., K.G. and H.B.; supervision, I.B. and H.S.; project administration, K.G.; funding acquisition, L.W. All authors have read and agreed to the published version of the manuscript.

Funding: This project was funded by the Central and Eastern Sydney Primary Health Network with in-kind support from the South Eastern Sydney Local Health District Multicultural Health Service. The article processing charge was funded by SESLHD Multicultural Health Service.

Institutional Review Board Statement: Ethics approval for evaluation of the group mindfulness program and the community partnerships was obtained from the SESLHD Human Research Ethics Committee (LNR/17/POWH/157), with external recognition from Western Sydney University Human Research Ethics Committee (RH12328). Evaluation of the workforce capacity building component was assessed by the SESLHD HREC as being a quality improvement or quality assurance activity not requiring independent ethics review.

Informed Consent Statement: Informed consent was obtained from all study participants.

Data Availability Statement: The data sets are not publicly available as they contain information that could potentially re-identify individuals but are available from LW upon reasonable request and with relevant ethical approval. Program materials are available from HS.

Acknowledgments: We thank all the health services and community partners that have contributed to implementation and evaluation of the CALD Mindfulness Program, as well as all the program participants. We thank Hanan Youssef for assistance with the community partner interviews.

Conflicts of Interest: The authors declare no conflict of interest. The funders had no role in the design of the study; in the collection, analyses, or interpretation of data; in the writing of the manuscript, or in the decision to publish the results.

Appendix A

Group session 1: Introduction and Debriefing
Aim: To discuss signs of stress and vulnerabilities experienced by participants, identify helpful and unhelpful stress responses and provide a set of motivating and practical stress management skills.
Video: Mindfulness in Challenging Times.
Mindfulness practice: Grounding exercise with sensory awareness.
Mnemonic: HOPEFUL + L, a set of cognitive and practical tips to stay afloat during stressful times:

> Hang on to helpful thoughts and let go of unhelpful catastrophic ones.
> Optimism is crucial to our survival and the key to courage in times of adversity.
> Pray, reflect, practice mindfulness/relaxation and self-care.
> Exercise daily, keep active to stay healthy and fit.
> Filter and limit exposure to social media and electronic devices—which is quickly becoming a primary reason for stress today.
> Understand and accept that there are circumstances completely beyond our control
> Lead a normal life as much as the circumstances permit: work, study, read, cook, clean, play, etc.
> Live day by day and remember that change is constant and inevitable.

Group session 2: Stress Experiences and Responses, Mindfulness
Aim: To educate participants about stress from an evolutionary perspective, introduce mindfulness concepts and explore their cultural and spiritual applicability and provide a set of mindfulness skills.
Mindfulness practice: Mindfulness breathing exercise.
Mnemonic: Five 'A's of mindfulness—awareness, acknowledgement, actions, acceptance and appreciation:

> Awareness of our thoughts, feelings and reactions and what is going on around you.
> Acknowledge and embrace our fears without judgment.
> Actions to change what we can—problem solve.
> Acceptance of what is beyond our control.
> Appreciate and invest into the resources and support we have.

Group session 3: Mindfulness Based Stress Reduction Strategies

Aim: To promote participants' awareness of the interconnectedness of thoughts, feelings and behaviours, differentiate themselves from their thoughts, introduce mindfulness-based stress management skills.
Mindfulness practice: Leaves on a stream exercise, body scan exercise.
Mnemonic: BE PRESENT, a set of mindfulness-based stress management skills and practices to help reduce distress:

Breathe—be mindful of the breath.
Engage in one mind—focus regularly.
Practice mindfulness whenever and wherever you can.
Remember the influence of our thoughts on our feelings and behaviours.
Engage your five senses to ground yourself.
Stop and reflect on current experience of situation.
Exercise and stay fit—A healthy mind is in a healthy body and vice versa.
Never give up—It can take time to learn new skills, keep practising.
Take time out for yourself—Include yourself in the cycle of care.

Group Session 4: Loving Kindness and Self-Compassion, Review
Aim: To define sense of self, emphasise self-care practices through loving kindness and self-compassion and review stress management skills learnt throughout the program.To reflect and recap topics and discussions from previous sessions summed up in a Chinese proverb (below) highlighting the impact of habitual thoughts, feeling and behaviours and their successive effect on many aspects of our lives.
Mindfulness practice: Loving kindness and self-compassion exercise.
Mnemonic: REFLECTION, a program summary:

Re-think life; reassess your thoughts, attitudes, choices, reactions and priorities. Changing the world is not entirely up to you, work on changing yourself.
Everyone experiences mental health vulnerabilities when facing life changes—no one is immune.
Focus on your strength and invest your energy into building your resilience and just be grateful.
Life is a journey with planned humps along the way. Embrace them, as they are just part of the deal.
Evolve, adapt and learn to grow from difficult times as they usually bring with them powerful lessons.
Commit to long-term changes with healthy thinking and maintain a robust lifestyle.
Take one day at a time, stay focused, connected and be hopeful. Change is imminent.
Include yourself into the circle of care and embed self-compassion in your daily practices.
Open your mind and heart during uncertain times to be able to forgo the life you planned and to partake in the life that is waiting for you.
Never underestimate your capabilities in making a difference—"The potential for greatness lives within each of us".

"Be careful of your thoughts, for your thoughts become your words. Be careful of your words, for your words become your actions. Be careful of your actions, for your actions become your habits. Be careful of your habits, for your habits become your character. Be careful of your character, for your character becomes your destiny.". Chinese Proverb.

Appendix B. Comparison of the Face-to-Face and Online Group Programs

Features	Face-to-Face Program	Online Program
No. of sessions	5	4
Mental health outcome measures	K10+ and DASS21	K10+
Co-facilitators	Bilingual mental health clinician and bilingual community worker	Bilingual mental health clinician and bilingual community worker
PowerPoint to present information	Yes	Yes
Access to audio resources	CD, USB or web link	Web link
Participant handbook and handouts	Yes	No
Focus of the first session	Introduction to mindfulness	Identifying and normalising stress responses, especially related to COVID-19
Education on stress and the stress response	Yes	Yes
Training in mindfulness-based stress management strategies	Yes	Yes
Definition of self, emphasising self-care through loving kindness and self-compassion	Yes	Yes
Education on judgement and self-judgement and managing painful emotions	Yes	No
Weekly contact between sessions	Yes	Yes
Criteria for referral	K10 score > 30 DASS21 'severe' or 'extremely severe' Clinician facilitator judgement Participant request	K10 score > 30 Clinician facilitator judgement
Advertising	Health and community networks, flyers, social media, and word-of-mouth	Social media, community networks and word-of-mouth
Venue	Community venues, e.g., migrant resource centre and mosque and church facilities	Home
Catering	Refreshments provided	Not applicable
Childcare	Provided as needed	Not applicable

Appendix C. CALD Mindfulness Audio and Video Resources

Audio and video resources developed through of the CALD Mindfulness Program are available on the NSW Health Multicultural Health Communications Service website. https://www.mhcs.health.nsw.gov.au/about-us/campaigns-and-projects/current-campaigns/mindfulness-program-audio-resources (accessed on 30 January 2022).

Audio resources include:

- Arabic Mindfulness Exercises—6 exercises plus an introduction https://www.mhcs.health.nsw.gov.au/about-us/campaigns-and-projects/current-campaigns/mindfulness-program-audio-resources/arabic (accessed on 30 January 2022)
- Bangla Mindfulness Exercises—6 exercises plus an introduction https://www.mhcs.health.nsw.gov.au/about-us/campaigns-and-projects/current-campaigns/mindfulness-program-audio-resources/bangla (accessed on 30 January 2022)
- English Mindfulness Exercises—6 exercises plus an introduction https://www.mhcs.health.nsw.gov.au/about-us/campaigns-and-projects/current-campaigns/mindfulness-program-audio-resources/english (accessed on 30 January 2022)

- Mandarin Mindfulness Exercises—6 exercises plus an introduction https://www.mhcs.health.nsw.gov.au/about-us/campaigns-and-projects/current-campaigns/mindfulness-program-audio-resources/mandarin (accessed on 30 January 2022)
- Nepali Mindfulness Exercises—6 exercises plus an introduction https://www.mhcs.health.nsw.gov.au/about-us/campaigns-and-projects/current-campaigns/mindfulness-program-audio-resources/nepali (accessed on 30 January 2022)

Audio track titles and duration are indicated in the table below.

Track	Language & Duration (min)				
	Arabic	Bangla	English	Mandarin	Nepali
Introduction	3.36	4.29	3.55	3.44	4.05
Grounding Exercise with Sensory Awareness	6.48	9.33	6.55	6.54	7.33
Mindful Breathing	10.26	11.17	9.12	9.04	9.49
Leaves on a Stream	11.59	12.31	10.10	10.35	10.45
Body Scan	13.51	14.26	13.40	11.57	11.44
Practicing Loving Kindness and Self-Compassion	12.40	12.33	10.26	10.53	9.59
Sitting with Difficult Emotions	17.41	17.10	15.22	15.09	15.04

Video resources include:

- Mindfulness in Challenging Times in Arabic (6:14 min) https://www.youtube.com/watch?v=M2CneDhvYTI (accessed on 30 January 2022)
- Mindfulness in Challenging Times in Bangla (6:16 min) https://www.youtube.com/watch?v=DHGhPpSUtVI (accessed on 30 January 2022)
- Mindfulness in Challenging Times in English (6:18 min) https://www.youtube.com/watch?v=8pnrlhR_rvY (accessed on 30 January 2022)

References

1. Organisation for Economic Co-operation and Development. *International Migration Outlook 2020*; OECD Publishing: Paris, France, 2020. [CrossRef]
2. United Nations High Commissioner for Refugees. Global Trends: Forced Displacement in 2019; UNHCR, 2020. Available online: www.unhcr.org/globaltrends2019 (accessed on 30 January 2022).
3. Jupp, J. *The Australian People: An Encyclopedia of the Nation, its People and Their Origins*; Cambridge University Press: Cambridge, UK, 2001.
4. Australian Bureau of Statistics. 2071.0—Census of Population and Housing: Reflecting Australia—Stories from the Census, 2016; Cultural Diversity in Australia, 2016. Commonwealth of Australia: Canberra, 2017. Available online: https://www.abs.gov.au/ausstats/abs@.nsf/Lookup/by%20Subject/2071.0~{}2016~{}Main%20Features~{}Cultural%20Diversity%20Article~{}60 (accessed on 30 January 2022).
5. Phillips, J.; Simon-Davies, J. Migration—Australian Migration Flows and Population; Parliamentary Library Research Publications: Canberra, 2016. Available online: https://www.aph.gov.au/About_Parliament/Parliamentary_Departments/Parliamentary_Library/pubs/BriefingBook45p/MigrationFlows (accessed on 30 January 2022).
6. Australian Government. Australian Governments' Multicultural Statement: Multicultural Australia–United, Strong, Successful; Commonwealth of Australia: Canberra, 2018. Available online: https://www.homeaffairs.gov.au/about-us/our-portfolios/multicultural-affairs/about-multicultural-affairs/our-statement (accessed on 30 January 2022).
7. NSW Ministry of Health. NSW Plan for Healthy Culturally and Linguistically Diverse Communities: 2019–2023; NSW Ministry of Health, 2019. Available online: https://www1.health.nsw.gov.au/pds/Pages/doc.aspx?dn=PD2019_018 (accessed on 30 January 2022).
8. World Health Organization. *Promoting Mental Health: Concepts, Emerging Evidence, Practice (Summary Report)*; WHO: Geneva, Switzerland, 2004.
9. Minas, H.; Kakuma, R.; Too, L.S.; Vayani, H.; Orapeleng, S.; Prasad-Ildes, R.; Turner, G.; Procter, N.; Oehm, D. Mental health research and evaluation in multicultural Australia: Developing a culture of inclusion. *Int. J. Ment. Health Syst.* **2013**, *7*, 23. [CrossRef]
10. Kirmayer, L.J.; Narasiah, L.; Munoz, M.; Rashid, M.; Ryder, A.G.; Guzder, J.; Hassan, G.; Rousseau, C.; Pottie, K. Common mental health problems in immigrants and refugees: General approach in primary care. *CMAJ* **2011**, *183*, E959–E967. [CrossRef] [PubMed]
11. Renzaho, A.M.; Dhingra, N.; Georgeou, N. Youth as contested sites of culture: The intergenerational acculturation gap amongst new migrant communities–Parental and young adult perspectives. *PLoS ONE* **2017**, *12*, e0170700. [CrossRef]

12. Ferdinand, A.S.; Paradies, Y.; Kelaher, M. Mental health impacts of racial discrimination in Australian culturally and linguistically diverse communities: A cross-sectional survey. *BMC Public Health* **2015**, *15*, 401. [CrossRef]

13. Silove, D.; Ventevogel, P.; Rees, S. The contemporary refugee crisis: An overview of mental health challenges. *World Psychiatry* **2017**, *16*, 130–139. [CrossRef] [PubMed]

14. Walther, L.; Kröger, H.; Tibubos, A.N.; Ta, T.; von Scheve, C.; Schupp, J.; Hahn, E.; Bajbouj, M. Psychological distress among refugees in Germany: A cross-sectional analysis of individual and contextual risk factors and potential consequences for integration using a nationally representative survey. *BMJ Open* **2020**, *10*, e033658. [CrossRef] [PubMed]

15. National Mental Health Strategy. National Mental Health Policy 2008; Commonwealth of Australia: Canberra, 2009. Available online: https://www.health.gov.au/sites/default/files/documents/2020/11/national-mental-health-policy-2008.pdf (accessed on 30 January 2022).

16. Tilford, S. Mental health promotion. In *Mental Health Promotion: A Lifespan Approach*; Cattan, M., Tilford, S., Eds.; Open University Press McGraw-Hill: Maidenhead, UK, 2006.

17. National Mental Health Strategy. The Fifth National Mental Health and Suicide Prevention Plan; Commonwealth of Australia: Canberra, 2017. Available online: https://www.mentalhealthcommission.gov.au/monitoring-and-reporting/fifth-plan/5th-national-mental-health-and-suicide-prevention (accessed on 30 January 2022).

18. Department of Health. Reform and System Transformation—A 5-Year Horizon for Primary Health Networks, 2019. Available online: https://www.health.gov.au/resources/publications/reform-and-system-transformation-a-5-year-horizon-for-prima ry-health-networks (accessed on 30 January 2022).

19. Department of Health. Primary Health Networks (PHN) Primary Mental Health Care Guidance–Stepped Care, 2019. Available online: https://www.health.gov.au/resources/publications/primary-health-networks-phn-primary-mental-health-care-guid ance-stepped-care (accessed on 30 January 2022).

20. Department of Health. Primary Health Networks (PHN) Primary Mental Health Care Guidance–Psychological Therapies Provided by Mental Health Professionals to Underserviced Groups, 2019. Available online: https://www.health.gov.au/resource s/publications/primary-health-networks-phn-primary-mental-health-care-guidance-psychological-therapies-provided-by-m ental-health-professionals-to-underserviced-groups (accessed on 30 January 2022).

21. Department of Health. Australian Government Response to Contributing Lives, Thriving Communities–Review of Mental Health Programmes and Services; Commonwealth of Australia, Canberra, 2015. Available online: https://www.health.gov.au/resource s/publications/review-of-mental-health-programmes-and-services (accessed on 30 January 2022).

22. Creswell, J.D. Mindfulness interventions. *Annu. Rev. Psychol.* **2017**, *68*, 491–516. [CrossRef]

23. Janssen, M.; Heerkens, Y.; Kuijer, W.; van der Heijden, B.; Engels, J. Effects of mindfulness-based stress reduction on employees' mental health: A systematic review. *PLoS ONE* **2018**, *13*, e0191332. [CrossRef]

24. Blignault, I.; Saab, H.; Woodland, L.; Comino, E. Evaluation of the acceptability and clinical utility of an Arabic-language Mindfulness CD in an Australian community setting. *Transcult. Psychiatry* **2019**, *56*, 552–568. [CrossRef]

25. Blignault, I.; Saab, H.; Woodland, L.; O'Callaghan, C. Cultivating mindfulness: Evaluation of a community-based mindfulness program for Arabic-speaking women in Australia. *Curr. Psychol.* **2021**, 1–12. [CrossRef]

26. Blignault, I.; Saab, H.; Woodland, L.; Manan, H.; Kaur, A. Effectiveness of a community-based group mindfulness program tailored for Arabic and Bangla-speaking migrants. *Int. J. Ment. Health Syst.* **2021**, *15*, 32. [CrossRef] [PubMed]

27. NSW Health Multicultural Health Communications Service Website. Available online: https://www.mhcs.health.nsw.gov.au/a bout-us/campaigns-and-projects/current-campaigns/mindfulness-program-audio-resources (accessed on 30 January 2022).

28. Central and Eastern Sydney PHN. 2018 Needs Assessment; CESPHN, 2018. Available online: https://www.cesphn.org.au/docu ments/planning-strategy-and-evaluation/2398-2018-needs-assessment-report/file (accessed on 30 January 2022).

29. Central and Eastern Sydney PHN. Strategic Plan 2019–2021; CESPHN, 2019. Available online: http://www.cesphn.org.au/imag es/Central_and_Eastern_Sydney_PHN_Strategic_Plan-2019-2021.pdf (accessed on 30 January 2022).

30. South Eastern Sydney Local Health District. Vulnerable and Priority Populations in South Eastern Sydney Local Health District, Analysis of ABS Census Data, Population Profile; SESLHD, 2018. Available online: https://seslhd.health.nsw.gov.au/sites/defau lt/files/groups/PICH/Priority%20Populations/Population%20Profile_vulnerable%20and%20priority%20populations_SESL HD_ABS%20Census%202016.pdf (accessed on 30 January 2022).

31. Department of Home Affairs. Australia's Offshore Humanitarian Program: 2018–2019. Available online: https://www.homeaffa irs.gov.au/research-and-stats/files/australia-offshore-humanitarian-program-2018-19.pdf (accessed on 30 January 2022).

32. Cruickshank, K. Arabic-English Bilingualism in Australia. In *Encyclopedia of Language and Education*; Hornberger, N.H., Ed.; Springer: Boston, MA, USA, 2008. [CrossRef]

33. Department of Home Affairs. Bangladesh-born Community Information Summary. Available online: https://www.homeaffairs. gov.au/mca/files/2016-cis-bangladesh.PDF (accessed on 30 January 2022).

34. Hayes, S.C.; Hofmann, S.G. The third wave of cognitive behavioral therapy and the rise of process-based care. *World Psychiatry* **2017**, *16*, 245–246. [CrossRef] [PubMed]

35. Kessler, R.C.; Andrews, G.; Colpe, L.J.; Hiripi, E.; Mroczek, D.K.; Normand, S.L.; Walters, E.E.; Zaslavsky, A.M. Short screening scales to monitor population prevalences and trends in non-specific psychological distress. *Psychol. Med.* **2002**, *32*, 959–976. [CrossRef] [PubMed]

36. Lovibond, S.H.; Lovibond, P.F. *Manual for the Depression Anxiety Stress Scales*, 2nd ed.; Psychology Foundation of Australia: Balwyn, VIC, Australia, 1995.
37. Australian Mental Health Outcomes and Classification Network: Kessler 10+. Available online: https://www.amhocn.org/publi cations/kessler-10 (accessed on 30 January 2022).
38. *IBM SPSS Statistics for Windows*; Version 27; IBM Corp.: Armonk, NY, USA, 2021.
39. Bhugra, D.; Gupta, S. *Migration and Mental Health*; Cambridge University Press: Cambridge, UK, 2011.
40. Tobin, M. Developing mental health rehabilitation services in a culturally appropriate context. *Aust. Health Rev.* **2000**, *23*, 177–184. [CrossRef] [PubMed]
41. Krstanoska-Blazeska, K.; Thomson, R.; Slewa-Younan, S. Mental illness stigma and associated factors among Arabic-speaking religious and community leaders. *Int. J. Environ. Res. Public Health* **2021**, *18*, 7991. [CrossRef]
42. Rabie, S.; Bantjes, J.; Gordon, S.; Almirol, E.; Stewart, J.; Tomlinson, M.; Rotheram-Borus, M.J. Who can we reach and who can we keep? Predictors of intervention engagement and adherence in a cluster randomized controlled trial in South Africa. *BMC Public Health* **2020**, *20*, 275. [CrossRef]
43. Ranjbar, N.; Erb, M.; Mohammad, O.; Moreno, F.A. trauma-informed care and cultural humility in the mental health care of people from minoritized communities. *Focus* **2020**, *18*, 8–15. [CrossRef]
44. Woodland, L.; Blignault, I.; O'Callaghan, C.; Harris-Roxas, B.F. A framework for conducting culturally competent health research in a multicultural society. *Health Res. Policy Syst.* **2021**, *19*, 24. [CrossRef]
45. Thomas, J.; Furber, S.; Grey, I. The rise of mindfulness and its resonance with the Islamic tradition. *Ment. Health Relig. Cult.* **2017**, *20*, 973–985. [CrossRef]
46. Williams, R. Cultural safety: What does it mean for our work practice? *Aust. N. Z. J. Public Health* **1999**, *23*, 213–214. [CrossRef]
47. Olson, R.E.; Mutch, A.; Lisa Fitzgerald, L.; Hickey, S. The Social and Cultural Determinants of Health. In *Culture, Diversity and Health in Australia: Towards Culturally Safe Health Care*; Dune, T., McLeod, B., Williams, R., Eds.; Routledge: Abingdon, UK, 2021.
48. Bower, M.; Smout, S.; Ellsmore, S.; Donohoe-Bales, A.; Sivaprakash, P.P.; Lim, C.; Gray, M.; Francis, A.; Grager, A.; Riches, J. *COVID-19 and Australia's Mental Health*; Australia's Mental Health Think Tank: Sydney, Australia, 2021.
49. Fisher, J.R.; Tran, T.D.; Hammarberg, K.; Sastry, J.; Nguyen, H.; Rowe, H.; Popplestone, S.; Stocker, R.; Stubber, C.; Kirkman, M. Mental health of people in Australia in the first month of COVID-19 restrictions: A national survey. *Med. J. Aust.* **2020**, *213*, 458–464. [CrossRef] [PubMed]
50. Mahoney, A.; Elders, A.; Li, I.; David, C.; Haskelberg, H.; Guiney, H.; Millard, M. A tale of two countries: Increased uptake of digital mental health services during the COVID-19 pandemic in Australia and New Zealand. *Internet Interv.* **2021**, *25*, 100439. [CrossRef] [PubMed]
51. Abraham, A.; Jithesh, A.; Doraiswamy, S.; Al-Khawaga, N.; Mamtani, R.; Cheema, S. Telemental health use in the COVID-19 pandemic: A scoping review and evidence gap mapping. *Front. Psychiatry* **2021**, *12*, 748069. [CrossRef]
52. El-Morr, C.; Ritvo, P.; Ahmad, F.; Moineddin, R. Effectiveness of an 8-week web-based mindfulness virtual community intervention for university students on symptoms of stress, anxiety, and depression: Randomized controlled trial. *JMIR Ment. Health* **2020**, *7*, e18595. [CrossRef] [PubMed]
53. Kwon, C.Y.; Kwak, H.Y.; Kim, J.W. Using mind-body modalities via telemedicine during the COVID-19 crisis: Cases in the Republic of Korea. *Int. J. Environ. Res. Public Health* **2020**, *17*, 4477. [CrossRef] [PubMed]
54. Williams, R.; Dune, T.; McLeod, K. Principles of cultural safety. In *Culture, Diversity and Health in Australia: Towards Culturally Safe Health Care*; Dune, T., McLeod, K., Williams, R., Eds.; Routledge: Abingdon, UK, 2021; pp. 55–72.
55. Rodriguez, M.; Eisenlohr-Moul, T.A.; Weisman, J.; Rosenthal, M.Z. The use of task shifting to improve treatment engagement in an internet-based mindfulness intervention among Chinese university students: Randomized controlled trial. *JMIR Form. Res.* **2021**, *5*, e25772. [CrossRef]
56. Greenhalgh, T.; Robert, G.; Macfarlane, F.; Bate, P.; Kyriakidou, O. Diffusion of innovations in service organizations: Systematic review and recommendations. *Milbank Q.* **2004**, *82*, 581–629. [CrossRef] [PubMed]
57. McMurray, A. *Community Health and Wellness: A Socioecological Approach*, 3rd ed.; Mosby Elsevier: Sydney, Australia, 2007.

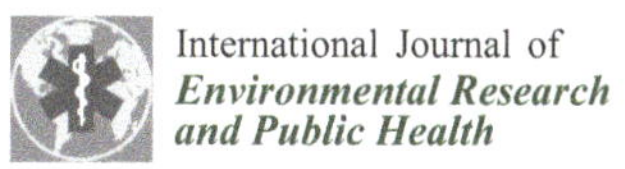
International Journal of
Environmental Research and Public Health

MDPI

Article

Impact of a Pilot Peer-Mentoring Empowerment Program on Personal Well-Being for Migrant and Refugee Women in Western Australia

Shelley Gower [1], Zakia Jeemi [2], Niranjani Wickramasinghe [2], Paul Kebble [3], David Forbes [2] and Jaya A R Dantas [2,*]

1 Curtin School of Nursing, Curtin University, Perth 6102, Australia; shelley.gower@curtin.edu.au
2 Curtin School of Population Health, Curtin University, Perth 6102, Australia; zakia.jeemi@curtin.edu.au (Z.J.); niranji_w@yahoo.com (N.W.); davideforbes@msn.com (D.F.)
3 Faculty of Health Sciences, Curtin University, Perth 6102, Australia; paul.kebble@curtin.edu.au
* Correspondence: jaya.dantas@curtin.edu.au

Abstract: The Empowerment and Peer Mentoring of Migrant and Refugee Women study (EMPOWER) examined the effectiveness of a participatory, peer mentoring program specifically tailored for migrant and refugee women to build ability, confidence, and knowledge to seek employment, a known contributor to mental health and wellbeing. Female migrant mentors ($n = 21$) supported five cohorts of mentees ($n = 32$), predominantly from Middle Eastern and Asian backgrounds, over a period of 3–12 months each between September 2019 and November 2021. The program consisted of both individual mentoring and group workshops facilitated by content experts and the research team. The mental health and wellbeing outcomes for the mentees were explored through individual interviews with both mentors and mentees. Results indicate the program helped participants develop social connections, self-esteem, self-efficacy, and personal health and safety skills. There are ongoing mental health needs in this cohort related to competing priorities and trauma. The development of trusting, respectful relationships with mentors who are committed and flexible is essential for positive wellbeing outcomes. Peer mentoring programs for migrant and refugee women can enhance mental health and wellbeing outcomes and facilitate independence. Mentors need resources to provide appropriate mental and physical health support for some groups.

Keywords: mentoring; refugees; migrants; women; empowerment; mental health; employability

Citation: Gower, S.; Jeemi, Z.; Wickramasinghe, N.; Kebble, P.; Forbes, D.; Dantas, J.A.R. Impact of a Pilot Peer-Mentoring Empowerment Program on Personal Well-Being for Migrant and Refugee Women in Western Australia. *Int. J. Environ. Res. Public Health* **2022**, *19*, 3338. https://doi.org/10.3390/ijerph19063338

Academic Editors: Shameran Slewa-Younan and Greg Armstrong

Received: 1 February 2022
Accepted: 9 March 2022
Published: 11 March 2022

Publisher's Note: MDPI stays neutral with regard to jurisdictional claims in published maps and institutional affiliations.

1. Introduction

1.1. Global Migration Movements

The issue of global migration is significant, with over 281 million people having migrated world-wide, according to the International Migration 2020 highlights [1]. The UNHCR estimates that of this number, 33.72 million were forced to migrate due to civil conflict, internal crises, persecution, human rights violations, and climate-based disasters, with millions of civilians also facing internal displacement [1].

Australia's humanitarian program offers resettlement to people who have been found to be refugees according to the 1951 Refugee Convention or are in need of resettlement due to evolving humanitarian situations overseas [2]. In 2019–20, the number of offshore Humanitarian Program visas was set at 18,750 for people from countries such as Iraq, Democratic Republic of Congo, Syria, Myanmar, Afghanistan, and Eritrea [3]. In 2020, the Federal Government announced it would reduce the annual refugee intake to 13,750 places as part of the COVID-19 Economic Recovery Plan [4].

1.2. Employment and Mental Health

Migrants' sense of belonging to their new country is enhanced through labour force participation and is a recognised key factor in successful settlement [5,6]. For women, who may have lower access to resources, the ability to have an independent income is crucial in enabling them to become autonomous decision-makers within the family and to foster social inclusion. The lack of employment opportunities may result in isolation and loneliness [7,8]. The subsequent impact on socio-economic status can affect mental health outcomes, with a strong correlation between socio-economic status and poor mental health [9].

Resettled refugees have higher rates of unemployment than other migrant groups [10]. For refugee women in particular, employment is often temporary, or in lower-paid and lower-status roles than Australian-born women [11,12]. Skilled migrant women have lower employment rates and are less likely to be employed in positions commensurate with their qualifications than their male counterparts, or with locally born people [13], and this experience may impact negatively on their mental health.

1.3. Challenges Faced by Refugees and Migrants Seeking Employment

Employment policies for migrants and refugees vary between countries and visa types [14]. Employment rights for those with a skilled migrant or refugee visa are stronger than for those seeking asylum or on humanitarian visas [15]. In Australia, migrants, including temporary migrants such as those on student and work visas and refugees on humanitarian visas, have the right to work [16]. However, the difficulties faced by refugees and migrants in Australia seeking employment are well established and include language difficulties, racism, and discrimination [17], skills atrophy, and non-recognition of skills and qualifications [18–20]. Family commitments are highlighted both in Australia and internationally as presenting a particular barrier to workforce participation for both refugee and migrant women, including those who are highly skilled [13]. A reluctance to use formal childcare [8] as well as traditional cultural values around the carer's role [21] limit options. A lack of networks and experience, potentially limited prior education, and employer attitudes towards cultural dress also act as barriers [10,22,23]. Poor English language competency can limit one's ability to meet job requirements, increase social isolation and loneliness, and restrict access to further education [8,24].

1.4. Employment-Focussed Programs and Interventions for Unskilled Migrant Women

Previous programs that have offered social networking, work experience, and mentoring for unskilled migrants have been offered successfully in the eastern states of Australia but have not been undertaken in Western Australia and are not always specifically targeted at women [25–27]. Similarly, government initiatives to enhance employment outcomes for refugees do not have a specific focus on women [28].

1.5. Peer Support and Mentoring Programs

Peer mentoring demonstrates a belief in the value of the individual and expresses a commitment to ongoing development, capacity building, and the expectation of contributing to one's own life through empowerment. It recognises potential, enhances growth, and encourages discovery [29]. Peer mentoring is a reciprocal process through which a more experienced individual encourages and assists a less experienced individual in developing skills, knowledge, and attitudes to be more successful. Community participation promotes a sense of belonging and improves health and well-being, while social support and peer mentoring have a protective influence on health [30].

1.6. Community-Based Participatory Research and Personal Empowerment

Community-based participatory research (CBPR) approaches are increasingly used to implement effective interventions through social and community action, the outcomes of which have included policy and practice changes, increased community capacity, and improvements in health inequities [30]. Wallerstein [31] defines 'empowerment' as "a social action process that promotes participation of people, organizations and communities towards the goals of individual and community control, political efficacy, improved quality of life and social justice" (p. 198). The ability for CBPRs to empower communities, democratise knowledge, and create social change is well-recognised [32,33]. Studies that have utilised community-based participatory approaches (CBPAs) have reported sound engagement of community stakeholders in intervention development [34].

Between 2015 and 2017, we undertook another CBPR project—The Photovoice Project—with our community partner Ishar. A recommendation from that project was the need for mentoring programs for refugee and migrant women. This project arose from that recommendation and need. The Empowering and Peer Mentoring of Migrant and Refugee Women (EMPOWER) program was co-designed with our community partner and is a participatory, peer mentoring program with refugee and migrant women to build confidence, improve knowledge to seek employment, and improve psychosocial well-being.

1.7. Aim

This study qualitatively examined the effectiveness of a co-designed, pilot participatory peer support intervention from the perspective of program participants. The intervention sought to have holistic impacts, such as building empowerment and improving well-being. The following objectives guided the study:

1. To develop a participatory peer mentoring program with refugee women themselves, using their existing strengths, the social capital available, and noting the systemic and structural barriers they face;
2. To identify areas where additional support is required by refugee women in employment seeking, skill development, and personal empowerment;
3. To evaluate the program and its perceived influence on refugee women's personal empowerment, confidence, skill development, and health and well-being.

2. Materials and Methods

This study used a community-based participatory approach (CBPA) to develop the peer mentoring program and respond to challenges that emerged throughout the project.

2.1. Community Partners

In keeping with the CBPA the research team engaged with several Western Australian community organisations to help guide the project and assist with recruiting of participants. These were Ishar Multicultural Women's Health Services (Ishar) (https://www.ishar.org.au/, accessed on 10 March 2022), Centacare Employment and Training (https://www.centacarewa.com.au/, accessed on 10 March 2022), the Indian Society of Western Australia (ISWA), the Sri Lankan Cultural Society Western Australia, United in Diversity (https://www.uidwa.org.au/, accessed on 10 March 2022) and a community contact from the Mongolian Community in WA.

2.2. Development of the Mentoring Program

The content and focus of the mentoring program were developed through a multiphase process of consultation with women in the CALD community and other community representatives. A mixed methods community assessment to identify current gaps, needs, expectations, skills, and knowledge of refugee and migrant women regarding employment-seeking was undertaken with 34 women at Ishar, the results of which further informed the content and focus of the mentoring program. Secondly potential mentors provided input based on their own personal experiences in resettling and establishing connections in Australia. Lastly, representatives from local government councils provided input on maintaining sustainability.

The questionnaire and focus group data from the community assessment showed women felt they needed support with developing basic computer literacy, knowledge of legal rights and responsibilities at work, building confidence and a social network, and overcoming known barriers such as family responsibilities. Some wariness also emerged in the focus group discussions. The women reported they had been offered job preparation programs in the past that had not been fruitful.

Informal discussions with key stakeholders from the supporting community organization revealed that the disappointment expressed by participants was likely due to mismatched goals and expectations between program providers and participants regarding the provision of actual employment. Job-readiness programs do not guarantee employment and there may have been misunderstandings about this by the participants. This information highlights the importance of building a trusting and respectful relationship with the women throughout the program.

From these findings, and to maintain the flexibility to cater to individual needs, the mentoring program was culturally informed, holistic, and designed to build social capital and concepts of community participation, links to community groups and resources, emotional and social support, sense of belonging, and responsibility. In our study the needs of refugee and migrant women were different depending on their cultural background and previous educational and employment opportunities. There was deliberate flexibility in the program to allow the mentors to address and meet the varied needs of the mentees. While a suggested list of 12 topic areas was provided, mentors had the discretion and flexibility to modify the discussions and areas of focus to be of most relevance to the mentee. The anticipated outcomes were an improvement in employment skills, reduced isolation, and improvements in overall health and well-being. The final program format consisted of individual mentoring sessions approximately twice per month and group workshops covering English for employment, employment skills, and financial management. The EMPOWER program was delivered between September 2019 and November 2021, lasting between 3 and 12 months each time (Table 1). Each cohort was recruited through different community partners.

Table 1. Table of participant cohorts and workshops delivered.

Group Duration	Participants	Workshops Delivered	Attendance
Group 1 commenced September 2019	10 mentees 9 mentors	English for Employment Employment Skills Financial Management	9 mentees 10 mentees 10 mentees
Group 2 commenced March 2020	6 mentees 5 mentors [1]	English for Employment Employment Skills Financial Management	5 mentees 4 mentees 5 mentees
Group 3 commenced between August 2020	8 mentees 7 mentors [1]	Financial Management and Starting a New Business [2] Employment Skills [2,3]	5 mentees 7 mentees
Group 4 commenced between April–August 2021	5 mentees 1 mentor		
Group 5—group mentoring sessions held between September and October 2021	4 mentees [4] 2 mentors	Session One [3] Session Two [3] Session Three [3]	4 mentees 4 mentees 3 mentees

[1] A mentor from Groups 2 and 3 also participated in Group 1. [2] Groups 3 and 4 had workshops delivered at the same time. Participants in these groups also did not require an English for Employment workshop. [3] Workshops and sessions were delivered in mixed, in-person (face-to-face) and videoconference format. [4] One of the mentees also participated in Group 3.

2.3. Participant Recruitment

2.3.1. Mentors

The community partners identified potential mentors from their network of service providers who provide support to refugee and migrant women in the community. Other mentors were identified from the researchers' personal networks and from participation in previous research projects led by the researchers. Inclusion criteria for mentors were female migrants who had established themselves in the Australian workforce and were willing to meet with a mentee approximately twice per month. There was variation in the cultural and employment backgrounds of the mentors too, and each mentor was therefore able to respond to the different needs of their mentee. A total of 21 mentors (Table 1) were recruited and trained by the research team via a 3 h training program on communication and listening skills, mentor responsibilities, problem solving and goal setting, confidentiality, and accessing external specialist counselling support for mentees who had experienced trauma.

2.3.2. Mentees

Inclusion criteria were initially limited to refugee or humanitarian entrants only, but this was broadened to migrant women from non-humanitarian backgrounds with limited English and employability skills as our preliminary stakeholder meetings with Ishar and other community members identified them to be a similar group in need. Skilled women, including international students, who had been disproportionately isolated and impacted by lost employment opportunities during the COVID-19 pandemic were also included. This resulted in a non-homogenous sample with maximum variation, which enabled exploration of different cultural perspectives [35]. Using a recruitment flyer, the community partners promoted the project through their networks. All interested participants were provided with contact information for the research team to ask further questions.

An opening event was held for each cohort where mentor-mentee pairs were introduced, program resources were distributed, and clear expectations and intentions for the program were established. Mentees were invited to discuss their goals, both as a group and with their mentors. Translators were available as necessary. In keeping with CBPR, additional mentees were included in the program after it had commenced, as the need arose. A total of 32 mentees participated in the program along with 21 mentors across 5 cohorts (Table 1).

2.3.3. Matching Mentors and Mentees

As much as possible, mentors and mentees were matched according to prior work, if any, or education background and area of employment interest. Initially, a deliberate choice was made to match mentors and mentees who spoke different languages to encourage English conversation. However, when some participants withdrew and others did not attend the launch events, some rearrangement of the pairings was necessitated. As a result, the decision to keep language groups separate was overturned.

2.4. Ethical Considerations

Ethical approval was sought and obtained from the Curtin University Human Research Ethics Committee (HRE2018-0310). All potential participants were informed at recruitment that participation was voluntary, that any relationship between them and the community partners would not be affected by their decision to participate or not participate, that they would receive a small stipend for participation, and that all personal information would be stored confidentially. Participants provided informed consent to participate in the study and for their data to be used in the research.

A code of ethics to guide conduct and behaviour between mentors and mentees was developed in consultation with community partners to facilitate a welcoming, respectful, and non-judgemental environment. Assistance was provided on an individual basis where possible to alleviate known barriers to participation such as transport [36]. Lastly, safeguards were provided for maintaining confidentiality throughout the project, including discreet use of photographs, which were only taken with consent of the participants. Written consent was obtained from mentees for participation in the program, the use of photographs, and involvement in evaluation activities such as completion of questionnaires and interviews. An orientation was provided to mentors with regard to the project, the mentoring process and the need for confidentiality and professionalism towards mentees.

2.5. EMPOWER Program Content

The EMPOWER pilot program was specifically tailored to provide migrant and refugee women with the ability, confidence, and knowledge to seek employment. The individual peer mentoring session topics included but were not limited to the following topics: (1) goal setting and identifying strengths, (2) Australian workplace environment, (3) interpersonal skills, self-care, and financial management, (4) legal rights and responsibilities at work, (5) interview skills, (6) developing a work search plan, (7) networking, and 8) starting your own business. Mentors and mentees were also asked to follow a set of guidelines including that mentors were not to assume a role of advocacy on their mentee's behalf, and were not to have inappropriate expectations of mentees such as those that might be expected of an employee. At all times mentors were required to treat the mentees fairly and with sensitivity, dignity, respect, and in a non-discriminatory manner.

To supplement the individual mentoring, workshops were developed and delivered by EMPOWER staff and associated providers. Each workshop was approximately 2 h in length and was a combination of written and spoken activities, allowing for different learning styles and levels of English competency. The workshop topics were English for Employment, Employment Skills (job applications and interview skills), Financial Management and Starting a New Business (Table 1). Workshops were adjusted to suit the needs of each cohort, in keeping with the CBPR's flexible approach, and as such content differed slightly between groups.

2.6. Interruptions Due to COVID-19 Public Health Measures

In February–March 2020, the COVID-19 Pandemic impacted Western Australia, with lockdowns imposed across Australia and included the public health measures of widespread closure of businesses, schools, universities, and other settings. The government mandated social distancing, online education, working from home, and social distancing [37]. With approximately one million Australians losing their jobs due to the closure of businesses during the COVID 19 pandemic, seeking employment became particularly difficult for migrant women. In addition, they were isolated and often carried the burden of home schooling children. As a result, the focus of the EMPOWER program during this period was to maintain the relationships between the mentors and mentees with an emphasis on social and emotional support, and mentors were encouraged to communicate online.

2.7. Data Collection and Analysis

Qualitative data were collected using mentors' progress journals, email correspondence from mentors and mentees, and individual semi-structured interviews with mentees and mentors. The online journals were submitted regularly by mentors who responded to open-ended questions about successes, challenges and general reflections on the mentoring process and outcomes for participants. Individual interviews with 15 mentors and 10 mentees were conducted between June 2020 and January 2022. Most of the participants had attended at least 2 workshops and completed at least 8 individual mentoring sessions. As the mentoring was conducted on a needs basis not all mentees attended all available workshops. Any relevant content missed was covered in the individual sessions. Interviews were undertaken at community partner sites, or by telephone, and were audiotaped and transcribed verbatim. The triangulation achieved by using multiple data collection methods provided rich, deep information and increased the trustworthiness of the study [38].

2.8. Data Analysis

Thematic analysis of the qualitative data provided information on the mechanisms by which the program had influenced mental health and wellbeing. Audio recordings were transcribed verbatim. Four members of the research team used Braun and Clarke's inductive thematic analysis technique to conduct the initial coding, undertaking continual interpretation and identification of specific themes and subthemes [38]. Within each transcript meaning units were identified and these became the initial codes. Codes were then condensed into themes. After the initial coding, continual discussion between the authors helped to refine the themes and clarify points of difference. This investigator triangulation enhanced the credibility of the findings. Initially 16 codes were identified across 8 themes and a coding framework was developed. Upon re-reading the transcripts and reading associated literature the following changes were made: 'cultural understandings' was condensed into the 'social connection' theme; 'confidence' and 'identifying strengths' were initially coded as separate themes but were combined with 'trusting self' to make 'self-esteem'; occupational outcomes such as 'paid employment', 'volunteering' and 'education' were condensed into 'self-efficacy' to reflect the focus on mental wellbeing. Continual review of the coding framework over several meetings led to the finalization of themes [39].

Care was taken to ensure the analysis continued to accurately represent the views of the participants [40].

3. Results

Twenty-one mentors of average age 46.05 (SD = 12.26) years, residing in Australia for average 19.12 (15.97) years mentored 32 mentees of average age 41.66 (8.79) years, of which 25% have resided in Australia for 0–2 years or 3–5 years and 37.5% have resided for 10 or more years (Table 2). 25% of mentees arrived in Australia on a student visa, 21.9% on a partner visa, and 78.1% have a university degree. The most common languages spoken by mentees were Arabic (n = 7) and Sinhalese (n = 5) and for mentors, Hindi (n = 6) (Table 2).

Table 2. Characteristics of participants.

Mentors		Mentees	
Total Mentors	21	Total Mentees	32
Country of Origin	N	Country of Origin	N
Australia [1]; Bangladesh [1]; Egypt [1]; England [1]; France [1]; Italy [1]; Lebanon [1]; Mongolia [1]; Nepal [1]; Serbia [1]; Singapore [1]	11	Bangladesh [1]; China [1]; Ethiopia [1]; Lebanon [1]; Libya [1]; Lithuania [1]; Pakistan [1]; Scotland [1]; Somalia [1]; Thailand [1]; Togo	11
India	8	Egypt	3
Sri Lanka	2	India	2
		Iran	2
		Iraq	2
		Malaysia	2
		Mongolia	3
		Philippines	2
		Sri Lanka	5
Age in years		Age in years	
Mean (SD)	46.05 (12.26)	Mean (SD)	41.66 (8.79)
Range	26–70	Range	25–62
Years in Australia		Years in Australia	
Mean (SD)	19.12 (15.97)	0–2	8
Range	2.5–63	3–5	8
		6–9	4
		10 or more years	12
Highest Level of Education	N	Highest Level of Education	N
Technical and Further Education (TAFE)/Technical College	2	Never attended school	1
University	19	7–9 years of schooling	2
		12 or more years of schooling	2
		Trade or technical qualification beyond school	2
		University degree	25

Table 2. *Cont.*

Mentors		Mentees	
Main Language Spoken	N	Main Language Spoken	N
Arabic	2	Amharic [1]; Bangladeshi [1]; Ewe [1]; Farsi [1]; Lithuanian [1]; Mandarin [1]; Persian [1]; Scottish [1]; Somali [1]; Tagalog [1]; Tamil [1]; Thai [1]; Urdu [1]	13
Bangladeshi [1]; French [1]; Italian [1]; Malayalam [1]; Mandarin [1]; Mongolian [1]; Nepali [1]; Serbian [1]; Sinhalese [1]; Tamil [1]; Urdu [1]	11	Arabic	7
English	2	English	3
Hindi	6	Mongolian	2
		Sinhalese	5
		Telugu	2
Industry of Employment	**N**	**Visa Category (top 3)**	**N**
Aged Care and Disability	1	Partner	7
Community Services	6	Refugee	4
Finance	1	Student	8
Government	1	Other	13
Hospital	2		
Self-employed/Freelance	6		
Tertiary Education	4		
		Employment status pre-program	**N**
		Employed	9
		Unemployed	23

[1] Count of one i.e., $N = 1$.

Thematic analysis revealed that whilst this project aimed to enhance employability, there were also other clear positive perceived influences on the mental health and wellbeing of the mentees. Overall, participants believed the program had worked well, with positive outcomes for themselves and the mentees, even if those outcomes were not employment related.

The following four themes were identified: social connection, self-esteem, self-efficacy, and personal health and safety (Table 3). However, specific areas of poor mental health and wellbeing also emerged and highlighted areas of ongoing need.

Table 3. Perceived impact of peer mentoring program on mental health of refugee and migrant women.

Theme	Sub-Theme
Social Connection	Reducing isolation Building social networks Cultural understandings
Self-esteem	Confidence Identifying strengths Trusting self
Self-efficacy	Simple financial management Legal rights Time management Occupation and engagement
Personal health and safety	COVID-19 information Cyber safety
Ongoing needs	Overwhelmed with stressors Desire for mental health support

3.1. Social Connection

3.1.1. Reducing Isolation

For some mentor-mentee pairs, social support was deemed a greater need than employment advice. Simple social interaction outside the home was part of the support provided, and social connection became a significant outcome. In some cases, the mentorship inspired the mentee to make more of an effort to be social in her own group. In other cases, strong friendships developed within the pairs. The social connection also provided a safe space for the mentees to acknowledge and discuss their feelings.

"I think it has resulted in [Mentee] not being isolated in her home." (Mentor 3)

"My mentor [name] has helped with me a lot in different way and never let me down, even we became friends now." (Mentee 1)

"I'm not scared to speak to new people so that's the best thing that [Mentor] gave it to me." (Mentee 8)

3.1.2. Building Social Networks

For mentees with limited English skills, the mentors provided opportunities for socialising in ways that would also improve the mentee's language skills. For mentees with particular disadvantages, the opportunity to mix with people outside their current support groups was also deemed valuable. For mentees that were more skilled and had developed their own networks, the focus was primarily on employment networks.

"The opportunity for someone like [Mentee] to link in with people who can give her support and to have a little bit of a network of other people who are not just people with a DV background. Because I think with the current group, everyone having DV issues, you know it doesn't, it doesn't necessarily give her the same opportunities." (Mentor 8)

"[Mentee] was able to practice English conversation and expand her network." (Mentor 3)

"My network is now bigger than before. Now I know what the meaning of network, it helped a lot to have people around you." (Mentee 2)

3.1.3. Cultural Understandings

Mentees expressed interest in learning about Australian lifestyles, cultural customs, and workplace culture. Mentors were able to discuss this and suggest activities that would enhance community integration. Mentees reported that they felt cultural barriers had been lessened.

"[Mentee] expressed interest in the events being held in Perth during the Christmas season. So, the exposure to the Australian way of life and you encourage her to experiment and enjoy that aspect." (Mentor 4)

"[Mentor] Helpful for guidance, because we don't know most of the things, how we going with the Australian culture." (Mentee 9)

3.2. Self-Esteem

The mentoring process enables mentees to build inner strength and self-worth. Mentees recognised their varied life experiences that enabled them during difficult situations. Exposure to a wider network built confidence. There was satisfaction with what had, for most, been an uplifting and inspiring experience. Mentors described this as a sense of 'hope and positivity'.

3.2.1. Confidence

Mentees identified that they had previously been lacking in confidence, but through mentor support had developed the confidence to engage socially and pursue their goals. Mentors described the building of confidence as being one of their initial priorities with the mentees. This, at times, requires considerable effort.

"I was very scared and intimidated but this program just boosted my confidence basically." (Mentee 3)

"Because I was so nervous before and when I see white people I'm like oh my God, they're just going to, you know, judge me. So, after this program I'm not scared to speak to new people so that's the best thing." (Mentee 8)

"The most difficult part was getting that interaction going because a lot of occasions I felt that it's the one-way street." (Mentor 1)

3.2.2. Identifying Strengths

Identifying mentees' strengths was a common outcome. Often the mentees were not aware of their own strengths prior to the program and seemed surprised when they emerged through discussion.

"[Mentee] completed the Strengths Exploration Worksheets which was a revelation to her of her many strengths." (Mentor 4)

"Our discussion has reinforced for her, how strong and self-reliant she is." (Mentor 8)

3.2.3. Trusting Self

The development of self-awareness and trust was identified by mentees as being useful for not only pursuing career goals but also enhancing their ability to socialise.

"I learnt a lot about myself, I know how to discover more things in my personality that I can use it for my career." (Mentee 2)

"After Empower session I think I started to trust myself more, even I realised how other people may accept me." (Mentee 1)

3.3. Self-Efficacy

Skills that enhanced and enabled self-efficacy and independence were also developed. A number of mentees became engaged in ventures that gave them purpose and focus, including paid employment, volunteering roles, and commencing courses of study.

3.3.1. Simple Financial Management

"I shared some resources on managing finances. We talked through just basic stuff like the Barefoot Investor was an easy book to read." (Mentor 9)

"Especially the lady was there with bank. How to save money, we do it twice I think. It was very nice." (Mentee 6)

3.3.2. Legal Rights Knowledge

Some mentors provided explanations of superannuation and employee rights in their discussions to help mentees working in precarious roles and foster independence.

"It's not just finding a job it's helping her understand how superannuation works, what her rights are within that." (Mentor 5)

3.3.3. Time Management

Cultural differences in time management arose in some discussions around workplace culture. Mentors identified a need for time management skills for mentees who needed to combine family responsibilities with employment.

"We discussed the importance of managing time not only at the workplace but also at home and in our daily life." (Mentor 7)

3.3.4. Occupation and Engagement

In alignment with the primary focus of the program, a number of mentees attained positions in paid employment, volunteering, or courses of study. Some mentees found positions in areas they desired, others moved to new fields or considered entrepreneurship. Mentors enabled mentees to achieve their goals by assisting with CVs and applications for work and study.

> *"[Mentor] actually went through my CV and helped me around that. So that was a really good outcome so finally I was able to get a job."* (Mentee 7)

> *"She [Mentee] even started working, it's a small role but it's a very good step."* (Mentor 2)

> *"She [Mentee] has just recently joined Certificate IV in accounting and she's well on track of you know progressing further."* (Mentor 3)

> *"I'm studying now fashion design on TAFE, I'll finish my certificate 4."* (Mentee 2)

> *"I'm enrolled to do interpreting diploma."* (Mentee 3)

> *"She [Mentor] gave me proper guidance regarding finding a job, how to make a proper CV and cover letter. And once finishing that internship … I left and found a job."* (Mentee 9)

3.4. Personal Health and Safety

The outbreak of the COVID-19 pandemic created anxiety in this cohort, particularly those with limited English skills. Mentors were able to provide clear health information in culturally appropriate ways that enabled mentees to manage lockdowns safely.

3.4.1. COVID Information

> *"I thought talking about COVID 19 and giving information to [Mentee] is very important. So, we spent our whole session just talking on this topic."* (Mentor 7)

3.4.2. Cyber Safety

Mentors identified a lack of understanding of cyber safety in some mentees. By educating the mentees about the safe use of personal data online, the mentors were able to prevent harm and ensure the maintenance of privacy and dignity.

> *"I told [Mentee] she should be very careful while using emails, internet or social media. She said she uses emails and Facebook a lot but she didn't know it can be unsafe to share personal information on it."* (Mentor 7)

3.5. Ongoing Needs
3.5.1. Overwhelmed with Stressors

Some mentees were managing multiple daily challenges and commitments. These included minimal financial independence, unwell extended family members, and childcare responsibilities that impeded their capacity to look for and commit to employment. Often, mentors had to assist mentees in addressing these competing priorities before moving on to the process of job seeking.

> *"Minimal family support and no childcare support available."* (Mentor 1)

> *"She had personal health problems and some financial difficulties."* (Mentor 11)

Complex physical and mental health issues, domestic violence situations, family law court matters, and mentees trying to help family members in danger in their home countries all contributed significantly to mental health concerns. One mentor felt conflicted by her role of helping with employment and wondered whether she should have been advocating for social services instead. Mentees also faced significant financial issues that took priority over, and sometimes precluded, seeking employment. The skills and training required to obtain employment, such as a driver's license or completing a training course, are out of reach for some mentees due to the financial cost.

> *"How do I help a mentee who cannot pay the rent?"* (Mentor 9)

> *"Difficult situation as her mother has disappeared back home and she cannot go back to look for her as her ex-husband will not sign for her children to have passports."* (Mentor 8)

"I observed that she is quite depressed and isolated. She has very low self-esteem and also she has some health issues." (Mentor 7)

3.5.2. Desire for Mental Health Support

A number of mentees expressed a desire for more mental health support. Specific assistance was requested with managing loss, health issues, and parenting in a new culture.

"Some people are depressing and like you know, mental, mental health part. If you guys can cover those areas, that would be great." (Mentee 8)

"I think mental health is important for us like migrant, how to raise a kid for migrant, even I think about psychology sessions. It will be very good if you provide a program." (Mentee 1)

4. Discussion

The EMPOWER program utilized the motivation of the mentors and mentees to build confidence, connections, and skills with a focus on self-efficacy and job-readiness. Participants who completed the program reported improved social connection through reduced isolation, a greater personal and professional network, and attendance at community events that facilitated intercultural contact. Self-esteem was enhanced via improved self-confidence, the recognition of personal strengths, and greater self-awareness. Personal self-efficacy was built through improved knowledge of financial management, legal rights and responsibilities at work, and time management skills both at home and in the workplace. Several participants found positions in paid employment, volunteer roles, or commenced a course of study that enhanced their self-worth. There were several key components in the mentoring relationships that led to the following positive mental health outcomes: trust, support, flexibility, and commitment from mentors.

Mentors identified the development of trust as being critical in making the mentee feel secure, and strong personal connections were made. Trust is essential for an effective mentoring relationship [41] and may also influence mentoring behaviours [42]. Mentees who demonstrate a willingness to learn, openness, and an ability to set realistic goals are considered trustworthy by mentors who may be more willing to engage [42]. Positive emotional connections and attachments with mentees also enhance trust (Allen and Eby 2008) [43], and activities that encourage connection and understanding within pairs early in the mentoring relationship are recommended [42].

Support and encouragement were highly valued by the mentees, most of whom felt they could rely on their mentor despite difficult circumstances. The mentors' perseverance allowed mentees to develop their skills and identify abilities and goals [41,44]. Mentors respected and validated the lived experiences of the mentees, demonstrating acceptance and confirmation [44].

The mentoring process enables mentees to build self-awareness and develop a sense of trust in themselves. In some cases, this extended to greater trust in the broader Australian community. By acknowledging mentees' strengths, the EMPOWER program enabled mentees to confirm their inner identity and, at the same time, promoted a sense of place in Australia. This aligns with Adolfsson (2021), who studied migrants' sense of belonging in Sweden and found that 'multiple memberships between groups need not be contradictory but rather an expression of different spheres of inhabitance' [45]. A sense of belonging is a key component of mental health [45].

A sense of belonging is sometimes used interchangeably with the concept of integration. The term 'integration' has multiple levels of application and is used differently depending on the context. It can be a contentious term with negative connotations and is sometimes proposed as a solution to community discord [46]. However, Ager and Strang posit that integration can be both a goal and a process and identify 'indicators of integration' as access to the social determinants of health such as housing, education, and employment, as well as social relationships and connections [47]. In this study, by building social and cultural capital, the peer mentoring process empowered women to overcome isolation and hesitancy and acknowledge pre-existing strengths that enabled greater participation in society.

As per the participatory, holistic, and inclusive design of the program, mentors tailored their support based on the individual needs, abilities, opportunities, and agency of the women, using culturally appropriate and sensitive approaches. For some mentees, this could include helping them gain recognition of tertiary qualifications. For other mentees, a much simpler level of support was required, such as helping them compile a list of known skills, reviewing CVs and providing an opportunity and avenue to discuss their hopes and challenges. Better outcomes were identified in mentees with a degree of pre-existing agency, such as holding formal qualifications, having sound English language skills, and an adequate level of self-confidence. Mentees with those assets made the most progress towards achieving employability. Agency has been shown to assist migrants with the navigation of unpredictable and precarious employment environments [48,49]. In a study of Polish migrants in the UK, Szewcayk, (2013) [49] found that graduates used their personal agency to create career trajectories for themselves in response to changeable employment markets. The use of this personal capital was necessary to manage the unpredictability of their employment journeys. Similarly, May (2019) [48] found that undocumented asylum seekers in France used agency to make the most of the limited opportunities available to them, although structural factors ultimately restricted their options. In the current study, mentors were able to build on the existing agency of the mentees with a targeted approach to help achieve specific goals. Unskilled mentees with limited language skills faced greater hurdles and presented more challenges to the mentors, who sometimes needed to work hard to overcome initial barriers and build trust. Not all mentors were successful in establishing relationships, primarily due to the considerable barriers faced by the most vulnerable mentees.

Some mentees were managing significant stressors. These include financial problems, physical and mental health issues, and difficult family situations. Mentors need to be committed and flexible to respond to mentees' needs, which may be complex. Personal and emotional issues have been shown to hamper the mentoring process [50], and mentors need resources and support to learn new strategies and direct mentees to appropriate resources. When mentors can respond to challenges and obstacles, the mentoring relationship is more positive [41]. When mentors can understand their mentee's worldview and social environment, they are more able to assist the mentee to develop resilience and agency. Mentors in this study sometimes struggled with the complexities of the mentees' additional well-being and family needs outside the employment sphere. Mentors need support to refer mentees to professional services where necessary. Refugee and migrant women have been identified as experiencing higher rates of mental health problems than the mainstream Australian population. This may be a result of isolation due to childcare responsibilities, fewer opportunities for social activities, and a possible lack of language skills [16,51]. Separation from family overseas, and difficulties adapting to gender norms in the host country, are also identified as contributing to poor mental health [52].

For the more vulnerable mentees, the benefits of the program were social connection and a greater sense of belonging. The program was designed to enhance employability, but achievement of this goal is mitigated by both the personal attributes of the mentee and systemic barriers to employment, such as a lack of work experience and discrimination [10,53,54]. Not all mentees made progress towards finding employment. Program organizers and mentors must be clear in their communications about setting realistic goals and focusing on empowerment and building self-efficacy. Mentee expectations must be identified and managed where necessary to enhance the development of trust and connection.

4.1. Limitations and Strengths

A strength of this research was the connection that the authors had to various community organizations, allowing for access that would otherwise be difficult to attain. The community organizations assisted with recruitment and provided venues for workshops. A limitation of this study is the small sample size; therefore, the results presented are not generalizable; however, as this was a qualitative study, the depth of information, transferability, and credibility of the study were important.

Another limitation was the impact of COVID on the project, which made it difficult for mentors and mentees to meet in person. Difficulties in recruiting and retaining refugee women from different ethnic backgrounds made it necessary to expand our sampling inclusion criteria to non-refugee women. However, this is in keeping with the community-based participatory approach, which is flexible to meet the needs of participants and respond to emerging challenges. Non-refugee migrant women face similar challenges to refugee women regarding employment, and these were exacerbated by COVID-19.

4.2. Recommendations

Our study and the findings highlighted some recommendations for future mentoring programs. These include providing trauma-informed training to mentors and an orientation program for mentees to improve their skills in interacting and working with a mentor for mutual benefit. Mentoring programs for refugee and migrant women also need to acknowledge and work with the systemic, structural, and practical barriers to success faced by this cohort of women. Recommendations for policy include offering peer mentoring programs as a non-pharmacological mental health support and intervention for refugee and migrant women that enhances psychosocial well-being. Recommendations for research include having longitudinal studies over time to assess program effectiveness and influence on wellbeing. Future studies could evaluate the effectiveness of a work experience and internship program on employment and mental health outcomes of this cohort.

5. Conclusions

The EMPOWER peer mentoring program aims to enhance employability and networks for vulnerable refugee and migrant women. The pilot program provided opportunities for social connection, built mentees' confidence and self-worth, and improved self-efficacy. Mentees with pre-existing agency had better employability outcomes. The most vulnerable mentees sometimes faced barriers to full participation in the program. Mentors with lived experience of migration were critical to providing validation and acknowledgment of the mentees' stories. Ongoing trauma and mental health issues have caused some ongoing barriers to employment, and further resources are needed in this area. With adequate training and support, peer mentors can promote the mental health of refugee and migrant women through improvements in community participation. Despite the challenges of resettlement and integration, there remains a strong sense of community and family connection among refugee and migrant women, as well as a desire to learn new skills, gain further education, and contribute economically to their new homeland.

Author Contributions: Conceptualization, J.A.R.D., S.G., and Z.J.; methodology, J.A.R.D., S.G., and Z.J.; software, S.G. and Z.J.; validation, S.G. and Z.J.; formal analysis, S.G., Z.J., N.W., and P.K.; investigation, S.G., Z.J., and J.D; resources, J.A.R.D., P.K., and D.F.; data curation, S.G. and Z.J.; writing—original draft preparation, S.G. and Z.J.; writing—review and editing, S.G., Z.J., N.W., P.K., D.F., and J.A.R.D.; visualization, Z.J.; supervision, J.A.R.D.; project administration, S.G. and Z.J.; funding acquisition, J.A.R.D. All authors have read and agreed to the published version of the manuscript.

Funding: This research was funded by Healthway, the Health Promotion Foundation of Western Australia, [Grant number 31973—2018 to 2021].

Institutional Review Board Statement: The study was conducted according to the guidelines of the Declaration of Helsinki and approved by the Human Research Ethics Committee of Curtin University (protocol code HRE2018-0310 and 31 May 2018).

Informed Consent Statement: Written consent was obtained from all subjects involved in the study. Information about the study was provided in written form and explained by interpreters and mentors.

Data Availability Statement: The datasets produced and analyzed for this study are not publicly available but are available from the corresponding author on reasonable request.

Acknowledgments: The authors would like to thank our community partners and all participants.

Conflicts of Interest: The authors declare no conflict of interest. The funder had no role in the design of the study; in the collection, analyses, or interpretation of data; in the writing of the manuscript, or in the decision to publish the results.

References

1. United Nations Department of Economics and Social Affairs. International Migration 2020 Highlights. 2021. Available online: https://www.un.org/en/desa/international-migration-2020-highlights (accessed on 3 December 2021).
2. Australian Government Department of Home Affairs. About the Refugee and Humanitarian Program. 2021. Available online: https://immi.homeaffairs.gov.au/what-we-do/refugee-and-humanitarian-program/about-the-program (accessed on 3 December 2021).
3. Australian Government Department of Home Affairs. Australia's Offshore Humanitarian Program: 2019–20. 2020. Available online: https://www.homeaffairs.gov.au/research-and-stats/files/australia-offshore-humanitarian-program-2019-20.pdf (accessed on 3 December 2021).
4. Tudge, A.; Dutton, P. Securing and Uniting Australia as part of the Government's Economic Recovery Plan. Joint Media Release; 2020. Available online: https://minister.homeaffairs.gov.au/alantudge/Pages/Securing-and-Uniting-Australia-as-part-of-the-Government%E2%80%99s-economic-recovery-plan-.aspx#:~{}:text=Securing%20and%20Uniting%20Australia%20as%20part%20of%20the%20Government\T1\textquoterights%20economic%20recovery%20plan,-06%20October%202020&text=As%20Australia%20faces%20the%20single,the%20pandemic%20and%20protect%20Australians (accessed on 25 January 2022).
5. Warfa, N.; Curtis, S.; Watters, C.; Carswell, K.; Ingleby, D.; Bhui, K. Migration experiences, employment status and psychological distress among Somali immigrants: A mixed-method international study. *BMC Public Health* **2012**, *12*, 749. [CrossRef] [PubMed]
6. Wood, N.; Charlwood, G.; Zecchin, C.; Hansen, V.; Douglas, M.; Pit, S.W. Qualitative exploration of the impact of employment and volunteering upon the health and wellbeing of African refugees settled in regional Australia: A refugee perspective. *BMC Public Health* **2019**, *19*, 1–15. [CrossRef] [PubMed]
7. Cheung, S.Y.; Phillimore, J. Gender and Refugee Integration: A Quantitative Analysis of Integration and Social Policy Outcomes. *J. Soc. Policy* **2016**, *46*, 211–230. [CrossRef]
8. Nilan, P.; Samarayi, I.; Lovat, T. Female Muslim Jobseekers in Australia: Liminality, Obstacles and Resilience. *Int. J. Asian Soc. Sci.* **2012**, *2*, 682–692.
9. Hynie, M. The Social Determinants of Refugee Mental Health in the Post-Migration Context: A Critical Review. *Can. J. Psychiatry* **2017**, *63*, 297–303. [CrossRef]
10. Van Kooy, J. Refugee women as entrepreneurs in Australia. *Forced Migr. Rev.* **2016**, *53*, 71–73.
11. Women's Health West. Promoting Economic Participation and Equity for Women from Refugee and Migrant Backgrounds. Melbourne: Women's Health West. 2016. Available online: https://whwest.org.au/wp-content/uploads/2016/05/WHW-economic-participation-report-LOW.pdf (accessed on 19 October 2021).
12. Koyama, J. Constructing Gender: Refugee Women Working in the United States. *J. Refug. Stud.* **2014**, *28*, 258–275. [CrossRef]
13. Riaño, Y. Highly Skilled Migrant and Non-Migrant Women and Men: How Do Differences in Quality of Employment Arise? *Adm. Sci.* **2021**, *11*, 5. [CrossRef]
14. OECD/UNHCR. Engaging with Employers in the Hiring of Refugees: A 10-Point Multi-Stakeholder Action Plan for Employers, Refugees, Governments and Civil Society. 2018. Available online: https://www.oecd.org/els/mig/UNHCR-OECD-Engaging-with-employers-in-the-hiring-of-refugees.pdf (accessed on 24 February 2022).
15. Lu, Y.; Gure, Y.; Frenette, M. The long-Term Labour Market Integration of Refugee Claimants Who Became Permanent Residents in Canada, Analytical Studies Branch Research Paper Series, 11F0019M-455. 2020. Available online: https://www150.statcan.gc.ca/n1/en/pub/11f0019m/11f0019m2020018-eng.pdf?st=gpmFPfvN (accessed on 24 February 2022).
16. Newman, A.; Nielsen, I.; Smyth, R.; Hirst, G.; Dunwoodie, K.; Kemp, H.; Nugent, A. A Guide for Employers: Supporting Access to Employment for People from a Refugee or Asylum Seeking Background. 2018. Available online: https://deakincreate.org.au/wp-content/uploads/sites/96/2019/02/DEA_GuideforEmployers_RefugeesAsylumSeekers_AMEND01.WEB_.pdf (accessed on 24 February 2022).
17. Ziersch, A.; Due, C.; Walsh, M. Discrimination: A health hazard for people from refugee and asylum-seeking backgrounds resettled in Australia. *BMC Public Health* **2020**, *20*, 1–14. [CrossRef]
18. Campbell, S.C. 'What's a sundial in the shade?': Brain waste among refugee professionals who are denied meaningful oppor-tunity for credential recognition. *Emory Law J.* **2018**, *68*, 139–181.
19. Nichles, L.; Nyce, S. Towards greater visibility and recruitment of skilled refugees. *Forced Migr. Rev.* **2018**, *58*, 36–37.
20. Cameron, R.; Farivar, F.; Dantas, J. The unanticipated road to skills wastage for skilled migrants: The non-recognition of overseas qualifications and experience (ROQE). *Labour Ind. J. Soc. Econ. Relat. Work.* **2019**, *29*, 80–97. [CrossRef]
21. Baranik, L.E. Employment and attitudes toward women among Syrian refugees. *Pers. Rev.* **2020**, *50*, 1233–1252. [CrossRef]

22. Gaillard, D.; Hughes, K. Key considerations for facilitating employment of female Sudanese refugees in Australia. *J. Manag. Organ.* **2014**, *20*, 671–690. [CrossRef]
23. Correa-Velez, I.; Barnett, A.G.; Gifford, S. Working for a Better Life: Longitudinal Evidence on the Predictors of Employment Among Recently Arrived Refugee Migrant Men Living in Australia. *Int. Migr.* **2013**, *53*, 321–337. [CrossRef]
24. Casimiro, S.; Hancock, P.; Northcote, J. Isolation and Insecurity: Resettlement Issues Among Muslim Refugee Women in Perth, Western Australia. *Aust. J. Soc. Issues* **2007**, *42*, 55–69. [CrossRef]
25. Brotherhood of St. Laurence. Stepping Stones to Small Business. 2017. Available online: https://www.bsl.org.au/services/refugees-immigration-multiculturalism/stepping-stones/ (accessed on 3 December 2021).
26. New South Wales Government. Refugee Employment Support Program. 2021. Available online: https://education.nsw.gov.au/skills-nsw/students-and-job-seekers/low-cost-and-free-training-options/support-for-refugees-asylum-seekers.html (accessed on 18 October 2021).
27. Refugee Council of Australia. Bright Ideas. 2019. Available online: https://www.refugeecouncil.org.au/our-work/publications/bright-ideas/ (accessed on 11 October 2021).
28. New South Wales Government. Refugee Health Policy. 2021. Available online: https://www.health.nsw.gov.au/multicultural/Pages/refugee-health-policy.aspx (accessed on 8 May 2021).
29. Wisconsin Healthy and Ready to Work. *The Power of Peer Mentoring*; University of Wisconsin: Madison, WI, USA, 2006.
30. Wallerstein, N.; Duran, B. Community-Based Participatory Research Contributions to Intervention Research: The Intersection of Science and Practice to Improve Health Equity. *Am. J. Public Health* **2010**, *100*, S40–S46. [CrossRef]
31. Wallerstein, N. Health and safety education for workers with low-literacy or limited-english skills. *Am. J. Ind. Med.* **1992**, *22*, 751–765. [CrossRef]
32. Masuda, J.R.; Creighton, G.; Nixon, S.; Frankish, J. Building Capacity for Community-Based Participatory Research for Health Disparities in Canada: The Case of "Partnerships in Community Health Research". *Health Promot. Pract.* **2011**, *12*, 280–292. [CrossRef]
33. Themba, M.N.; Minkler, M. Influencing policy through community based participatory research. In *Community-Based Participatory Research for Health*; Wallerstein, M.M.N., Ed.; Jossey-Bass: San Francisco, CA, USA, 2003; pp. 349–370.
34. Finlayson, T.L.; Asgari, P.; Hoffman, L.; Palomo-Zerfas, A.; Gonzalez, M.; Stamm, N.; Rocha, M.-I.; Nunez-Alvarez, A. Formative Research: Using a Community-Based Participatory Research Approach to Develop an Oral Health Intervention for Migrant Mexican Families. *Health Promot. Prac.* **2016**, *18*, 454–465. [CrossRef]
35. Creswell, J.W. *Qualitative Inquiry and Research Design: Choosing Among Five Approaches*, 3rd ed.; SAGE Publishing: Thousand Oaks, CA, USA, 2013.
36. Stewart, M.; Simich, L.; Shizha, E.; Makumbe, K.; Makwarimba, E. Supporting African refugees in Canada: Insights from a support intervention. *Health Soc. Care Community* **2012**, *20*, 516–527. [CrossRef] [PubMed]
37. Government of Western Australia. COVID-19 Coronavirus: Community Advice. 2022. Available online: https://www.wa.gov.au/government/covid-19-coronavirus/covid-19-coronavirus-community-advice (accessed on 25 January 2022).
38. Braun, V.; Clarke, V. *Successful Qualitative Research: A Practical Guide for Beginners*, 1st ed.; SAGE Publishing: London, UK, 2013.
39. O'Connor, C.; Joffe, H. Intercoder Reliability in Qualitative Research: Debates and Practical Guidelines. *Int. J. Qual. Methods* **2020**, *19*. [CrossRef]
40. Polit, D.F.; Beck, C.T. *Essentials of Nursing Research: Appraising Evidence for Nursing Practice*, 9th ed.; Lippincott Williams & Wilkins: Philadelphia, PA, USA, 2018.
41. Boddy, J.; Agllias, K.; Gray, M. Mentoring in social work: Key findings from a women's community-based mentoring program. *J. Soc. Work. Pract.* **2012**, *26*, 385–405. [CrossRef]
42. Leck, J.D.; Orser, B. Fostering trust in mentoring relationships: An exploratory study. *Equal. Divers. Incl. Int. J.* **2013**, *32*, 410–425. [CrossRef]
43. Allen, T.D.; Eby, L.T. Mentor commitment in formal mentoring relationships. *J. Vocat. Behav.* **2008**, *72*, 309–316. [CrossRef]
44. Levesque, L.L.; O'Neill, R.M.; Nelson, T.; Dumas, C. Sex differences in the perceived importance of mentoring functions. *Career Dev. Int.* **2005**, *10*, 429–443. [CrossRef]
45. Adolfsson, C. 'I'm Not *Swedish* Swedish': Self-Appraised National and Ethnic Identification among Migrant-Descendants in Sweden. *Genealogy* **2021**, *5*, 56. [CrossRef]
46. Kirkwood, S.; McKinlay, A.; McVittie, C. 'Some People It's Very Difficult to Trust': Attributions of Agency and Accountability in Practitioners' Talk About Integration. *J. Community Appl. Soc. Psychol.* **2014**, *24*, 376–389. [CrossRef]
47. Ager, A.; Strang, A. *Indicators of Integration: Final Report; Research DaSD, Report No. 28*; Home Office: London, UK, 2004.
48. May, P. Exercising agency in a hostile environment: How do refused asylum seekers find work? *Ethnicities* **2019**, *20*, 1049–1070. [CrossRef]
49. Szewczyk, A. Continuation or Switching? Career Patterns of Polish Graduate Migrants in England. *J. Ethn. Migr. Stud.* **2013**, *40*, 847–864. [CrossRef]
50. Ludwig, S.; Stein, R.E. Anatomy of mentoring. *J. Pediatr.* **2008**, *152*, 151–152. [CrossRef] [PubMed]
51. Jarallah, Y.; Baxter, J. Gender disparities and psychological distress among humanitarian migrants in Australia: A moderating role of migration pathway? *Confl. Health* **2019**, *13*, 13. [CrossRef] [PubMed]

52. Lumbus, A.; Fleay, C.; Hartley, L.K.; Gower, S.; Creado, A.; Dantas, J.A.R. "I want to become part of the Australian community": Challenging the marginalisation of women resettled as refugees in Australia—Findings from a photovoice project. *Aust. J. Soc. Issues* **2021**. [CrossRef]
53. Khawaja, N.; Khawaja, S. Acculturative Issues of Muslims in Australia. *J. Muslim Ment. Health* **2016**, *10*, 43–53. [CrossRef]
54. Hsieh, Y.-J.T. Learning language and gaining employment: Problems for refugee migrants in Australia. *Equal. Divers. Inclusion: Int. J.* **2021**, *40*, 1013–1031. [CrossRef]

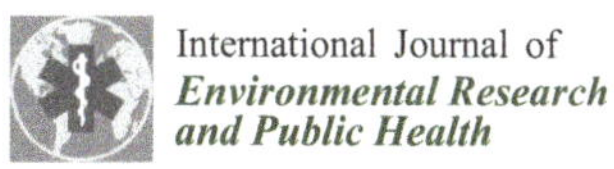

International Journal of
*Environmental Research
and Public Health*

MDPI

Article

Physical Activity Experiences of South Asian Migrant Women in Western Australia: Implications for Intervention Development

Alexis Pullia [1,2], Zakia Jeemi [1], Miguel Reina Ortiz [2] and Jaya A. R. Dantas [1,*]

[1]   Curtin School of Population Health, Curtin University, Perth 6102, Australia;
     alexispullia123@gmail.com (A.P.); zakia.jeemi@curtin.edu.au (Z.J.)
[2]   College of Public Health, University of South Florida, Tampa, FL 33612, USA; miguelreina@usf.edu
*   Correspondence: jaya.dantas@curtin.edu.au

Abstract: The benefits of physical activity are widely recognised; however, physical activity uptake remains low in South Asian populations. South Asian migrant women face health risks as they adapt to new cultures, and these risks are often intensified through their limited participation in physical activity as one of the behaviours that promote positive health outcomes. Three focus group discussions with sixteen South Asian migrant women aged between 33 and 64 years, with a median age of 48 years and who live in Western Australia, were conducted. Thematic analysis of the transcribed qualitative data was completed to explore and uncover South Asian women's experiences with physical activity, as well as their motivation, beliefs, attitudes, and knowledge about physical activity. Five major themes emerged after coding and analysing the data. The themes included the women's knowledge of physical activity, their general attitudes and beliefs surrounding physical activity, the advantages and disadvantages of participation in physical activity, their experiences with physical activity, and the barriers, challenges, and facilitators surrounding physical activity. Recommendations are proposed to increase physical activity among this group to improve overall health and wellbeing and implications for intervention development are discussed.

Keywords: South Asian; migrants; women; physical activity

Citation: Pullia, A.; Jeemi, Z.; Reina Ortiz, M.; Dantas, J.A.R. Physical Activity Experiences of South Asian Migrant Women in Western Australia: Implications for Intervention Development. *Int. J. Environ. Res. Public Health* **2022**, *19*, 3585. https://doi.org/10.3390/ijerph19063585

Academic Editors: Greg Armstrong and Shameran Slewa-Younan

Received: 1 February 2022
Accepted: 15 March 2022
Published: 17 March 2022

Publisher's Note: MDPI stays neutral with regard to jurisdictional claims in published maps and institutional affiliations.

1. Introduction

The number of foreign-born, permanent residents in Australia has continued to increase, as historically, more people migrate to then emigrate from the country [1]. In 2020, there were more than 7.6 million migrants living in Australia [1]. The rise in migration to Australia has only increased Australia's diverse population, both culturally and linguistically [2]. Migration from South Asia, especially India to Australia, has increased in the last decade when compared to other dominant migrating populations, such as those from the United Kingdom and Europe [3]. In fact, the five countries with the highest immigration growth rates between 2006 and 2016 are Nepal (27.8%), Pakistan (13.2%), Brazil (12.1%), India (10.7%), and Bangladesh (8.9%). That is, 80% of these countries (four of these five countries) are in South Asia [3]. Furthermore, as of June 2020, India and Sri Lanka rank second and tenth, respectively, in the ranking of the Australian population by the top ten countries of birth [1]. It has been projected that by 2031, Asian populations will make up seven to nine percent of Australia's population [4].

1.1. Gender and Migration

Historically, it has been recognised that women and men have different social and cultural roles [5,6]. During migration, varying social and cultural roles of men and women negatively influence migrating women. Gender acts as a socio-cultural influence upon the resettlement of migrants globally [6]. Typically, males are regarded as highly skilled professionals that add value to society, while women are expected to reconstruct their family's domestic life [6]. This negatively impacts women's abilities to cope with community structures in their host country [6] and exacerbates the marginalisation of migrant women in society when compared to their male counterparts [7]. This process, in turn, impedes the ability of the newly migrated women to reinvent their gender identities [5,6]. Women generally experience more inequalities than men in relation to integration outcomes [8]. Jarallah and Baxter [9], explored the association between gender and psychological distress among an Australian population of humanitarian entrants and found that women reported significantly higher distress than men.

Overall, it has been shown that gender-specific measures, interventions, and programs are pertinent to female migrants' arrivals [5,6,8]. Cheung and Phillimore [8], argue that by creating gender-specific measures, it can be ensured that migrant women and children are embedded in society. With Australia being an immigrant nation [5], it is the country's duty to call upon public policymakers to assist migrant women with finding their voice through proper integration in their country of resettlement. Previous research has identified that explicit gender-sensitive changes in national policy and availability of support groups are some ways that women can become more active in society during resettlement [6,8].

1.2. Improving Health through Physical Activity

A global epidemiological transition is affecting both developed and developing countries, leading to an increase in the burden of disease attributable to non-communicable diseases [10]. Individuals are living increasingly sedentary lifestyles, which have significant impacts on the health and wellbeing of individuals and populations [11]. When the increase of chronic diseases and sedentary lifestyles are combined, there is an accumulated risk for negative health outcomes [12,13]. Thus, it is reasonable to say that there is a substantial public health concern for the negative health outcomes associated with both low levels of physical activity and a sedentary life [11,12,14].

The impacts of both health-related changes are depicted globally in the leading causes of death worldwide, specifically cardiovascular disease, cancer, respiratory disease, diabetes, and dementia [15]. Notably, in Australia, coronary heart disease (CHD), dementia, cerebrovascular disease, lung cancer, and chronic obstructive pulmonary dis-ease are the top five leading causes of death [16]. Risk factors that contribute to the leading causes of death globally and in Australia include unhealthy diet, physical inactivity, and tobacco use [12].

Addressing physical inactivity has been found to be the most economical and effective manner of preventing the leading causes of death, especially cardiovascular disease [11,12,17,18]. Low levels of exercise and insufficient moderate and vigorous levels of physical activity [10,11] are modifiable through behaviour change that begins with minimal financial investment and time [11]. For decades, on a global level, the benefits of sport and physical activity have been observed and used for the empowerment of women and children, social justice, and to achieve gender equality [19]. Today, in developed countries, physical activity is present in government policies due to its significance related to health care systems and the economy [20]. More specifically, Bailey et al. [17], discusses the human capital model that combines the benefits of physical activity in public policy to support the fact that physical activity has the capacity to deliver valuable returns in the form of physical, emotional, individual, social, intellectual, and financial capital.

The Australian Government Department of Health provides national guidelines and recommendations to address sedentary behaviour and to encourage physical activity [21]. Despite these recommendations, Australians are not fulfilling their weekly or daily physical activity requirements. According to the Australian Institute of Health and Welfare, data from the 2017–18 National Health Survey (2017–2018) show 55% of adults did not participate in sufficient physical activity with women more frequently found to be insufficiently active (59%) when compared to men (50%) [22]. This poses a public health concern because research has demonstrated that risk factors related to obesity change very little from childhood to adulthood [17].

1.3. Physical Activity Interventions for South Asian Women and Immigrants

Previous research has identified that there are various barriers that South Asian women face when participating in physical activity [23–25]. Babakus and Thompson [23] reported that these difficulties include both cultural and structural barriers. Namely, South Asian women justify that partaking in physical activity takes time away from their families and communities and is described as a selfish act. This is further compounded by gender roles within South Asian culture which often state that a woman's focus should be on family and to perform domestic duties [23,25]. Thus, women do not receive the necessary support needed to be physically active [25]. Cultural and structural barriers, inappropriate interventions, and facilities have acted as barriers to the participation of this population in physical activity [23]. Thus, using physical activity as a protective measure against noncommunicable chronic diseases has been extremely low in this population [23–25]. It has also been noted that a lack of education and understanding surrounding physical activity, the recommended levels, and its benefits inhibit one's choice and ability to successfully engage in physical activity [23].

South Asians, including women, are significantly burdened by chronic diseases [26–28]. When compared to their Caucasian counterparts, South Asians face CHD, diabetes, abdominal adiposity, and corresponding complications at younger ages [24,29]. A study of 16,287 urban South Asian adults reported on the prevalence and risk factors associated with having two or more chronic conditions and found that multiple chronic conditions affected nearly 10% of South Asians and each additional chronic condition carried a progressively higher risk of mortality [30]. In an Indian study conducted by Eapen et al. [24], it was found that there was an approximate 50% decrease in risk for CHD when the study participants partook in 30 to 45 min of moderate physical activity per day. Other studies have further exhibited that physical activity has had positive outcomes on abdominal adiposity, LDL (low-density lipoprotein), HDL (high-density lipoprotein), diabetes, and hypertension [24]. It is thus imperative that South Asian women engage in physical activity due to the high prevalence of metabolic syndrome and cardiovascular disease (CVD) within the population [24].

Nonetheless, South Asian women are motivated to take care of their health and bodies to decrease their risk of disease and illness [23]. Kandula et al. [25] reported that women were more likely to participate in physical activity if exercise interventions and programs were culturally appropriate, included only women, and were held in an established community setting. In addition to this, women were more motivated to engage in physical activity if children were allowed to participate [25]. Thus, it is necessary that physical activity interventions consider socio-cultural factors to ensure the effectiveness and acceptability of the intervention [25].

The importance of physical activity remains one of the least expensive and most effective preventive treatments for combating chronic disease [18]. Furthermore, research has shown the positive relationship between physical activity and mental health [31], and that physical activity, even at lower levels, has been shown to be positively associated with mental health wellbeing [32]. Sport and physical activity are powerful instruments for mobilisation and advocacy and can be used as a means for enhancing personal empowerment, combating discrimination, and achieving gender equality [19]. Increasing participation in physical activity forms a core objective across a range of government policies in most developed countries. The broad development of physical activity has become a policy target because of its significance for health care systems and economies [20].

1.4. Global Physical Activity Programs and Interventions

Researchers affiliated with The Waikato Institute of Technology and the University of Waikato in New Zealand focused on physical activity intervention efforts among refugee

Somali women relocated to Hamilton, New Zealand [33]. Through in-person interaction with the study participants and face-to-face interviews with the women, researchers explored the barriers and intricate social and cultural dynamics involving physical activity among these refugee women [33]. From these interactions and interviews, the researchers implemented several interventions, including exercise classes and a trial-run membership to a local, women-only fitness centre [33]. While there were no data-driven indicators of the success, the intervention efforts provided researchers with viable information regarding physical activity barriers and the importance of taking a cultural approach to intervention implementation.

Wieland et al. [34], used a community-based participatory approach to analyse immigrant and refugee women in Rochester, Minnesota. In order to combat the decline in physical activity and poor nutrition intake for those who are post-immigration, researchers utilised community-based participatory research (CBPR) to create socially and culturally driven exercise and nutrition plans [34]. Forty-five women of Hispanic, Somali, Cambodian, and non-immigrant African American descent participated in this six-week program [34]. According to a physical activity class satisfaction questionnaire, upon completion of the six-week program, participants were more likely to exercise regularly, and report a higher quality of life and self-efficacy regarding diet and exercise [34]. Researchers have attributed these positive results to the socio-cultural dynamics of the program [34]. They also noted that this type of approach is more useful for refugees and immigrants displaced to Westernised settlements with no structure for maintaining diet and exercise [34].

Two additional studies utilising the CBPR approach to implement interventions include studies conducted by Marinescu et al. [35], and Dave et al. [36]. Marinescu et al. [35], utilised focus groups to evaluate and gather information regarding culture and community to specifically analyse the "Be Active Together" program directed at Muslim women in Seattle communities. This program supported physical activity and specifically provided outreach to women in public housing communities across the country [35]. From the feedback provided by the Muslim women, researchers were able to implement physical activity protocols and interventions driven by cultural insight provided by the Muslim women of these communities [35].

Dave et al. [36], interviewed South Asian immigrants in Chicago to assess physical activity barriers at various life stages. Researchers found that barriers differed depending on the life stage these women were experiencing. For older women, ailments such as chronic disease posed the largest threat to decreased physical activity [36]. In contrast, for younger women, the negative perception of being "too skinny" largely deterred these women from physical exercise [36]. In the case of women who start families or have children, researchers saw a sharp decline in physical activity, as these women saw a shift in their priorities and responsibilities to raise their families [36]. In any case, women across all ages expressed the need to consider cultural, religious, and life stages when creating physical activity interventions [36].

Another study looked at South Asian immigrant mothers at risk of type 2 diabetes in settlements located in Chicago [25]. Researchers specifically targeted women displaying risk factors for type 2 diabetes who had children between the ages of 6 and 14, in order to develop a socio-cultural physical activity intervention. The intervention ran for 16 weeks and included an exercise class two times per week, the use of Fitbits for objective exercise tracking, and educational classes on healthy eating [25]. Additionally, children were offered an exercise class alongside their mothers at the same time as their mother's workout class [25]. The women who attended at least 80% of these workout classes lost approximately five pounds and showed a significant increase in exercise-related confidence [25]. Researchers found that this multifaceted exercise intervention structure, coupled with the cultural significance of having their children engage in physical activity alongside the mothers, was an extremely beneficial component to the intervention's success [25].

Culturally and linguistically diverse (CALD) women from South Asia find it difficult to properly acclimate to new cultures and establish a sense of identity and belonging.

Empirical evidence has found that these barriers significantly impact their health and wellbeing and limit their participation in physical activity. Due to this, South Asian women are at risk for chronic diseases, including the development of abdominal adiposity, diabetes, and CVD. However, it has been demonstrated that physical activity interventions and programs have lessened the impact of and risk for chronic diseases in this population, while also acting as positive influences on social inclusion and physical and mental health.

The main objectives of this study were:

1. Explore the beliefs, attitudes, and knowledge that South Asian women have regarding physical activity;
2. Understand the experiences that South Asian women have had when partaking in physical activity and the types of activities they engage in;
3. Understand the barriers and facilitators that South Asian women have with partaking in physical activity.

2. Materials and Methods

2.1. Context and Study

This study is the initial part of the larger SAMBA (South Asian Mothers and Children Being Active) study (2018–2021). This study was undertaken in WA and was the first stage of a larger health promotion intervention study focussing on physical activity and psychosocial wellbeing in migrant women from South Asia and the Middle East.

2.2. Participant Recruitment

Participants were recruited from South Asian communities through snowball and purposive sampling with the help of a key informant, who is a member of the South Asian women's community, and with the help of already recruited South Asian women. Women who did not meet the current recommendations for physical activity requirements were targeted. Thus, women that did not meet the recommendations of 150 to 300 min of moderate-intensity physical activity or 75 to 150 min of vigorous-intensity physical activity per week outlined in Australia's Physical Activity and Sedentary Behaviour Guidelines for Adults (18–64 years) [37], were invited to participate in the study.

2.3. Ethics and Informed Consent

The Curtin University Human Research Ethics Committee (HRE2018-0351) provided approval for the larger project of which this research was a component. Reciprocal ethics were obtained from the University of South Florida Institutional Review Board (Pro00035741). Participants provided informed consent to participate in the study and for their data to be used in the research. Informed consent was obtained from the participants before the focus group discussions.

2.4. Focus Group Discussions

This study was based on CBPR approaches and was guided by the health behaviour model [38].

Three semi-structured focus group discussions were conducted in order to assess South Asian women's general experiences with physical activity, knowledge of physical activity, attitudes, and beliefs surrounding physical activity, as well as the facilitators, barriers, and challenges they encounter when trying to participate in physical activity. A semi-structured interview guide was used to guide the focus group discussions and the items on the guide were grounded in the health behaviour model [38]. Thus, providing rich qualitative data to further comprehend if and why challenges related to the synergistic and multifaceted relationship between health behaviours, determinants of health, as well as gender and cultural issues surrounding South Asian women have a large effect on the amounts of physical activity these women are partaking in.

A total of 16 female participants between the ages of 33 and 64 years were recruited to partake in the focus group discussions. There were four to six women per focus group. The focus groups were audio-recorded with the participants' consent and lasted one hour to one and a half hours.

All focus group discussions were transcribed verbatim, and the qualitative data gathered from the focus groups were analysed through an inductive approach from drawing quotes and themes using thematic content analysis in order to identify and establish themes and codes [39]. The thematic analysis was conducted by the first author and the themes and codes generated were then discussed with and reviewed by the other authors. The results of this study helped guide further focus group discussions and individual interviews, which led to the development of the SAMBA physical activity intervention for CALD women.

3. Results

3.1. Demographic Data

There was a total of three focus group discussions that included a total of 16 South Asian migrant women aged between 33 and 64 years with a median age of 48 years. The focus groups included women from five of the eight countries belonging to the World Bank's South Asia Geographic Region [40]; namely, Sri Lanka, India, Bhutan, Nepal, and Pakistan. Focus group one encompassed five women from India and one woman from Pakistan. Focus group two included six women from Sri Lanka and focus group three was comprised of four women from Nepal and one woman from Bhutan. The number of years the women have resided in Western Australia was between 4 years and 32 years, with a median period of 12 years. All the women spoke English in addition to other languages, specifically Hindi (N = 11), Marathi (N = 2), Gujarati (N = 2), Urdu (N = 1), Farsi (N = 1), Hazaraghi (N = 1), Dari (N = 1), Tamil (N = 3), Marwadi (N = 1), Punjabi (N = 1), Sinhalese (N = 4), and Nepali (N = 5). Interpreters were not needed for the focus groups.

The women had varying levels of education that included no schooling, technical school, college, or university, and post-graduate studies. There were also variations in employment status. Nine women worked full-time, where one Nepali woman stated she had her own business, three worked part-time, two identified as homemakers where one woman stated she was only on maternity leave, and two were retired. The participants came from the following religious groups: Hindu (N =8), Buddhist (N = 4), Christian (N = 2), Muslim (N = 1), and Tamil (N = 1). Furthermore, 15 of the 16 women were married, with only one woman identifying as being separated from her former husband (Table 1).

Table 1. Demographic characteristics of study participants.

Characteristic	Count
Age in Years	N
32–38	3
39–45	3
46–52	7
53–59	1
60–66	2
Previous Country of Residence	N
Sri Lanka	5
India	5
Bhutan	1
Nepal	4
Pakistan	1
Number of Years in Western Australia	N
1–5	2
6–10	5
11–15	2
16–20	3
21–25	1
26–30	1
31–35	2

Table 1. *Cont.*

Characteristic	Count
Education	N
No School	1
Technical school	2
College or University	9
Post-Graduate	4
Employment Status	N
Full-Time	9 *
Part-Time	3
Homemaker	2 **
Retired	2
Marital Status	N
Married	15
Separated	1

* Including one participant who owns a business with her husband ** Including one participant who is on maternity leave.

Regardless of the prior country of residence and employment status, the women across all the focus groups identified themselves as wives, mothers, homemakers, caregivers, cooks, and cleaners within their households. Many of the women stated that they lived with immediate and extended family. Those living with their immediate family stated that they lived with their husbands, children, and parents. The women living with their extended family mentioned they lived with their in-laws and/or nephews.

3.2. Themes

The overarching themes that were drawn from the analysis of the focus groups included the women's (Table 2):

(1) Knowledge of physical activity with a subtheme of knowledge of frequency and duration of physical activity;
(2) General attitudes and beliefs towards physical activity, including impacts on mental health and wellbeing;
(3) Advantages and disadvantages of physical activity;
(4) Experiences with physical activity with subthemes of past physical activity, current physical activity, the difference in physical activity levels, justification for activities, preferred physical activities; and
(5) Barriers and facilitators to participating in physical activity with subthemes of barriers and challenges and facilitators.

Table 2. Table of themes drawn from the analysis.

Themes	Subthemes
Knowledge of physical activity	Frequency and duration of physical activity
General attitudes and beliefs toward physical activity	
Advantages and disadvantages of physical activity	
Experiences with physical activity	Past physical activity Current physical activity Difference in physical activity levels Justifications for activities Preferred physical activities
Barriers, challenges, and facilitators surrounding physical activity	Barriers and challenges Facilitators

3.2.1. Theme 1: Knowledge of Physical Activity

None of the women could completely articulate the definition of physical activity. Women mentioned that physical activity involved the movement of hands and legs, an increase in breathing and heart rate, and noted that it is completed to make muscles stronger. They also mentioned that physical activity could also be relaxing and not rigorous. The examples of physical activity that the women provided included yoga, meditation, chores, mowing the lawn, walking, going to the gym, running, cycling, dancing, and Zumba.

Subtheme 1.1: Frequency and duration. There were some differences in how often physical activity should be completed by the participants. Some women thought physical activity should be done every day. Other women believed physical activity should be completed anywhere between two and five times a week for approximately 45 min to one hour. Interestingly, one woman explicitly stated that physical activity was not meant to be completed every day of the week. Women further mentioned that the frequency of physical activity was dependent on the age of the woman.

3.2.2. Theme 2: General Attitudes and Beliefs towards Physical Activity and Wellbeing

All the women believed that physical activity was beneficial and necessary to maintain their health. They also exhibited positive attitudes toward physical activity. They understood that there were both mental and physical benefits to participating in physical activity. The women believed that physical activity was required for health and needed to be completed. All focus groups emphasised that physical activity needed to be enjoyable and fun. A woman from focus group one further explained this by stating,

"Indian woman, Focus Group One: . . . I'm not learning new things. I'm just keep going doing the same thing. So, it's all the same maybe they get bored."

In addition, the women stressed the importance of finding the "right exercise" to engage in. This alluded to the awareness that the frequency and types of exercise an individual can vary over the life course, especially if one is older, sick, a mother, or has experienced injury or is recovering from an injury. The women also discussed that members of their community, including friends and family, liked physical activity and believed it to be important.

3.2.3. Theme 3: Advantages and Disadvantages of Physical Activity

The women acknowledged various health benefits attached to physical activity. Notably, they mentioned benefits which included taking care of their individual health, weight loss, maintaining fitness, preventing disease and heart conditions, inner happiness, flexibility, strengthening muscles, the flow of oxygen in the body, and a fresh mind. Women also stated that physical activity was good for one's lungs, liver, breathing, and brain. Moreover, some of the women said that another benefit would be a boost in personal self-confidence. Various disadvantages of physical activity were also mentioned. These included being sore and not wanting to exercise again until the soreness subsided, as well as being too tired afterward, which impeded priorities, such as household duties, family, and cooking. A woman in focus group one specifically stated,

"Indian woman, Focus Group One: Even if I had time, I'd rather not go for it [physical activity], because my body will ache."

Additional disadvantages included potential exercise-induced injuries and general pain and discomfort during and after physical activity. The women stated that other disadvantages would be over-exercising, selecting the incorrect activities to participate in—especially if one has a medical condition—and the underlying distress of not completing a physical activity in the correct way. All the women shared that physical activity provided them with improved health, increased happiness and contentment, and improved physical and mental wellbeing.

3.2.4. Theme 4: Experiences with Physical Activity

During the focus groups, women were asked about their experiences with physical activity prior to migration and after migration. *Subtheme 4.1: Past physical activity.* All women in the study self-reported that they did not participate in regular physical activity, as per recommendations at the time of the study. Some of the women connected physical activity to past work-related activities and responsibilities as an employee. These activities included fieldwork and walking around an office space. In all focus groups, domesticated housework was mentioned as a type of physical activity, since the women stated it was physically taxing. The women connected physical activity to work-related activities and housework because completing these activities kept them moving with little time for sedentary behaviours.

Activities, such as walking in their home countries to get to public transport and cycling when public transport was unavailable, were also noted as past physical activities. Other past activities that the women participated in were yoga and meditation, badminton, hiking, fast-paced walking, swimming, and qigong. Using treadmills and stationary bikes at the gym were also mentioned. A woman also stated she used to participate in dance fitness classes led by an instructor but stopped because she found them too strenuous.

Subtheme 4.2: Current physical activity. Across all groups, walking and yoga were found to be the most prevalent types of physical activity the women were engaging in. When engaging in these activities, the duration of walking would last between 5 and 50 min, while yoga would last at least 45 min and up to 60 min. Meditation was mentioned as a type of physical activity in two groups. A woman mentioned that she line-danced two to three times per week, and another disclosed she participated in Bollywood dance classes a few times a week. Dancing and cycling were also mentioned, in addition to physical activity classes specifically tailored to older adults' physical abilities and skills. Women mentioned that having a busy social life was part of physical activity, as it required frequent movement. One woman stated that she recently joined a gym and was trying to attend regularly.

Subtheme 4.3: Differences in physical activity level. Across all groups, most of the women mentioned a decrease in activity when they compared their current physical activity level to their past activity level. Women stated that age was an influential factor for varying levels of physical activity. These women expressed that, as women age, physical activity decreases overall, especially high-intensity activities because the body changes with age and health issues and complications can present. Therefore, these factors generally decrease participation in an activity and the level at which a woman can sustain an activity for an extended period. Women in two discrete groups agreed that they were more active in their home countries since they either did not have access to a personal vehicle or had limited access to public transportation for travel. This required them to walk more, which inherently increased their frequency and duration of physical activity. A woman also mentioned that walking in Australia is less strenuous than it was in her home country because the weather reached higher temperatures, which led to discomfort.

Subtheme 4.4: Justifications for activities. Many reasons were discussed as to why the study participants were partaking in their current activities. Women stated that they engaged in their current physical activities to benefit their physical and mental health. They also mentioned that they participated in the activities because they wanted to look good in regard to body image. Across all groups, the idea of social support was given as a reason for partaking in physical activity. Participants found that completing activities with family or friends in a group setting was easier, more fun, and more enjoyable than doing physical activity alone. There was also a sense of increased self-efficacy when completing activities in groups. To elaborate on self-efficacy, one woman stated,

> *"Indian woman, Focus Group One: . . . there are a bunch of mums who have kids and they're able to do, why not me??"*

Women also mentioned that the activities they participated in were convenient for them and that members of their family encouraged them to engage in those specific physical activities. Women in another group discussed that age, as well as injuries and pain, were decisive factors in terms of the activities they chose to participate in. Women in this group also expressed that engaging in their physical activities made them 'feel good' and less irritable, improved their mental health, helped with weight loss, and empowered them. Women in another group voiced how they believed the activities they engaged in were the safest activities for them, fit within cultural boundaries and appropriateness, and were also easy to perform and matched their abilities. To further explain this, one woman stated,

> *"Nepali woman, Focus Group Three: I would not run, because I cannot run for long and cannot run far. So, I would not do it, and it makes me self-conscious since I cannot do it well."*

Women also discussed how they had become comfortable with the activities that they are completing, due to repeated participation in the activity.

Subtheme 4.5: Preferred physical activities. Women preferred to participate in low-intensity exercises and activities, such as walking and yoga. In contrast, they were less inclined to participate in activities that were perceived as being rigorous or complex. The focus groups specifically yielded qualitative information stating that the women would not participate in activities utilising dumbbell weights, because the activity was too rigorous, and they did not want to be in pain or injure themselves.

> *"Indian woman, Focus Group One: Oh, I would least likely do those dumbbells, and other rigorous activities, I can't do it."*

The women also stated they would not participate in vigorous running and jogging because they did not want to risk injury. Women also mentioned that they were less likely to participate in swimming for physical activity than other types of physical activity. They stated that they felt insecure about their underdeveloped level of skill and expressed fears of drowning. This was compounded by the idea that they believed it was too late in life for them to learn new or unfamiliar skills to carry out certain activities.

> *"Sri Lankan woman, Focus Group Two: I'm too old to learn how to swim you need to get those skills when you are younger. It's harder to learn properly when you are older."*

Another woman also expressed her battle with her skill level when discussing participation in fitness classes she attended, which can be linked to feelings of inadequacy.

> *"Indian woman, Focus Group One: . . . I don't like [name of dance-based fitness class] and aerobics. I'm not coordinated, my body is not made for that. I tried, it just doesn't work for me."*

3.2.5. Theme 5: Barriers, Challenges, and Facilitators Related to Participation in Physical Activity

The barriers and challenges faced by the migrant women from South Asia in regard to taking part in physical activities were explored in this theme. *Subtheme 5.1: Barriers and challenges.* Across all groups, time, cost, and lifestyle factors, including stress, were expressed as barriers and challenges. Participants felt that there was not enough time in the day to adequately participate in physical activity. Most of the women were employed full-time, and were also primarily responsible for activities, including tending to children and the house and cooking meals for the family. Participants also gave priority to frequent community and cultural activities, many of which do not traditionally involve physical activity. In addition, women also stated that not having a group of friends or social network to complete a physical activity with, soreness, and the presence of men while engaging in physical activity were all barriers and challenges that made it difficult for them to participate in physical activity. Women in two discrete groups expressed tiredness and a lack of motivation to engage in physical activity as challenges. Similarly, one woman stated she would rather prioritise sleep than do physical activity.

All focus groups also identified fear of judgement from others, their personal insecurities, shyness, self-consciousness, and embarrassment surrounding their skills and abilities for physical activity as barriers to participation and expressed how this impacted their personal wellbeing. This is best presented through the words of one woman,

"Indian woman, Focus Group One: I don't know if it's my own insecurity, like I'm being judged every time I take a wrong step. I feel like I'm being judged for that, which I'm sure people don't care. They're not even looking at you. I think it's just a built-in insecurity really are they looking?"

Facilitators that help women make informed decisions about physical activity were also examined. *Subtheme 5.2: Facilitators.* In order to make physical activity easier and not burdensome for South Asian women to complete, a variety of factors need to be considered. Participants stated that a physical activity class or facility located near their places of residence with group classes later in the evening would be extremely beneficial and convenient. Participants explained that this would allow them to complete their household tasks and outstanding priorities before engaging in physical activity and becoming tired since energy is needed to fulfil daily work, cooking, and caretaking. It would also allow them to take part in physical activity with friends and other migrant women, developing social support and group motivation. Furthermore, an affordable gym or recreation facility membership or free services would encourage women to participate in physical activity more often. One group stated that women-only facilities or classes would be advantageous and accommodating for reasons related to culture, as well as self-consciousness. It was also discussed that low-cost or free childcare would be beneficial because a woman's husband is traditionally tired after working a long day. Therefore, the women do not want to concern the husband or other members of the family with childcare. The idea of allowing children to attend physical activity classes alongside their mothers also emerged, was positively accepted, and thought of as fun.

4. Discussion

This qualitative study drew on the experiences and knowledge of South Asian migrant women residing in Western Australia. The thematic analysis of focus group discussions found that the South Asian women included in this study face various internal and external influences when participating in physical activity. Relevant topics discussed during the discussions included the women's knowledge of physical activity, their general attitudes and beliefs about physical activity, advantages and disadvantages of physical activity, experiences with physical activity, and the barriers, challenges, and facilitators surrounding physical activity.

Notably, the barriers that these women faced can be described as determinants of health that are embedded within the levels of the social-ecological model, specifically the individual, interpersonal, organisational, and community levels. Interestingly, even though there was a diverse sample of women from five South Asian countries, all the women discussed similar socio-cultural influences to participating in physical activity. Thus, solidifying that the influences, which reside within the social-ecological model of health, can persist in various CALD populations.

On comparing the results of this study to previous literature [5,6,23,33,35], we identified several themes that CALD migrant women populations face. Participants in this study understood and valued the importance of the positive association between physical activity and physical and mental health wellbeing and identified various personal, social, and environmental barriers and facilitators to participation. Influences of participation in physical activity, found in this study and also presented and discussed in previous research, included work, culture, gender, cost, time, family, health status, and environmental factors [41,42]. However, the participants in this study did not find language, religion, dress, or social isolation as influencing their participation in physical activity.

4.1. Strengths and Limitations

A limitation of the study is the small and heterogeneous sample size. Therefore, the results presented are not generalizable to other CALD populations. However, being a qualitative study, depth, transferability, and credibility were of importance. A strength of this study was providing South Asian migrant women with a voice to share their thoughts about physical activity and wellbeing. The sharing of experiences revealed challenges and successes the women had faced during resettlement and provided rich data on what physical activity program could be designed and would interest the women. Interviewer bias may be another limitation of this study. In order to avoid this bias, the focus groups were semi-structured, and prompts were frequently utilised after multiple questions to stimulate discussion. Future studies should improve by recruiting a larger sample size that includes women from the South Asian countries that were not represented in this study. In addition, matching the number of participants from each country between groups could increase the generalizability of the results, something that was not possible in this study due to time constraints in recruitment. For future studies, the sample size could be expanded to women who also meet the weekly physical activity recommendations to allow for comparisons and identify factors of participation. Individual interviews, rather than focus group discussions, may reflect country contexts and cultural differences better and allow for a more in-depth exploration of the physical activity experiences of South Asian women.

4.2. Recommendations

Failing to address socio-cultural influences within this population significantly hinders the population's ability to partake in physical activity. Therefore, based on this study, it is recommended that targeted and sustained funding for future programs and interventions targeting this population include an educational component. Including an educational component in a program or intervention would dispel any confusion concerning the recommended duration and frequency of physical activity, and would describe the benefits of physical activity, and address age-appropriate exercise, provide strategies for motivation and sustained participation in physical activity, as well as provide information on activities for women who have underlying health conditions. Providing the women with opportunities to increase their knowledge also has the potential to lead to individual and group empowerment and increase motivation and self-efficacy. Similarly, the study documented that the women are capable of learning new skills, even later in life.

Additionally, physical activity programs should be made fun and enjoyable for the women versus being constructed as rigorous and repetitive. A program's emphasis on women-only group classes would likely result in higher and sustained engagement instead of constructing a program to cater to individual-level participation in physical activity. Furthermore, group classes should be held at a mutually convenient time and close to the women's homes. Allowing children to participate in physical activity alongside their mothers would also be beneficial because it would be more fun for the women, and they would not need to find supplemental childcare. Finally, it is recommended that CBPR methods are employed as an effective means to further consider the social, cultural, and environmental determinants of health when implementing public health measures to improve physical and mental health and wellbeing for populations globally.

CBPR is increasingly utilised in public health to connect educational opportunities with social action, especially regarding chronic disease prevention [43–45]. CBPR offers the opportunity for public health professionals to engage with communities to further understand complexities on a local level within populations and complexities on a macro-level, which are often overlooked but contribute to unsustainable interventions and programs [45]. Since CBPR engages the community, beneficiaries, and stakeholders, while considering a community's knowledge, attitudes, beliefs, and cultural practices, it also ensures that the objectives and goals of a study are sensible, relevant, and consistent with the target population's needs [46].

CPBR offers the ability to address health disparities and inequities, as well as environmental and social justice [43,47]. Subsequently, this has empowered communities to take charge of the determinants affecting their health and form community coalitions [45].

Therefore, it is expected that interventions and programs utilising CBPR will elicit greater positive impacts, long-term benefits, reduce community resistance to participation, and meet a community's needs [47].

The results of this study helped guide further focus group discussions and individual interviews, which led to the development of the SAMBA physical activity intervention using CBPR methods. The SAMBA study was a pilot physical activity intervention study conducted with CALD women from South Asian and Middle Eastern backgrounds in Western Australia.

5. Conclusions

This study contributes to prior research and uncovers new findings within the Western Australian context and challenges related to the synergistic and multifaceted relationship between health behaviours, determinants of health, as well as gender and cultural factors surrounding South Asian migrant women and physical activity. Specifically, it exemplifies that physical activity participation within the South Asian women population in Western Australia is low. It additionally provides insights into the various influences that affect the participation rates of migrant South Asian women in physical activity. Therefore, this study offers important socio-cultural information for the development of successful and sustainable physical activity interventions for South Asian women. By providing formative research for the development of culturally sensitive physical activity programs, which can ultimately contribute to higher physical activity participation rates and a greater quality of life for this population, can, in turn, improve the mental health and physical wellbeing for migrant women and their families.

Author Contributions: Conceptualization, J.A.R.D.; methodology, J.A.R.D. and A.P.; software, A.P. and J.A.R.D.; formal analysis, A.P. and J.A.R.D.; investigation, A.P., Z.J. and J.A.R.D.; resources, J.A.R.D.; data curation, A.P., Z.J. and J.A.R.D.; writing—original draft preparation, A.P., J.A.R.D. and Z.J.; writing—review and editing, A.P., Z.J., M.R.O. and J.A.R.D.; visualization, A.P.; supervision, J.A.R.D. and M.R.O.; project administration, Z.J. and J.A.R.D.; funding acquisition, J.A.R.D. All authors have read and agreed to the published version of the manuscript.

Funding: This research is part of a larger study funded by Healthway, the Health Promotion Foundation of Western Australia. [Grant number 31974—2018 to 2021].

Institutional Review Board Statement: The study was conducted according to the guidelines of the Declaration of Helsinki, and approved by the Human Research Ethics Committee of Curtin University (protocol code HRE2018-0351, 13 June 2018) with reciprocal approval from the University of South Florida Institutional Review Board (protocol code Pro00035741, 18 June 2018).

Informed Consent Statement: Informed consent was obtained from all subjects involved in the study. Participants provided informed consent to participate in the study and for their data to be used in the research.

Data Availability Statement: The datasets produced and analyzed for this study are available from the corresponding author on reasonable request.

Acknowledgments: We would like to thank our community partners and all participants for their time and support of the study.

Conflicts of Interest: The authors declare no conflict of interest. The funder had no role in the design of the study; in the collection, analyses, or interpretation of data; in the writing of the manuscript, or in the decision to publish the results.

References

1. Australian Bureau of Statistics. Migration, Australia, 2019–2020 Financial Year. 2021. Available online: https://www.abs.gov.au/statistics/people/population/migration-australia/latest-release (accessed on 3 December 2021).
2. Australian Bureau of Statistics. Census of Population and Housing: Reflecting Australia—Stories from the Census, 2016 (No. 2071.0). 2017. Available online: https://www.abs.gov.au/ausstats/abs@.nsf/Lookup/by%20Subject/2071.0~2016~Main%20Features~Cultural%20Diversity%20Article~60 (accessed on 19 October 2021).

3. Australian Bureau of Statistics. Migration, Australia, 2015–2016 (No. 3412.0). 2017. Available online: https://www.abs.gov.au/ausstats/abs@.nsf/previousproducts/3412.0main%20features32015-16 (accessed on 3 December 2021).

4. Parliament of Australia. Asian Immigration: Current Issues Briefs 1996–1997. Available online: https://www.aph.gov.au/sitecore/content/Home/About_Parliament/Parliamentary_Departments/Parliamentary_Library/Publications_Archive/CIB/CIB9697/97cib16 (accessed on 19 October 2021).

5. Casimiro, S.; Hancock, P.; Northcote, J. Isolation and Insecurity: Resettlement Issues Among Muslim Refugee Women in Perth, Western Australia. *Aust. J. Soc. Issues* **2007**, *42*, 55–69. [CrossRef]

6. Koyama, J. Constructing Gender: Refugee Women Working in the United States. *J. Refugee Stud.* **2014**, *28*, 258–275. [CrossRef]

7. Hunt, T.A. Transcending polarization? Strategic identity construction in young women's transnational feminist networks. *Women's Stud. Int. Forum* **2013**, *40*, 152–161. [CrossRef]

8. Cheung, S.Y.; Phillimore, J. Gender and Refugee Integration: A Quantitative Analysis of Integration and Social Policy Outcomes. *J. Soc. Policy* **2017**, *46*, 211–230. [CrossRef]

9. Jarallah, Y.; Baxter, J. Gender disparities and psychological distress among humanitarian migrants in Australia: A moderating role of migration pathway? *Confl. Health* **2019**, *13*, 13. [CrossRef]

10. Begg, S.; Vos, T.; Barker, B.; Stevenson, C.; Stanley, L.; Lopez, A.D. *The Burden of Disease and Injury in Australia 2003*; Australian Institute of Health and Welfare: Canberra, ACT, Australia, 2007.

11. Tremblay, M.S.; Colley, R.C.; Saunders, T.J.; Healy, G.N.; Owen, N. Physiological and health implications of a sedentary lifestyle. *Appl. Physiol. Nutr. Metab.* **2010**, *35*, 725–740. [CrossRef]

12. World Health Organization. Noncommunicable Diseases. 2021. Available online: https://www.who.int/news-room/fact-sheets/detail/noncommunicable-diseases (accessed on 30 November 2021).

13. Knight, J.A. Physical inactivity: Associated diseases and disorders. *Ann. Clin. Lab. Sci.* **2012**, *42*, 320–337.

14. Owen, N.; Sparling, P.B.; Healy, G.N.; Dunstan, D.W.; Matthews, C.E. Sedentary behavior: Emerging evidence for a new health risk. *Mayo Clin. Proc.* **2010**, *85*, 1138–1141. [CrossRef]

15. Ritchie, H.; Roser, M. *Causes of Death*; University of Oxford: Oxford, UK, 2018.

16. Australian Institute of Health and Welfare. Deaths. 2017. Available online: https://www.aihw.gov.au/reports/life-expectancy-death/deaths-in-australia/contents/leading-causes-of-death (accessed on 3 December 2021).

17. Bailey, R.; Hillman, C.; Arent, S.; Petitpas, A. Physical activity: An underestimated investment in human capital? *J. Phys. Act. Health* **2013**, *10*, 289–308. [CrossRef]

18. Bonow, R.O.; Smaha, L.A.; Smith, S.C.; Mensah, G.A., Jr.; Lenfant, C. World Heart Day 2002: The international burden of cardiovascular disease: Responding to the emerging global epidemic. *Circulation* **2002**, *106*, 1602–1605. [CrossRef]

19. Beutler, I. Sport serving development and peace: Achieving the goals of the United Nations through sport. *Sport Soc.* **2008**, *11*, 359–369. [CrossRef]

20. Breuer, C.; Pawlowski, T. Socioeconomic perspectives on physical activity and aging. *Eur. Rev. Aging Phys. Act.* **2011**, *8*, 53–56. [CrossRef]

21. Australian Government Department of Health. Australia's Physical Activity and Sedentary Behaviour Guidelines. Available online: https://www1.health.gov.au/internet/main/publishing.nsf/Content/health-pubhlth-strateg-phys-act-guidelines (accessed on 10 October 2019).

22. Australian Institute of Health and Welfare. Insufficient Physical Activity. 2020. Available online: https://www.aihw.gov.au/reports/australias-health/insufficient-physical-activity (accessed on 3 December 2021).

23. Babakus, W.S.; Thompson, J.L. Physical activity among South Asian women: A systematic, mixed-methods review. *Int. J. Behav. Nutr. Phys. Act.* **2012**, *9*, 150. [CrossRef]

24. Eapen, D.; Kalra, G.L.; Merchant, N.; Arora, A.; Khan, B.V. Metabolic syndrome and cardiovascular disease in South Asians. *Vasc. Health Risk Manag.* **2009**, *5*, 731–743.

25. Kandula, N.R.; Dave, S.; De Chavez, P.J.; Marquez, D.X.; Bharucha, H.; Mammen, S.; Dunaif, A.; Ackermann, R.T.; Kumar, S.; Siddique, J. An Exercise Intervention for South Asian Mothers with Risk Factors for Diabetes. *Transl. J. Am. Coll. Sports Med.* **2016**, *1*, 52–59.

26. Kanaya, A.M.; Wassel, C.L.; Mathur, D.; Stewart, A.; Herrington, D.; Budoff, M.J.; Ranpura, V.; Liu, K. Prevalence and correlates of diabetes in South Asian Indians in the United States: Findings from the metabolic syndrome and atherosclerosis in South Asians living in America study and the multi-ethnic study of atherosclerosis. *Metab. Syndr. Relat. Disord.* **2010**, *8*, 157–164. [CrossRef]

27. Bainey, K.R.; Jugdutt, B.I. Increased burden of coronary artery disease in South-Asians living in North America. Need for an aggressive management algorithm. *Atherosclerosis* **2009**, *204*, 1–10. [CrossRef]

28. Misra, A.; Khurana, L. Obesity-related non-communicable diseases: South Asians vs White Caucasians. *Int. J. Obes.* **2011**, *35*, 167–187. [CrossRef]

29. Misra, A.; Soares, M.J.; Mohan, V.; Anoop, S.; Abhishek, V.; Vaidya, R.; Pradeepa, R. Body fat, metabolic syndrome and hyperglycemia in South Asians. *J. Diabetes Complicat.* **2018**, *32*, 1068–1075. [CrossRef]

30. Singh, K.; Patel, S.A.; Biswas, S.; Shivashankar, R.; Kondal, D.; Ajay, V.S.; Anjana, R.M.; Fatmi, Z.; Ali, M.K.; Kadir, M.M.; et al. Multimorbidity in South Asian adults: Prevalence, risk factors and mortality. *J. Public Health* **2019**, *41*, 80–89. [CrossRef]

31. Tamminen, N.; Reinikainen, J.; Appelqvist-Schmidlechner, K.; Borodulin, K.; Mäki-Opas, T.; Solin, P. Associations of physical activity with positive mental health: A population-based study. *Ment. Health Phys. Act.* **2020**, *18*, 100319. [CrossRef]

32. Imai, A.; Kurihara, T.; Kimura, D.; Tanaka, N.; Sanada, K. Association between non-locomotive light-intensity physical activity and depressive symptoms in Japanese older women: A cross-sectional study. *Ment. Health Phys. Act.* **2020**, *18*, 100303. [CrossRef]
33. Guerin, P.B.; Diiriye, R.O.; Corrigan, C.; Guerin, B. Physical activity programs for refugee Somali women: Working out in a new country. *Women Health* **2003**, *38*, 83–99. [CrossRef] [PubMed]
34. Wieland, M.L.; Weis, J.A.; Palmer, T.; Goodson, M.; Loth, S.; Omer, F.; Abbenyi, A.; Krucker, K.; Edens, K.; Sia, I.G. Physical activity and nutrition among immigrant and refugee women: A community-based participatory research approach. *Women's Health Issues* **2012**, *22*, e225–e232. [CrossRef]
35. Marinescu, L.G.M.N.; Sharify, D.; Krieger, J.M.D.M.P.H.; Saelens, B.E.P.; Calleja, J.; Aden, A. Be Active Together: Supporting Physical Activity in Public Housing Communities Through Women-Only Programs. *Prog. Community Health Partnersh.* **2013**, *7*, 57–66. [CrossRef] [PubMed]
36. Dave, S.S.; Craft, L.L.; Mehta, P.; Naval, S.; Kumar, S.; Kandula, N.R. Life stage influences on U.S. South Asian women's physical activity. *Am. J. Health Promot. AJHP* **2015**, *29*, e100–e108. [CrossRef] [PubMed]
37. Australian Government Department of Health. Australia's Physical Activity and Sedentary Behaviour Guidelines for Adults (18–64 Years). Available online: https://www.health.gov.au/health-topics/physical-activity-and-exercise/physical-activity-and-exercise-guidelines-for-all-australians/for-adults-18-to-64-years (accessed on 10 May 2021).
38. Rosenstock, I.M. The health belief model: Explaining health behavior through expectancies. In *Health Behavior and Health Education: Theory, Research, and Practice*; The Jossey-Bass Health Series; Jossey-Bass: San Francisco, CA, USA, 1990; pp. 39–62.
39. Azungah, T. Qualitative research: Deductive and inductive approaches to data analysis. *Qual. Res. J.* **2018**, *18*, 383–400. [CrossRef]
40. The World Bank. South Asia. Available online: https://www.worldbank.org/en/region/sar (accessed on 20 January 2022).
41. Cortis, N. Social Inclusion and Sport: Culturally diverse women's perspectives. *Aust. J. Soc. Issues* **2009**, *44*, 91–106. [CrossRef]
42. Caperchione, C.M.; Kolt, G.S.; Tennent, R.; Mummery, W.K. Physical activity behaviours of Culturally and Linguistically Diverse (CALD) women living in Australia: A qualitative study of socio-cultural influences. *BMC Public Health* **2011**, *11*, 26. [CrossRef]
43. Cargo, M.; Mercer, S.L. The value and challenges of participatory research: Strengthening its practice. *Annu. Rev. Public Health* **2008**, *29*, 325–350. [CrossRef]
44. McLeroy, K.R.; Bibeau, D.; Steckler, A.; Glanz, K. An ecological perspective on health promotion programs. *Health Educ. Q.* **1988**, *15*, 351–377. [CrossRef]
45. Wallerstein, N.B.D.; Yen, I.H.P.M.P.H.; Syme, S.L.P. Integration of Social Epidemiology and Community-Engaged Interventions to Improve Health Equity. *Am. J. Public Health* **2011**, *101*, 822–830. [CrossRef]
46. Horowitz, C.R.; Robinson, M.; Seifer, S. Community-based participatory research from the margin to the mainstream: Are researchers prepared? *Circulation* **2009**, *119*, 2633–2642. [CrossRef]
47. Altman, D.G. Challenges in sustaining public health interventions. *Health Educ. Behav.* **2009**, *36*, 24–28, discussion 9–30. [CrossRef]

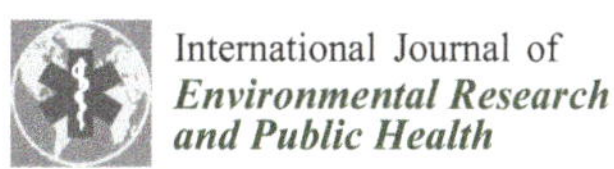

International Journal of
*Environmental Research
and Public Health*

MDPI

Article

Mental Illness Stigma and Associated Factors among Arabic-Speaking Religious and Community Leaders

Klimentina Krstanoska-Blazeska [1], Russell Thomson [2] and Shameran Slewa-Younan [1,3,*]

[1] Mental Health, Translational Health Research Institute, School of Medicine, Western Sydney University, Sydney, NSW 2560, Australia; klimentinakrstanoskablazeska@gmail.com
[2] Centre for Research in Mathematics and Data Science, Western Sydney University, Sydney, NSW 2560, Australia; russell.thomson@westernsydney.edu.au
[3] Centre for Mental Health, Melbourne School of Population and Global Health, University of Melbourne, Melbourne, VIC 3053, Australia
* Correspondence: s.younan@westernsydney.edu.au; Tel.: +61-2-4634-4579

Abstract: Evidence suggests that Arabic-speaking refugees in Australia seek help from informal sources, including religious and community leaders, when experiencing mental health issues. Despite their significant influence, there is scarce research exploring attitudes of Arabic-speaking leaders toward mental illness. The current exploratory study explored mental illness stigma and various factors among Arabic-speaking religious and community leaders. This study uses a subset of data from an evaluation trial of mental health literacy training for Arabic-speaking religious and community leaders. Our dataset contains the pre-intervention survey responses for 52 Arabic-speaking leaders (69.2% female; mean age = 47.1, SD = 15.3) on the ability to recognise a mental disorder, beliefs about causes for developing mental illness, and two stigma measures, personal stigma, and social distance. Being female was associated with a decrease in personal stigma. An increase in age was associated with an increase in personal stigma. Correct recognition of a mental disorder was associated with decreased personal stigma, and after adjusting for age and gender, significance was retained for the I-would-not-tell-anyone subscale. Endorsing the cause "being a person of weak character" was associated with an increase in personal stigma. There is an urgent need for future research to elucidate stigma to develop effective educational initiatives for stigma reduction among Arabic-speaking leaders.

Keywords: religious and community leaders; Arabic-speaking; refugees; stigma; mental illness

Citation: Krstanoska-Blazeska, K.; Thomson, R.; Slewa-Younan, S. Mental Illness Stigma and Associated Factors among Arabic-Speaking Religious and Community Leaders. *Int. J. Environ. Res. Public Health* **2021**, *18*, 7991. https://doi.org/10.3390/ijerph18157991

Academic Editor: Paul B. Tchounwou

Received: 16 June 2021
Accepted: 26 July 2021
Published: 28 July 2021

Publisher's Note: MDPI stays neutral with regard to jurisdictional claims in published maps and institutional affiliations.

1. Introduction

Arabic-speaking individuals represent a majority of the refugee population in Australia [1]. Indeed, Arabic was the top language spoken by humanitarian entrants who entered Australia between the years 2000 and 2014 with approximately 22% of humanitarian entrants speaking Arabic [2]. In the past five years, over half of the visas granted under Australia's Refugee and Humanitarian Program were to individuals born in Iraq or Syria fleeing their country due to persecution, violence, and human rights violations [1]. Pre-migration experiences characterised by exposure to traumatic events and post-migration stressors place refugees at higher risk of developing mental disorders, particularly post-traumatic stress disorder (PTSD) and depression [3,4]. A systematic review of the literature on PTSD in Iraqi refugees resettled in Western countries revealed a prevalence rate ranging from 8% to 37.2% for PTSD and ranging from 28.3% to 75% for depression [5]. The elevated prevalence rate for developing mental disorders among refugees surpasses the general Australian population [6] and endures five years or longer after resettlement [7].

Despite elevated rates of mental illness and psychological distress, resettled refugees in Australia demonstrate low uptake of mental health services [8,9]. Instead, Arabic-speaking individuals and refugees demonstrate a preference for informal sources of help such as family, friends, and religious leaders [10–12]. Several factors are suggested to contribute to low levels of professional help-seeking. One key concept related to help-seeking behaviours and attitudes is mental health literacy (MHL) which is defined as: "knowledge and beliefs about mental disorders which aid their recognition, management or prevention" [13] (p. 182). Poor levels of MHL, particularly low levels of mental illness recognition and treatment knowledge consistent with Western biomedical models, have been reported in Arabic-speaking refugees resettled in Australia and their community leaders [9,14]. Notably, reduced levels of MHL have been associated with stigma [15]. Stigma may be conceptualised as an interaction of negative cognitions, emotional reactions, and behaviours [16]. Mental health-related stigma is especially prominent and problematic in Arabic-speaking communities [14,17].

Central to MHL are beliefs about the causes of mental illness. Although there is some evidence Arabic-speaking individuals endorse beliefs about mental illness consistent with biomedical models (e.g., chemical imbalance), supernatural and religious attributions of mental illness prevail in Arab society, even among medical students, paediatric hospital staff, and mental health professionals [18–20]. Stigmatising beliefs include mental illness originating from evil supernatural forces [21] or caused by a lack of faith and sin [14]. Stemming from the belief of the supernatural or higher-order origin of mental illness, seeking informal help from religious leaders or traditional healers is often the norm [14,22].

To understand the pervasiveness of stigmatising attitudes toward mental illness and help-seeking in Arab society, cultural influences of collectivism and the significance of the family unit must be considered. It has been posited that in collectivistic cultures, "non-normal" behaviour is more obvious and less tolerated within the community [23,24]. Members of the public tend to react with discriminatory behaviours towards people with mental illness (PWMI), such as a desire to distance oneself from those with mental illness to avoid public stigma [16]. High levels of reluctance to associate with PWMI across a range of social situations and relationships, including friends, teachers, neighbours, and family members have been well-documented in studies conducted with Arabic-speaking individuals [21,25–27].

The presence of mental illness in the family unit typically brings dishonour, damaging reputation and social standing [10,28]. In turn, family members are commonly discouraged from seeking professional help [14]. Mental illness is particularly stigmatising for women [29] and it is common for women to experience feelings of shame and embarrassment about seeking help outside the family [30]. However, it has been suggested Arabic-speaking females are more likely to seek counselling from professionals compared to males, consistent with findings from the general Australian community [31], in addition to religious assistance [14].

1.1. Arabic-Speaking Religious and Community Leaders

If help is sought for mental health problems, approaching religious and community leaders or traditional healers are often the first points of contact [14,32]. Religious leaders are swiftly available, willing to help individuals experiencing a crisis, and seeking their assistance is considered a less stigmatising and shameful action compared to seeking professional help [14]. Immigration and separation from traditional support may also prompt individuals who have migrated to new countries to seek greater affiliation with religious and community leaders [14,33].

General practitioners in the Australian Arab community reported leaders significantly influence whether an individual seeks professional mental health care such as from a psychiatrist or a general practitioner [14]. Despite their paramount influence, to our knowledge, only two studies exploring the attitudes of Arabic-speaking religious and/or community leaders toward mental illness. A Ph.D. dissertation comprising two published papers involving religious leaders in Sydney revealed a majority of leaders endorsed "drug/alcohol addiction" (93.5%) and psychosocial issues (91.2–93.5%) as important causes of mental illness [34]. However, religious causes were also rated as important (57.1–84.7%).

Muslim leaders endorsed religious causes such as the "will of God" or "spiritual poverty" as more important causes for mental illness compared to Christian leaders [34]. One leader interviewed indicated a lack of confidence in the Western approach where the physical body is treated with medication often resulting in little improvement [14].

A recent study investigated Arabic-speaking Catholic male clerics' attitudes regarding mental health in Lebanon [35]. A majority (84.9%) believed they would recognise a patient with mental illness. However, this was not objectively measured using a vignette methodology. Concerning causal beliefs regarding mental illness, "traumatic childhood" and "drug/alcohol addiction" were endorsed as most important and 70% agreed chemical imbalance is a causal factor. Despite a majority denying religious causes, 20–30% endorsed the notion that "spiritual poverty" and "demonic possession" are causes. Stigmatising attitudes endorsed by a majority of clerics equated a person with mental illness to a young child in terms of the control and discipline s/he requires, conveyed PWMI should have restrictions placed on their individual rights, and "are a burden on society". Overall, the scarce research conducted to date seems to suggest Arabic-speaking leaders may hold stigmatising beliefs and attitudes, however, additional research is required. Moreover, an understanding of whether factors such as age and gender play a role in the stigmatising beliefs and attitudes toward mental illness held by Arabic-speaking leaders is important in developing targeted mental health promotion messages.

1.2. Current Study

The role of religious leaders in providing mental health care and facilitating help-seeking processes within immigrant communities is crucial [36–38]. To promote and facilitate the uptake of specialised mental health treatment for refugees, there is a critical need to explore stigma among Arabic-speaking leaders. If leaders have high levels of stigma themselves, this will negatively impact help-seeking and attitudes toward mental illness in the community. The aim of the current study is to explore relationships between measures of stigma and various factors in Arabic-speaking religious and community leaders. Drawing from the previous literature, it was hypothesised good MHL (i.e., correct problem recognition, knowledge of causes), will be associated with lower levels of stigma [32,39,40]. It was hypothesised being female and younger will be associated with lower levels of stigma [19,39,41].

2. Materials and Methods

2.1. Participants, Procedure, and Study Design

The present study is a subset of a dataset evaluating an MHL training course for Arabic-speaking religious and community leaders in South Western Sydney, Australia [42]. A total of 54 participants undertook a 6 h MHL training workshop (see Slewa-Younan and colleagues [42] for an overview of the intervention and power analysis). Of these individuals, 52 participants completed a self-report survey prior to and immediately following training but this study only utilised the pre-intervention survey responses. The training was advertised via religious centres and refugee service networks within South Western Sydney. Participants comprised volunteers who approached the workshop coordinator for enrolment. Individuals met eligibility criteria to participate if they were from an Arabic background, recognised themselves as religious or other community leaders, regularly communicated with Arabic-speaking refugee populations, and possessed a level of proficiency of the English language to ensure the understanding and the completion of the survey. The South Western Sydney Health Local District Research Ethics Committee (reference number 2019/ETH12040), jointly with Western Sydney University (H13411), provided approval of the research. Participants provided informed consent to participate in the study and for their data to be used in the research. Informed consent was obtained from participants when they attended the MHL training workshop and completed the pre-intervention survey. We would like to acknowledge that data from each participant in this study cannot be shared in order to comply with the protocols approved by the South

Western Sydney Local Health District and Western Sydney University Human Research Ethics Committees.

2.2. Measures

The survey utilised in the current study is based on a survey developed by Jorm and colleagues [13] to assess MHL and has been adapted for refugee populations and utilised in a previous study by Slewa-Younan and colleagues [9]. Socio-demographic characteristics were also collected.

2.3. Recognition of PTSD as Dawood's Main Problem

Previous studies have validated the use of a vignette for measuring MHL [43]. A culturally valid vignette portraying an Iraqi male refugee ("Dawood") was used to assess participants' ability to recognise Dawood's mental health problem as PTSD. Dawood's character met the 5th edition of the Diagnostic and Statistical Manual of Mental Disorders criteria for PTSD [44]. After participants read Dawood's story, they were presented with an open-ended question: "What, if anything, do you think is wrong with Dawood?". Open-ended responses correctly recognising Dawood's character as having PTSD were coded as "Yes" if they mentioned any of the following wording: "PTSD"; "post-traumatic stress disorder"; "post-trauma/tic-stress/disorder"; and "PTS". Responses that did not mention any of the aforementioned wording were coded as "No".

2.4. Stigmatising Attitudes

Stigmatising attitudes toward mental illness were assessed via a personal stigma scale and social distance scale. The personal stigma scale assessed participants' personal attitudes towards the character depicted in the vignette ("Dawood") using statements adapted from an Australian National Survey [43,45]. Participants responded to seven statements assessing personal stigma using a 5-point Likert-style scale (1 = strongly disagree to 5 = strongly agree). The personal stigma scale was made up of three subscales: Dangerous/unpredictable, Weak-not-sick, and I-would-not-tell-anyone. The Dangerous/unpredictable subscale comprised items about Dawood's dangerousness or unpredictability due to mental problems (e.g., "Dawood's problem makes him unpredictable"). The Weak-not-sick subscale comprised items about the legitimacy and controllability of Dawood's problems and the weakness of Dawood's character (e.g., "Dawood's problem is not a real medical illness"). The I-would-not-tell-anyone subscale comprised one item assessing if the participant would tell others if they had a problem like Dawood's ("You would not tell anyone if you had a problem like Dawood's"). The three subscales have been validated via structural equation modelling using data from a large Australian adult national survey [43] and utilised and validated in previous studies [46,47]. Higher scores for each subscale indicated higher levels of personal stigma.

The second measure of stigmatising attitudes toward mental illness comprised a Social Distance scale using statements developed by Link and colleagues [48]. The Social Distance scale assessed participants' willingness to participate in various hypothetical relationships (e.g., neighbour, friend, colleague) with Dawood [48,49]. Participants were asked whether they would be happy: "to move next door to Dawood"; "to spend an evening socialising with Dawood"; etc. Participants responded to five statements assessing Social Distance using a 5-point Likert-style scale (1 = strongly disagree to 5 = strongly agree). A total Social Distance score was calculated by summing up the responses to each item. Higher scores indicated a greater desire for social distance.

2.5. Beliefs about Causes for Developing Mental Illness

Participants answered a question about possible causes of Dawood's problem. Participants were asked: "How likely do you think each of the following is a factor in this sort of problem developing in anybody?". Eleven causes were presented including "Punishment from God", "Experiencing a traumatic event", and "Being a person with a weak character".

Participants rated each item as "very likely", "likely", or "not likely". For analysis purposes, responses for causes were recoded into 1 = "likely" ("likely" and "very likely" collapsed) and 0 = "not likely".

2.6. Statistical Analyses

Statistical analyses were performed using the Statistical Package for Social Sciences (SPSS 26.0 for Mac, IBM Corp., Armonk, NY, USA). Firstly, a non-parametric Kendall's Tau-b correlation was run to determine relationships between stigma scales. To test whether socio-demographic variables predicted stigma scale scores, standard multiple regression analyses with bootstrapping based on 1000 samples were performed with a stigma scale as the dependent variable and age and gender as independent variables. For the multiple linear regression models, percentage variance was presented based on R^2. To measure the effect of stigma on the ability to correctly identify PTSD as Dawood's main problem, four binary logistic regression analyses were undertaken with correct recognition of PTSD as the dependent variable and a stigma scale as the independent variable. Because age and/or gender predicted some stigma scales, logistic regression models were adjusted for age and gender thereafter.

To explore whether stigma affected the likelihood of endorsing a cause as "likely" for developing a problem like Dawood's, a series of binary logistic regression analyses were performed. For each logistic regression analysis, a cause (e.g., "Punishment from God") was entered as the dependent variable and a stigma scale (e.g., "Weak-not-sick") was entered as the independent variable. Because age and/or gender predicted some stigma scales, logistic regression models were adjusted for age and gender thereafter. Logistic regression results were presented as odds ratios. A $p < 0.05$ was considered statistically significant.

3. Results

Socio-demographic characteristics of participants are presented in Table 1. A majority of the stigma scales were significantly correlated (Table 2). To reduce the risk of collinearity, separate regression analyses were conducted when exploring associations between each stigma scale and socio-demographic variables, correct recognition of PTSD, and endorsement of a cause. Means and standard deviations for stigma scale scores were: Weak-not-sick (M = 7.5; SD = 3.2); I-would-not-tell-anyone (M = 2.0; SD = 1.1); Dangerous/unpredictable (M = 6.2; SD = 2.4); Social Distance (M = 9.3; SD = 2.3).

Table 1. Socio-demographic Characteristics.

Characteristics	Pre-Training (*n* = 52) *	
	N	Valid %
Gender		
Male	16	30.8
Female	36	69.2
Age (M, SD)	47.1 (15.3)	
Country of Origin (top 3)		
Iraq	18	33.3
Australia	13	24.1
Lebanon	8	14.8
Organisations represented by participants		
Churches/Mosques	17	32.7
Non-government organisation	21	40.4
Government organisation	14	26.9
Language spoken at home (top 3)		
Arabic	39	72.2
English	7	13
Assyrian	2	3.7
Marital Status		
Never married	7	13.7

Table 1. *Cont.*

Characteristics	Pre-Training (*n* = 52) *	
	N	Valid %
Married	35	68.6
Fiancée/partner	2	3.9
Divorced	6	11.8
Widowed	1	2
Education		
High school	3	5.6
Certificate	5	9.3
Diploma	5	9.3
Bachelor	31	57.4
Masters	6	11.1
For those born overseas		
Years in Australia (M, SD)	17.6 (10.9)	
Arrival status in Australia		
Refugee	7	19.4
Migrant	29	80.6
Religion		
Muslim	34	65.4
Christian	17	32.7

* Due to missing data may not add to 52.

Table 2. Kendall's Tau-b Correlations of Personal Stigma Subscales and Social Distance Scale.

Variable	I-Would-Not-Tell-Anyone	Weak-Not-Sick	Dangerous/Unpredictable
I-would-not-tell-anyone			
Weak-not-sick	0.43 ***		
Dangerous/unpredictable	0.50 ***	0.34 ***	
Social distance	0.18	0.20	0.33 **

*** $p < 0.001$; ** $p < 0.01$ (2-tailed).

3.1. Stigmatising Attitudes and Socio-Demographic Factors

Bootstrapping, a non-parametric resampling procedure, was used to test for statistical significance because the Kolmogorov–Smirnov test revealed the personal stigma subscales and Social Distance were not normally distributed ($p < 0.05$). For the regression analysis with Weak-not-sick as the dependent variable, gender (male = 1; female = 2) had a significant negative regression weight. Females were found to have lower Weak-not-sick scores compared to males, after controlling for age (Table 3). Age had a significant positive regression weight, indicating for a unit increase in age there was an increase in Weak-not-sick scores, after controlling for gender (Table 3). Age and gender explained 27.8% of the variation in the Weak-not-sick score. For the regression analysis with Social Distance as the dependent variable, bootstrapped coefficients revealed age had a significant positive regression weight, indicating for a unit increase in age there was an increase in Social Distance, after controlling for gender ($b = 0.04$, Bias = 0.00, Bootstrap SE = 0.02, 95% CI = 0.00, 0.08, $p = 0.042$). Age and gender explained 7.1% of the variation in the Social Distance score. Regression analyses with I-would-not-tell-anyone and Dangerous/unpredictable as dependent variables did not reveal significant differences. Age and gender explained 6.4% of the variation in the I-would-not-tell-anyone score. Age and gender explained 10.9% of the variation in the Dangerous/unpredictable score.

Table 3. Bootstrap coefficients for multiple linear regression model of socio-demographic predictors of Weak-not-sick subscale, with 95% percentile confidence intervals. Confidence intervals and standard errors are based on 1000 bootstrap samples.

Model	*B*	Bias	SE	*p*	95% CI (Lower, Upper)
Constant	7.27	−0.07	2.25	0.003	2.97, 12.00
Gender	−2.06	−0.01	0.91	0.036 *	−3.86, −0.08
Age	0.08	0.00	0.03	0.011 *	0.03, 0.13

Note. n = 50 due to missing data; *B* = Bootstrap regression coefficient; Bias = Bootstrap bias estimate; SE = Bootstrap standard error; CI (lower, upper) = confidence interval (lower limit, upper limit). * *p* Value is significant.

3.2. Stigmatising Attitudes and Recognition of PTSD as Dawood's Main Problem

Fifty-one percent of participants correctly identified PTSD. Logistic regression models revealed significant results for personal stigma subscales, but not for Social Distance. For every single level increase in I-would-not-tell-anyone, the odds of correctly identifying PTSD decreased by a factor of 0.44 (95% CI = 0.23, 0.84, p = 0.013). For every single level increase in Weak-not-sick, the odds of correctly identifying PTSD decreased by a factor of 0.82 (95% CI = 0.68, 0.99, p = 0.039). For every single level increase in Dangerous/unpredictable, the odds of correctly identifying PTSD decreased by a factor of 0.77 (95% CI = 0.59, 0.99, p = 0.042). After adjusting for age and gender, significant results were retained for I-would-not-tell-anyone (Table 4).

Table 4. Odds ratios of eight logistic regression analyses of predictors of correct recognition of PTSD and endorsement of a cause as "likely", adjusted for age and gender.

Variables	Problem Recognition (Dependent Variable)	Cause (Dependent Variable)
Personal stigma subscales and Social distance scale (independent variables)	Correct recognition of PTSD (95% CI lower, upper)	"being a person of weak character" (95% CI lower, upper)
I-would-not-tell-anyone subscale	0.48 * (0.25, 0.94)	2.52 * (1.17, 5.44)
Weak-not-sick subscale	0.88 (0.71, 1.10)	1.32 * (1.03, 1.68)
Dangerous/unpredictable subscale	0.83 (0.63, 1.10)	1.46 * (1.06, 2.02)
Social Distance scale	1.00 (0.77, 1.29)	0.99 (0.76, 1.30)

Note. Only causes that yielded statistically significant results are presented; Regressions presented are adjusted for age and gender; CI lower, upper = confidence interval lower limit, upper limit for odds ratio. * $p < 0.05$.

3.3. Stigmatising Attitudes and Beliefs about Causes for Developing Mental Illness

The cause "being a person of weak character" was endorsed as "likely" by 43.1% of participants. Logistic regression analyses for the cause "being a person of weak character" and personal stigma subscales revealed significant results. For every single level increase in I-would-not-tell-anyone, the odds of rating "being a person of weak character" as a "likely" cause increased by a factor of 2.49 (95% CI = 1.26, 4.95, p = 0.009). Additionally, for every single level increase in Weak-not-sick, the odds of rating "being a person of weak character" as a "likely" cause increased by a factor of 1.45 (95% CI = 1.16, 1.80, p = 0.001). Finally, for every single level increase in Dangerous/unpredictable, the odds of rating "being a person of weak character" as a "likely" cause increased by a factor of 1.58 (95% CI = 1.17, 2.14, p = 0.003). After adjusting for age and gender, significant results were retained (Table 4).

4. Discussion

This preliminary study sought to explore mental illness stigma and associated factors among Arabic-speaking leaders. As expected, females were shown to have lower Weak-not-sick scores compared to males. An increase in age of one year was associated with an increase in Weak-not-sick and Social distance scores. In terms of problem recognition, a central component of good MHL, the odds of correctly identifying PTSD decreased for every single level increase in personal stigma. After adjusting for age and gender, the odds of correctly identifying PTSD decreased for every single level increase in the I-would-not-tell-anyone subscale only. Finally, the odds of selecting "being a person of weak character" as a cause increased for every single level increase in personal stigma.

Female leaders were predicted to have lower Weak-not-sick scores compared to male leaders. This gender difference in the Weak-not-sick subscale has been reported in the general Australian adult population [43]. Further, females compared to males, have been shown to have lower stigmatising attitudes in a Lebanese sample [39] and a Slovakian sample [50]. In contrast to the current finding, Arabic-speaking males have been shown to have more positive attitudes toward mental illness compared to females (see Zolezzi and colleagues [21] for a systematic review). Thus, our findings contribute to the existing mixed results among Arabic-speaking individuals which appear to be less conclusive than Australian-based research [41].

Weak-not-sick was the sole subscale revealing gender differences which may reflect the intersectionality of mental illness stigma and male gender roles in Arab society. The expression of negative emotional experiences may threaten a male's capacity to perform their expected role as reliable and strong provider for the family unit [12]. Typically, disclosure of psychological problems is highly discouraged for males [12,51]. 'Dawood's' symptoms appear to have affected his ability to provide for his family as he was portrayed as withdrawing from the lives of his children and questioning his life. In one Egyptian study, a female displaying symptoms of depression elicited more acceptance as a family member than a male [26]. Therefore, male gender roles and expectations in Arab culture may have influenced specific attitudes toward mental illness in the current study.

An increase in age was associated with increased Weak-not-sick scores and a higher desire for social distance, after controlling for gender. Older age has been associated with more stigmatising attitudes toward mental illness [50,52] and an increased desire for social distance [53]. Although preliminary, these findings are especially interesting as a previous study with male Arab Catholic clerics in Lebanon was unable to detect a significant relationship between age and attitudes toward PWMI [35]. A relationship between stigmatising beliefs about the causes of mental illness in Muslim clerics compared to Christian clerics has been demonstrated [34]. Although the current study did not explore the relationship between religion, country of origin, and stigma, the socio-demographic characteristics of the current study's participants (e.g., majority of Muslim leaders) may have contributed to a difference in findings. This difference may also be related to our use of a vignette, allowing for a specific measure of personal stigma toward a character portrayed rather than general attitudes toward mental illness.

Correct recognition was associated with decreased levels of personal stigma. This is consistent with the finding that better attitudes toward mental illness was associated with more knowledge of mental illness in a Lebanese sample [39]. If a label of a specific disorder is placed, rather than placing a general label of "mental illness", this may activate knowledge of specific treatments or steps to take to treat the illness and relate to beneficial attitudes [15]. To our knowledge, this is the first study to explore the relationship between the ability to recognise a specific mental disorder and stigma in Arabic-speaking individuals. Our preliminary findings indicate a necessity for future research to further investigate this complex relationship of stigma in Arabic-speaking individuals and across various mental disorders. Our finding also suggests initiatives aimed at reducing mental illness stigma should consider incorporating training to improve the ability to recognise specific mental disorders, as these concepts may be related.

Personal stigma was associated with a negative belief that being a weak person is a cause for developing a problem like Dawood's. Similarly, the belief in a weak personality as a cause for various mental disorders was associated with higher scores on personal stigma in an Australian national survey [54]. Almost two-thirds of Iraqi individuals believed personal weakness is the cause of mental illness [55]. Endorsing weakness of character as a cause of mental illness is indicative of a dominant negative stereotype of mental illness and linked to low MHL [41,56]. This finding may be reflective of Arab cultural beliefs that link negative emotional expression with weakness, especially if such expression damages the family's social standing and elicits public stigma [10,57].

Among refugee men, self-stigma for seeking help was a significant barrier to seeking help from not only formal sources but also from informal community sources [58]. If an individual chooses to first seek help from a leader, it is crucial leaders are aware of the vulnerabilities associated with seeking help [59]. The knowledge that such individuals are likely in the process of navigating their self-worth and identity in the context of experiencing a mental illness in a patriarchal society and strong adherence to masculine ideals should be imparted in any educational initiatives.

4.1. Limitations and Strengths

The current study's limitations include a cross-sectional design which does not allow for causal explanations and the risk of social desirability as participants were leaders within the refugee community. Notably, the small sample size is a limitation in the current study, and future research with larger sample size is required to confirm the current findings. Participants were also individuals who actively sought MHL training. With regard to strengths, the use of a vignette allowed adaption to ensure a culturally sensitive measure to assess MHL. Research on MHL is primarily conducted using measures tapping into the Western biomedical conceptualisation of mental illness. Previous studies have resulted in conclusions of low MHL among culturally diverse populations including Arabic-speaking individuals despite lacking consideration of cultural perspectives on beliefs and treatment knowledge [12]. Evidently, the participants in our study reside in Western society. However, this does not entirely diminish the findings as contributing to our knowledge of MHL among culturally diverse populations.

4.2. Constraints on Generality

Arabic-speaking individuals are not a homogenous group and readers must keep the socio-demographic characteristics of the participants depicted in Table 1 in mind when generalising the findings. For example, our participants reside in Australia, a Western society, which may limit the generalisability of the current findings to Arabic-speaking leaders in Eastern societies. Further, refugee and humanitarian entrants in NSW have largely settled in the South Western Sydney local health district meaning the leaders in the current study may have higher exposure to refugees compared to leaders in other local health districts in NSW [60].

The results of the current study likely depend on the materials used. Our measure of MHL and stigmatising attitudes was limited to one vignette depicting a married male who is a father experiencing a specific mental disorder, PTSD. Readers should be cautious about generalising the findings as stigmatising attitudes and mental health literacy may vary depending on the character depicted in the vignette. For example, gender has been reported to moderate mental illness stigma [61]. Future research should utilise vignettes that depict individuals of various socio-demographic characteristics and types of mental illness. The findings of such studies will further inform specific target areas for reducing stigma through educational initiatives for Arabic-speaking leaders.

4.3. Clinical Implications

The mental health beliefs of the leaders in our study may represent a challenge to treatment adherence. Psychologists are encouraged to adopt a multilevel approach and collaborate with the client's family, religious, and community leaders. Psychologists should be willing to reach out to leaders within their client's community to develop insight into and a shared understanding of their client's worldview. Psychologists should be aware of the limitations of Western-based models underpinning cognitive-behavioural interventions when applied to Arabic-speaking individuals [62]. Such Western-based models may be different from the conceptualisations of mental illness Arabic-speaking refugees and their leaders possess. Challenging cognitive distortions and faulty beliefs posited to maintain symptoms of mental illness are core tools used in cognitive-behavioural therapy [63]. However, if clients are exposed to mental health beliefs from their leaders such as an experience of depression represents a test in life, an opportunity to cleanse and become more religious, as noted by a leader in Youssef and Deane's [14] study, challenging this thinking is likely to mismatch the client's worldview and they may feel misunderstood. Rather than challenging such beliefs, psychologists should be sensitive to these issues and deliver interventions that work alongside how Arabic-speaking refugee communities view and respond to mental illness, encompassing their cultural and religious beliefs.

5. Conclusions

Our preliminary findings lay the groundwork for future research by exploring factors associated with stigma among Arabic-speaking religious and community leaders. Leaders have immense potential to influence help-seeking and foster helpful attitudes toward mental illness. Our findings indicate an urgent need for future larger-scale research to further elucidate stigma, thereby, refining stigma reduction initiatives among Arabic-speaking leaders.

Author Contributions: Conceptualization, S.S.-Y.; Data curation, S.S.-Y.; Formal analysis, K.K.-B., R.T. and S.S.-Y.; Funding acquisition, S.S.-Y.; Investigation, S.S.-Y.; Methodology, S.S.-Y.; Project administration, S.S.-Y.; Supervision, S.S.-Y.; Writing–original draft, K.K.-B., R.T. and S.S.-Y.; Writing–review and editing, K.K.-B. and S.S.-Y. All authors have read and agreed to the published version of the manuscript.

Funding: This research was funded by the South Western Sydney Primary Health Network (SWSPHN) to Western Sydney University through the Fairfield City Health Alliance Health Literacy Working Group.

Institutional Review Board Statement: The study was conducted according to the guidelines of the National Statement on Ethical Conduct in Human Research (2007) and was approved by the South Western Sydney Health Local District Research Ethics Committee (reference number 2019/ETH12040), jointly with Western Sydney University (H13411) provided approval of the research on the 1 August 2019.

Informed Consent Statement: Informed consent was obtained from all of the subjects involved in the study. Participants provided informed consent to participate in the study and for their data to be used in the research. Informed consent was obtained from participants when they attended the MHL training workshop and completed the pre-intervention survey.

Data Availability Statement: We would like to acknowledge that data from each participant in this study cannot be shared in order to comply with the protocols approved by the South Western Sydney Local Health District and Western Sydney University Human Research Ethics Committees.

Acknowledgments: We would like to thank all of the participants from the Arabic-speaking community who participated in the study.

Conflicts of Interest: The authors declare no conflict of interest.

References

1. Department of Home Affairs. Australia's Offshore Humanitarian Program: 2018–19. Available online: https://www.homeaffairs.gov.au/research-and-stats/files/australia-offshore-humanitarian-program-2018-19.pdf (accessed on 22 July 2021).
2. Federation of Ethnic Communities' Councils of Australia. Australia's Growing Linguistic Diversity an Opportunity for a Strategic Approach to Language Services Policy and Practice. Available online: http://fecca.org.au/wp-content/uploads/2016/09/feccalanguagesreport.pdf (accessed on 21 July 2021).
3. Keyes, E.F. Mental health status in refugees: An integrative review of current research. *Issues Ment. Health Nurs.* **2000**, *21*, 397–410. [CrossRef]
4. Steel, Z.; Chey, T.; Silove, D.; Marnane, C.; Bryant, R.A.; Van Ommeren, M. Association of torture and other potentially traumatic events with mental health outcomes among populations exposed to mass conflict and displacement: A systematic review and meta-analysis. *JAMA* **2009**, *302*, 537–549. [CrossRef]
5. Slewa-Younan, S.; Uribe Guajardo, M.G.; Heriseanu, A.; Hasan, T. A systematic review of post-traumatic stress disorder and depression amongst Iraqi refugees located in Western countries. *J. Immigr. Minor. Health* **2015**, *17*, 1231–1239. [CrossRef]

6.   Australian Bureau of Statistics. National Survey of Mental Health and Wellbeing: Summary of Results. Report No. 4326.0. Available online: https://www.ausstats.abs.gov.au/ausstats/subscriber.nsf/0/6AE6DA447F985FC2CA2574EA00122BD6/$File/National%20Survey%20of%20Mental%20Health%20and%20Wellbeing%20Summary%20of%20Results.pdf (accessed on 22 July 2021).

7.   Bogic, M.; Njoku, A.; Priebe, S. Long-term mental health of war-refugees: A systematic literature review. *BMC Int. Health Hum. Rights* **2015**, *15*, 29. [CrossRef]

8.   De Anstiss, H.; Ziaian, T.; Procter, N.; Warland, J.; Baghurst, P. Help-seeking for mental health problems in young refugees: A review of the literature with implications for policy, practice, and research. *Transcult. Psychiatry* **2009**, *46*, 584–607. [CrossRef]

9.   Slewa-Younan, S.; Mond, J.; Bussion, E.; Mohammad, Y.; Uribe Guajardo, M.G.; Smith, M.; Milosevic, D.; Lujic, S.; Jorm, A.F. Mental health literacy of resettled Iraqi refugees in Australia: Knowledge about posttraumatic stress disorder and beliefs about helpfulness of interventions. *BMC Psychiatry* **2014**, *14*, 320. [CrossRef]

10.   Al-Darmaki, F.R. Attitudes towards seeking professional psychological help: What really counts for United Arab Emirates university students? *Soc. Behav. Personal.* **2003**, *31*, 497–508. [CrossRef]

11.   Al-Krenawi, A.; Graham, J.R. Social work and Koranic mental health healers. *Int. Soc. Work* **1999**, *42*, 53–65. [CrossRef]

12.   Byrow, Y.; Pajak, R.; Specker, P.; Nickerson, A. Perceptions of mental health and perceived barriers to mental health help-seeking amongst refugees: A systematic review. *Clin. Psychol. Rev.* **2020**, *75*, 101812. [CrossRef]

13.   Jorm, A.F.; Korten, A.E.; Jacomb, P.A.; Christensen, H.; Rodgers, B.; Pollitt, P. "Mental health literacy": A survey of the public's ability to recognise mental disorders and their beliefs about the effectiveness of treatment. *Med. J. Aust.* **1997**, *166*, 182–186. [CrossRef] [PubMed]

14.   Youssef, J.; Deane, F.P. Factors influencing mental-health help-seeking in Arabic-speaking communities in Sydney, Australia. *Ment. Health Relig. Cult.* **2006**, *9*, 43–66. [CrossRef]

15.   Jorm, A.F. Mental health literacy: Empowering the community to take action for better mental health. *Am. Psychol.* **2012**, *67*, 231–243. [CrossRef] [PubMed]

16.   Corrigan, P. How stigma interferes with mental health care. *Am. Psychol.* **2004**, *59*, 614–625. [CrossRef] [PubMed]

17.   El-Islam, M.F. Arab culture and mental health care. *Transcult. Psychiatry* **2008**, *45*, 671–682. [CrossRef] [PubMed]

18.   Al-Adawi, S.; Dorvlo, A.S.; Al-Ismaily, S.S.; Al-Ghafry, D.A.; Al-Noobi, B.Z.; Al-Salmi, A.; Burke, D.T.; Shah, M.K.; Ghassany, H.; Chand, S.P. Perception of and attitude towards mental illness in Oman. *Int. J. Soc. Psychiatry* **2002**, *48*, 305–317. [CrossRef]

19.   Hamdan-Mansour, A.M.; Wardam, L.A. Attitudes of Jordanian mental health nurses toward mental illness and patients with mental illness. *Issues Ment. Health Nurs.* **2009**, *30*, 705–711. [CrossRef]

20.   Slewa-Younan, S.; Nguyen, T.; Al-Yateem, N.; Rossiter, R.; Robb, W. Causes and risk factors for common mental illnesses: The beliefs of paediatric hospital staff in the United Arab Emirates. *Int. J. Ment. Health Syst.* **2020**, *14*, 35. [CrossRef]

21.   Zolezzi, M.; Alamri, M.; Shaar, S.; Rainkie, D. Stigma associated with mental illness and its treatment in the Arab culture: A systematic review. *Int. J. Soc. Psychiatry* **2018**, *64*, 597–609. [CrossRef]

22.   Al-Krenawi, A.; Graham, J.R.; Dean, Y.Z.; Eltaiba, N. Cross-national study of attitudes towards seeking professional help: Jordan, United Arab Emirates (UAE) and Arabs in Israel. *Int. J. Soc. Psychiatry* **2004**, *50*, 102–114. [CrossRef]

23.   Alhomaizi, D.; Alsaidi, S.; Moalie, A.; Muradwij, N.; Borba, C.P.C.; Lincoln, A.K. An exploration of the help-seeking behaviors of Arab-Muslims in the US: A socio-ecological approach. *J. Muslim Ment. Health* **2018**, *12*, 19–48. [CrossRef]

24.   Papadopoulos, C.; Foster, J.; Caldwell, K. 'Individualism-collectivism' as an explanatory device for mental illness stigma. *Community Ment. Health J.* **2013**, *49*, 270–280. [CrossRef]

25.   Abolfotouh, M.A.; Almutairi, A.F.; Almutairi, Z.; Salam, M.; Alhashem, A.; Adlan, A.A.; Modayfer, O. Attitudes toward mental illness, mentally ill persons, and help-seeking among the Saudi public and sociodemographic correlates. *Psychol. Res. Behav. Manag.* **2019**, *12*, 45–54. [CrossRef]

26.   Coker, E.M. Selfhood and social distance: Toward a cultural understanding of psychiatric stigma in Egypt. *Soc. Sci. Med.* **2005**, *61*, 920–930. [CrossRef] [PubMed]

27.   Tabassum, R.; Macaskill, A.; Ahmad, I. Attitudes towards mental health in an urban Pakistani community in the United Kingdom. *Int. J. Soc. Psychiatry* **2000**, *46*, 170–181. [CrossRef]

28.   Scull, N.C.; Khullar, N.; Al-Awadhi, N.; Erheim, R. A qualitative study of the perceptions of mental health care in Kuwait. *Int. Perspect. Psychol. Res. Pract. Consult.* **2014**, *3*, 284–299. [CrossRef]

29.   Savaya, R. The under-use of psychological services by Israeli Arabs: An examination of the roles of negative attitudes and the use of alternative sources of help. *Int. Soc. Work* **1998**, *41*, 195–209. [CrossRef]

30.   Abu-Ras, W.M. Barriers to services for Arab immigrant battered women in a Detroit suburb. *J. Soc. Work Res. Eval.* **2003**, *4*, 49–66.

31.   Parslow, R.A.; Jorm, A.F. Who uses mental health services in Australia? An analysis of data from the National Survey of Mental Health and Wellbeing. *Aust. N. Z. J. Psychiatry* **2000**, *34*, 997–1008. [CrossRef] [PubMed]

32.   Aloud, N.; Rathur, A. Factors affecting attitudes towards seeking and using formal mental health and psychological services among Arab Muslim populations. *J. Muslim Ment. Health* **2009**, *4*, 79–103. [CrossRef]

33.   Mackie, F. *Structure, Culture and Religion in the Welfare of Muslim Families: A Study of Immigrants Turkish and Lebanese Men and Women and their Families living in Melbourne*; Australian Government Publishing Service: Canberra, Australia, 1983.

34.   Youssef, J.; Deane, F.P. Arabic-speaking religious leaders' perceptions of the causes of mental illness and the use of medication for treatment. *Aust. N. Z. J. Psychiatry* **2013**, *47*, 1041–1050. [CrossRef] [PubMed]

35. Aramouny, C.; Kerbage, H.; Richa, N.; Rouhana, P.; Richa, S. Knowledge, attitudes, and beliefs of Catholic clerics' regarding mental health in Lebanon. *J. Relig. Health* **2020**, *59*, 257–276. [CrossRef] [PubMed]
36. Abu-Ras, W.; Gheith, A.; Cournos, F. The Imam's role in mental health promotion: A study at 22 Mosques in New York City's Muslim community. *J. Muslim Ment. Health* **2008**, *3*, 155–176. [CrossRef]
37. Ali, O.M.; Milstein, G.; Marzuk, P.M. The Imam's role in meeting the counseling needs of Muslim communities in the United States. *Psychiatr. Serv.* **2005**, *56*, 202–205. [CrossRef]
38. Slewa-Younan, S.; Rioseco, P.; Uribe Guajardo, M.G.; Mond, J. Predictors of professional help-seeking for emotional problems in Afghan and Iraqi refugees in Australia: Findings from the Building a New Life in Australia database. *BMC Public Health* **2019**, *19*, 1485. [CrossRef]
39. Abi Doumit, C.; Haddad, C.; Sacre, H.; Salameh, P.; Akel, M.; Obeid, S.; Akiki, M.; Mattar, E.; Hilal, N.; Hallit, S.; et al. Knowledge, attitude and behaviors towards patients with mental illness: Results from a national Lebanese study. *PLoS ONE* **2019**, *14*, 0222172. [CrossRef]
40. Kitchener, B.A.; Jorm, A.F. Mental health first aid training: Review of evaluation studies. *Aust. N. Z. J. Psychiatry* **2006**, *40*, 6–8. [CrossRef] [PubMed]
41. Reavley, N.J.; Morgan, A.J.; Jorm, A.F. Development of scales to assess mental health literacy relating to recognition of and interventions for depression, anxiety disorders and schizophrenia/psychosis. *Aust. N. Z. J. Psychiatry* **2014**, *48*, 61–69. [CrossRef]
42. Slewa-Younan, S.; Uribe Guajardo, M.G.; Mohammad, Y.; Lim, H.; Martinez, G.; Saleh, R.; Sapucci, M. An evaluation of a mental health literacy course for Arabic speaking religious and community leaders in Australia: Effects on posttraumatic stress disorder related knowledge, attitudes and help-seeking. *Int. J. Ment. Health Syst.* **2020**, *14*, 69. [CrossRef]
43. Yap, M.B.H.; Mackinnon, A.; Reavley, N.; Jorm, A.F. The measurement properties of stigmatizing attitudes towards mental disorders: Results from two community surveys. *Int. J. Methods Psychiatr. Res.* **2014**, *23*, 49–61. [CrossRef]
44. American Psychiatric Association. *Diagnostic and Statistical Manual of Mental Disorders*, 5th ed.; American Psychiatric Association: Arlington, VA, USA, 2013.
45. Griffiths, K.M.; Christensen, H.; Jorm, A.F.; Evans, K.; Groves, C. Effect of web-based literacy and cognitive-behavioural therapy interventions on stigmatising attitudes to depression: Randomised control trial. *Br. J. Psychiatry* **2004**, *185*, 342–349. [CrossRef] [PubMed]
46. Hart, L.M.; Morgan, A.J.; Rossetto, A.; Kelly, C.M.; Mackinnon, A.; Jorm, A.F. Helping adolescents to better support their peers with a mental health problem: A cluster-randomised crossover trial of teen mental health first aid. *Aust. N. Z. J. Psychiatry* **2018**, *52*, 638–651. [CrossRef]
47. Uribe Guajardo, M.G.; Kelly, C.; Bond, K.; Thomson, R.; Slewa-Younan, S. An evaluation of the teen and youth mental health first aid training with a CALD focus: An uncontrolled pilot study with adolescents and adults in Australia. *Int. J. Ment. Health Syst.* **2019**, *13*, 73. [CrossRef]
48. Link, B.; Phelan, J.; Bresnahan, M.; Stueve, A.; Pescosolido, B. Public conceptions of mental illness: Labels, causes, dangerousness, and social distance. *Am. J. Public Health* **1999**, *89*, 1328–1333. [CrossRef]
49. Lauber, C.; Nordt, C.; Falcato, L.; Rössler, W. Factors influencing social distance toward people with mental illness. *Community Ment. Health J.* **2004**, *40*, 265–274. [CrossRef] [PubMed]
50. Letovancovaá, K.; Kovalčíková, N.; Dobríková, P. Attitude of society towards people with mental illness: The result of national survey of the Slovak population. *Int. J. Soc. Psychiatry* **2017**, *63*, 255–260. [CrossRef] [PubMed]
51. Misra, T.; Connolly, A.M.; Majeed, A. Addressing mental health needs of asylum seekers and refugees in a London Borough: Epidemiological and user perspectives. *Prim. Health Care Res. Dev.* **2006**, *7*, 241–248. [CrossRef]
52. Aznar-Lou, I.; Serrano-Blanco, A.; Fernández, A.; Luciano, J.V.; Rubio-Valera, M. Attitudes and intended behaviour to mental disorders and associated factors in catalan population, Spain: Cross-sectional population-based survey. *BMC Public Health* **2015**, *16*, 127. [CrossRef] [PubMed]
53. Parcesepe, A.M.; Cabassa, L.J. Public stigma of mental illness in the United States: A systematic literature review. *Adm. Policy Ment. Health* **2013**, *40*, 384–399. [CrossRef] [PubMed]
54. Reavley, N.J.; Jorm, A.F. Association between beliefs about the causes of mental disorders and stigmatising attitudes: Results of a national survey of the Australian public. *Aust. N. Z. J. Psychiatry* **2014**, *48*, 764–771. [CrossRef] [PubMed]
55. Sadik, S.; Bradley, M.; Al-Hasoon, S.; Jenkins, R. Public perception of mental health in Iraq. *Int. J. Ment. Health Syst.* **2010**, *4*, 26. [CrossRef]
56. Corrigan, P.W.; Watson, A.C. The paradox of self-stigma and mental illness. *Clin. Psychol.* **2002**, *9*, 35 53. [CrossRef]
57. Vally, Z.; Cody, B.L.; Albloshi, M.A.; Alsheraifi, S.N.M. Public stigma and attitudes toward psychological help-seeking in the United Arab Emirates: The mediational role of self-stigma. *Perspect. Psychiatr. Care* **2018**, *54*, 571–579. [CrossRef]
58. Byrow, Y.; Pajak, R.; McMahon, T.; Rajouria, A.; Nickerson, A. Barriers to mental health help-seeking amongst refugee men. *Int. J. Environ. Res. Public Health* **2019**, *16*, 2634. [CrossRef] [PubMed]
59. Uribe Guajardo, M.G.; Slewa-Younan, S.; Santalucia, Y.; Jorm, A.F. Important considerations when providing mental health first aid to Iraqi refugees in Australia: A Delphi study. *Int. J. Ment. Health Syst.* **2016**, *10*, 54. [CrossRef] [PubMed]
60. Refugee Council of Australia. Humanitarian Entrants in New South Wales: A Resource for New South Wales Government Agencies. Available online: https://www.refugeecouncil.org.au/humanitarian-entrants-new-south-wales/ (accessed on 22 July 2021).

61. Wirth, J.H.; Bodenhausen, G.V. The role of gender in mental-illness stigma: A national experiment. *Psychol. Sci.* **2009**, *20*, 169–173. [CrossRef] [PubMed]
62. Christopher, J.C.; Wendt, D.C.; Marecek, J.; Goodman, D.M. Critical cultural awareness: Contributions to a globalizing psychology. *Am. Psychol.* **2014**, *69*, 645–655. [CrossRef]
63. Beck, J.S.; Beck, A.T. *Cognitive Behavior Therapy: Basics and Beyond*, 2nd ed.; Guilford: New York, NY, USA, 2011.

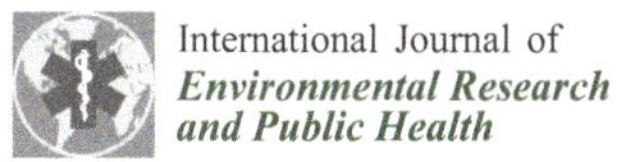

International Journal of
*Environmental Research
and Public Health*

Article

Professional Mental Health Help-Seeking Amongst Afghan and Iraqi Refugees in Australia: Understanding Predictors Five Years Post Resettlement

Ana-Marija Tomasi [1], Shameran Slewa-Younan [2,3], Renu Narchal [1] and Pilar Rioseco [4,*]

[1] School of Psychology, Western Sydney University, Sydney 2000, Australia;
    17690557@student.westernsydney.edu.au (A.-M.T.); R.Narchal@westernsydney.edu.au (R.N.)
[2] Mental Health, Translational Health Research Institute, School of Medicine, Western Sydney University,
    Sydney 2560, Australia; S.Younan@westernsydney.edu.au
[3] Centre for Mental Health, Melbourne School of Population and Global Health, University of Melbourne,
    Melbourne 3053, Australia
[4] Australian Institute of Family Studies, Melbourne 3006, Australia
* Correspondence: pilar.rioseco@aifs.gov.au

Abstract: The current longitudinal study sought to identify predictors of professional help seeking for mental health problems amongst Afghan and Iraqi refugees five years post-settlement utilising the Building a New Life in Australia dataset (BNLA). Data were collected via face-to-face or phone interviews across five waves from October 2013 to March 2018. Afghan and Iraqi born refugees numbering 1180 and over 18 years of age with a permanent humanitarian visa were included in this study. The results suggest differences in help-seeking behaviors amongst the two ethnic groups. Amongst the Afghan sample, older adults with high psychological distress were more likely to seek help, while living in regional Australia, not requiring interpreters, and knowing how to find out information about government services were related to lower likelihood of help-seeking. Within the Iraqi sample, poor overall health and knowing how to find out about services were related to a greater likelihood of help-seeking, while fewer financial hardships decreased the likelihood of help-seeking. Amongst those with probable PTSD, disability was associated with an increased likelihood of help-seeking while experiencing fewer financial hardships and living in regional Australia resulted in a lower likelihood of help-seeking in this group. These results have implications for promotional material and mental health interventions, suggesting that more integrated services tailored to specific characteristics of ethnic groups are needed.

Keywords: refugees; mental health; help-seeking; physical health; structural barriers; trauma exposure; PTSD; acculturation; discrimination; privacy

Citation: Tomasi, A.-M.;
Slewa-Younan, S.; Narchal, R.;
Rioseco, P. Professional Mental
Health Help-Seeking Amongst
Afghan and Iraqi Refugees in
Australia: Understanding Predictors
Five Years Post Resettlement. *Int. J.
Environ. Res. Public Health* **2022**, *19*,
1896. https://doi.org/10.3390/
ijerph19031896

Academic Editors: Yesim Erim and
David McDaid

Received: 2 December 2021
Accepted: 4 February 2022
Published: 8 February 2022

1. Introduction

The world is currently experiencing unprecedented challenges due to the rapid rise in displaced individuals worldwide, with numbers rising from 79.5 million at the end of 2019 [1] to 82.4 million in 2020, highlighting the magnitude of the growing problem [2]. In Australia, refugees from Afghanistan and Iraq have featured in the top five source countries for resettlement since 2016 [3]. Refugees are defined as individuals that are "unable or unwilling to return to their country of origin owing to a well-founded fear of persecution for reasons of race, religion, nationality, membership of a particular social group or political opinion" [4] (p. 3). Between 2018 and 2019 Australia became home to 18,750 refugees under the Humanitarian Visa Program with an additional 12,000 places allocated for individuals displaced by the conflict in Syria and Iraq [3]). Although, these numbers have been impacted by the current global pandemic, they are likely to be reinstated post COVID-19 with additional attention required for those affected by the current political upheaval in Afghanistan [5].

Resulting from exposure to significant trauma in the context of war, difficult migration journeys, and post-migration stressors, refugees often have high rates of psychological distress and mental health disorders [6–8]. A systematic literature review by Bogic et al. (2015) found that rates of depression ranged from 2.8% to 80%, rates of post-traumatic stress disorder (PTSD) ranged from 4.4 to 86%, and rates of anxiety ranged from 3% to 88%, with prevalence rates typically over 20% [9]. This is significantly higher than the rates of PTSD, anxiety, and depression reported within the general Australian population (4.4%, 13.1%, and 10.4%, respectively) [10,11].

Considering the high rates of mental health disorders, professional help-seeking, defined as seeking assistance from qualified mental health professionals to manage and treat these disorders, has been low [12,13]. For example, in Europe, a systematic review found that professional help-seeking amongst refugees and asylum seekers with mental health problems ranged from 8.8% to 26% [14]. Similarly, Australian research on Iraqi and Afghan refugees reported only 36–37% of participants received professional help for emotional problems [15]. Another study on Afghan refugees found that only 4.6% of participants with PTSD symptoms disclosed utilising specialist trauma and torture mental health services [16]. By comparison, within the general Australian population, 46% of individuals with mental health problems reported seeking professional help [17].

Anderson's health care utilisation model can be used to articulate factors that may influence an individual's utilisation of health care services [18]. The model proposed the following group of factors as influential: predisposing factors (socio-demographic characteristics), enabling factors (income, knowledge of health systems, travel, and waiting time), need (individuals health status), and external factors (community characteristics and interactions with health care providers) [19].

In line with Anderson's model, previous research has also identified demographic characteristics as influential in determining professional help-seeking [18,20,21]. Although inconsistent amongst refugee groups, age has been positively associated with professional help-seeking within the general population [22–24]. Similarly, females across both the general and refugee populations are more likely to discuss mental health, recognise symptoms and seek professional help [25]. Higher education has also been positively correlated with professional help-seeking within the general population, although this association has been inconsistent amongst refugees [15,26]. Proficiency in the host country's language has been considered a strong predictor of help-seeking across all populations [27,28]. For example, research on Latino and Asian Americans found that limited English-speaking proficiency resulted in delays in treatment, lower perceived need, and reduced utilisation of mental health services [27]. Research has also found variability in help-seeking rates and endorsement of traditional, informal and semi-formal sources of help amongst different ethnic groups [29,30].

Alongside demographic factors, structural barriers may impede utilisation of mental health services [31,32]. Structural barriers can include poor mental health literacy, defined by Jorm et al. (1997) as "the knowledge and beliefs about mental health disorders which aid their recognition, management or prevention" [33] (p. 182). Refugees often arrive to the host country with poor mental health literacy and limited understanding of the new health care system, available services, the role of mental health professionals, and pathways to obtaining health care [20,21,28]. This is further compounded by financial constraints resulting from not yet securing employment and having a multitude of unmet basic needs, thus reducing the importance placed on help-seeking for mental health problems [20,34,35]. Financial costs can also prevent refugees from seeking specialist services not covered by Medicare and restrain travel due to transportation expenses [21,34,36]. Other structural barriers may include difficulties with obtaining appointments, finding childcare, and taking time off work for those employed [21]. For refugees, extended waiting periods for appointments could be further exacerbated if interpreters are required and are difficult to obtain, especially for minority ethnic groups [28]. Once interpreters are secured, additional challenges may arise, including trusting interpreters and mental health professionals to keep information confidential [20].

Similarly, experiences of discrimination may also influence help-seeking [37]. Discrimination refers to unfair treatment due to ethnicity, age, gender, disability, sexual orientation, or marital status [38]. For example, a study on Tamil refugees in Canada found that 11% of participants experienced racial discrimination during encounters with health care professionals, resulting in decreased use of these services [39].

Acculturation is the process by which migrants adjust their values, beliefs, behaviors, and cultural practices to that of their host country's culture [40,41]. This process, therefore, involves learning the host nation's language, navigating new social systems, and familiarising oneself with new norms and ways of living [42]. Refugees' level of acculturation is likely to influence professional help-seeking. Research on Laotian and Cambodian refugees in America, for example, found that a higher level of acculturation to American mainstream culture was correlated with more positive attitudes towards help-seeking, greater openness when discussing psychological problems, and increased confidence in mental health professionals [25].

It should be noted that despite the increasing focus on help-seeking in refugee populations, findings remain inconsistent, and samples are often small, nonrandom, and are not representative of the population [15]. Additionally, most research has focused on recently arrived refugees, and limited longitudinal studies are available. Consequently, the following study utilises data from the Building a New Life in Australia database (BNLA) [43] to determine the predictors of professional help-seeking for mental health problems within two of the largest refugee groups in Australia: The Afghan and Iraqi population [3]. The BNLA study is the first and most comprehensive longitudinal cohort study in Australia to follow refugees and their families through the first five years of their resettlement journey. The research from the following study is necessary to inform policy makers and service providers on how to best support refugee populations and improve their overall mental health and wellbeing. Additionally, this research can also help clinicians better understand methods to promote engagement with the refugee population.

The aim of the current study was to identify the predictors of professional help-seeking ,for mental health problems amongst Afghan and Iraqi refugees five years post-resettlement. Informed by Anderson's model and previous literature, socio-demographic factors, mental health symptomology, general health, trauma exposure, structural barriers, acculturation, and trust and discrimination were included as predictors of interest [18]. Considering the Afghan and Iraqi sub-samples separately, the following was hypothesised:

1. Older age, female gender, higher levels of education, English-speaking proficiency, and residing in a major city would be associated with increased professional help-seeking;
2. Poor overall health and trauma exposure would be associated with greater levels of professional help-seeking;
3. Structural barriers including financial hardship, lack of knowledge about public transport and government services, not receiving an interpreter when needed, and not having an Australian driver's license would be associated with lower levels of professional help-seeking;
4. Greater acculturation to the mainstream Australian culture would be associated with greater levels of professional help-seeking;
5. Lower trust in government services and experiences of discrimination would be associated with lower levels of professional help-seeking;
6. Finally, amongst the combined Afghan and Iraqi sub-samples who met criteria for PTSD, the following is hypothesised: the association between poorer health, trauma exposure, structural barriers, acculturation, trust, discrimination, and professional help-seeking would be stronger.

2. Method

2.1. Participants

A total of 1180 adult participants from the BNLA database were included in this study, 773 were from Iraq and 407 were from Afghanistan. The full BNLA sample consisted of humanitarian migrants who arrived in Australia between May and December 2013 (offshore visa) or received their permanent visa during this time (onshore visa). Participants were recruited three to six months after being granted their permanent visa. Using the Australian Settlement Database, "migrating units"—a person or family named on the visa application—were randomly selected from 11 sites across Australia, including major cities and regional areas. These 11 sites were selected based on the number of eligible participants in each site and accounted for almost 92% of humanitarian arrivals in Australia at the time. The BNLA sample is representative of humanitarian migrants who arrived or were granted their permanent visa during this period.

2.2. Procedure

An ethics exemption was obtained from the Human Research Ethics Committee at Western Sydney University on the basis that the study would be using pre-existing data. Permission was granted from the Department of Social Services to access the BNLA dataset.

Participants for the BNLA study were recruited based on the principal applicant (PA) on the humanitarian visa. Once PA consented to participate, family members known as secondary applicants (SA) who were over the age of 15 and residing with the PA were also invited to participate. The BNLA dataset was collected annually across five waves from October 2013 to March 2018 via face-to-face (Waves 1, 3 and 5) or telephone interviews (Waves 2 and 4). Questionnaires were translated into 14 languages and consisted of settlement related measures.

2.3. Measures

2.3.1. Criterion

Professional Help-Seeking. This variable was assessed at Wave 5 using the following question: "In the last 12 months have you received help from a professional, such as a doctor, counsellor or psychologist to help you deal with emotional problems". Response options included "yes", "no, I didn't need it", and "no, I couldn't get it" and were coded into "yes" and "no" in line with previous research (earlier waves of the BNLA only included options "yes" and "no").

2.3.2. Predictors

Socio-Demographic Characteristics. Age, gender, country of birth, and highest completed education pre-arrival were all collected at Wave 1 and derived for the following waves. English-speaking proficiency and area of residence were collected at Wave 4. Country of birth acted as a proxy for nationality and only participants from the two largest source countries, Afghanistan and Iraq, were included in this study. Location was categorised into "major cities" or "regional Australia". Education was categorised into "never attended school", "9 years or less of school", "10 or more years of school" and "post-school education", whilst English-speaking proficiency was categorised into "not at all", "not well" and "well/very well".

General Health. At Wave 4, participants were asked *"Overall, how would you rate your health during the past 4 weeks?"*. Responses were recorded on a 6-point Likert scale ranging from "excellent" to "very poor" but recoded into "good", "fair", and "poor". The question *"Do you have a disability, injury or health condition that has lasted or is likely to last 12 months or more?"* was also asked in Wave 4 with response options "yes" and "no".

Mental Health. The Kessler Screening Scale for Psychological Distress (K6) and the PTSD-8 Scale were collected at Wave 4 [44,45]. K6 is a six-item measure assessing psychological distress and possible presence of mental illness within the last four weeks. Responses were recorded on a 5-point Likert scale ranging from "none of the time" to "all the time". Total scores ranged from six to thirty with higher scores suggesting greater psychological distress. The PTSD-8 is an eight-item scale derived from the Harvard Trauma Questionnaire (HTQ) to assess for symptoms of PTSD within the last week. Participants who answered "sometimes" or "most of the time" to at least one item in the three categories of symptoms (intrusions, avoidance, and hypervigilance) were deemed to have probable PTSD. Both scales have been validated cross-culturally [46,47].

Exposure to Traumatic Events. Participants at Wave 3 were provided with a list of nine possibly traumatic events and asked to select the ones they experienced prior to arrival in Australia. Examples included the following: combat exposure and torture. Responses were recoded into five categories ranging from "no response" to "4 or more events".

Structural Barriers. Questions available in the BNLA dataset that constituted structural barriers included financial hardship, knowledge of transport and government services, availability of interpreters when needed, and having a current driver's licence. *(1)* Financial hardship was assessed using the item *"In the last 12 months have any of the following happened to you because you didn't have enough money"*. Eight response options were provided (e.g., could not pay the rent or mortgage payments on time) and later recoded into five categories ranging from "no financial hardship" to "4+ hardships"; *(2)* ability to use public transport and find out about government services was measured using the question *"We are interested to know how you are getting on with things like transport, accessing information and other day to day activities. If you had to, would you know how to . . . use public transport, find out what government services and benefits are available"*. Responses were indicated on a 4-point Likert scale ranging from "would know very well" to "wouldn't know at all"; *(3)* Receiving interpreting assistance was measured using the item *"In the last 12 months, how often were you able to get interpreting assistance when you needed it?"*. Responses were recorded on a 4-point Likert scale ranging from "always" to "never", and a response option of "haven't needed interpreting assistance" was also included. *(4)* Finally, *"Do you have a current Australian driver's licence (including provisional licence)?"* was asked and response options included "yes" and "no". Data from Wave 4 were used for all variables.

Acculturation. Several questions from the survey were utilised as proxies for acculturation. Firstly, length of residency was obtained from the difference between time of arrival and interview date and was derived for the following waves. Responses were recoded into "2 years", "3 years", and "4+ years". Secondly, community support was measured at Wave 4 using the item *"Do you feel that you have been given support/comfort in Australia from (a) Your national or ethnic community (b) Your religious community (c) Other community groups"*. Response options included "yes", "sometimes", and "no". Support from own religious and ethnic community were combined into one variable "support from own community". Thirdly, friends in Australia were assessed at Wave 4 using the question *"Would you say your friends in Australia are . . . (a) mostly from my ethnic religious community (b) mostly from other ethnic religious communities (c) a mixture (d) Do not have any friends in Australia yet"*. Responses were recoded into "mostly own ethnic/religious", "mostly other community/mixture" and "no friends in Australia yet". Finally, endorsing the item *"getting used to life in Australia"* on the question *"have any of the following been a source of stress in your life in the last 12 months"* indicated possible acculturative stress and was measured at Wave 4. Response options included "not selected" and "selected".

Discrimination. At Wave 4, participants were asked "In the last 12 months, do you think you have been discriminated against, stopped from doing something or been hassled or made to feel inferior, because of your ethnicity, religion or skin color?". Response options included "yes" and "no".

Trust. Assessed at Wave 4 with the question "Now thinking about government services (e.g., Medicare, Centrelink, public housing), have you experienced any of the following in the last 12 months? . . . was afraid that my information would not be kept private". Response options included "no", "yes", "haven't used government services", and "no response".

2.4. Statistical Analysis and Design

Employing a longitudinal design, statistical analyses were conducted using SPSS version 28.0. The last observation carried forward a method that was utilised when data were unavailable at Wave 4 [48]. Missing data were removed on an analysis-by-analysis basis or a non-response category was included for sensitive questions where missing data were expected. Descriptive analyses included frequencies and proportions for categorical variables and means and standard deviations for continuous variables. Initially, multivariable logistic regressions were conducted separately for the Afghan and Iraqis in blocks of variables based on Anderson's model: socio-demographics, health, trauma, structural barriers, acculturation, trust, and discrimination [18]. Following this, full models were created including theoretically relevant and statistically significant variables from each block. For parsimony, final models excluded the least significant variables once controlling for all relevant variables from the blocks [49]. Finally, a multivariable logistic regression was conducted with the PTSD sub-sample and only variables in the full model were utilised due to the limited sample size. Given that more than one member of a family could be included in the sample, models were adjusted for clustering at the household level.

3. Results

3.1. Participant Descriptives

Table 1 presents participants' descriptive statistics.

Table 1. Descriptive statistics of predictor variables by country of birth, PTSD sample and total sample.

Variables		Afghanistan % (N = 407) (n; SE)	Iraq % (N = 773) (n; SE)	PTSD % (N = 281) (n; SE)	Total % (N = 1180) (n; SE)
Socio-demographics					
	Age	38.72 (379; 0.600)	43.51 (743; 0.536)	45.14 (281; 0.679)	41.89 (1122; 0.414)
Gender	Male	56.3 (229)	52.5 (406)	45.9 (129)	53.8 (635)
	Female	43.7 (178)	47.5 (367)	54.1 (152)	46.2 (545)
Married/Partnered	No	31.7 (120)	31.0 (229)	31.3 (88)	31.3 (349)
	Yes	68.3 (258)	69.0 (509)	68.7 (193)	68.7 (767)
Education Level	Never attended School	40.6 (164)	6.0 (55)	11.5 (32)	17.9 (210)
	9 years or less	45.5 (184)	39.5 (304)	44.6 (124)	41.6 (488)
	10 years or less	11.4 (46)	32.0 (246)	22.3 (62)	24.9 (292)
	Post-school education	2.5 (10)	22.5 (173)	21.6 (60)	15.6 (183)
Location	Major cities	86.1 (327)	99.6 (740)	94.7 (266)	95.0 (1067)
	Regional Australia	13.9 (53)	0.4 (3)	5.3 (15)	5.0 (56)
English Proficiency	Not at all	18.9 (71)	14.3 (105)	21.0 (59)	15.8 (176)
	Not well	44.4 (167)	45.4 (334)	49.8 (140)	45.1 (501)
	Well/Very well	36.7 (138)	40.2 (296)	29.2 (82)	39.1 (434)
Health					
Self-rated Health	Good	70.6 (266)	51.2 (377)	29.2 (82)	57.8 (643)
	Fair	15.1 (57)	26.0 (191)	32.4 (91)	22.3 (248)
	Poor	14.3 (54)	22.8 (168)	38.4 (108)	19.9 (222)
Kessler6 Total Score		11.37 (377; 0.294)	13.07 (735; 0.237)	18.43 (0.374)	12.49 (1112; 0.187)
PTSD	Unlikely to have PTSD	85.4 (321)	69.2 (507)	-	74.7 (828)
	May have PTSD	14.6 (55)	30.8 (226)	100 (281)	25.3 (281)
Long Term Illness/Disability	Yes	28.5 (106)	43.0 (305)	61.5 (169)	38.0 (411)
	No	71.5 (266)	57.0 (405)	38.5 (106)	62.0 (671)
Trauma Exposure					
Traumatic Events	No response	22.7 (82)	8.0 (56)	7.2 (19)	13.0 (138)
	1	35.7 (129)	21.6 (152)	24.2 (64)	26.4 (281)
	2	15.0 (54)	15.2 (107)	10.2 (27)	15.1 (161)
	3	8.0 (29)	18.6 (131)	15.5 (41)	15.0 (160)
	4 or more	18.6 (67)	36.6 (257)	42.8 (113)	30.5 (324)
Structural Barriers					
Financial Hardship	0	62.3 (236)	52.7 (389)	35.7 (100)	56.0 (625)
	1	12.4 (47)	22.6 (167)	28.2 (79)	19.2 (214)
	2	10.0 (38)	11.9 (88)	14.3 (40)	11.3 (126)
	3	6.9 (26)	7.7 (57)	13.2 (37)	7.4 (83)
	4 or more	8.4 (32)	5.0 (37)	8.6 (24)	6.2 (69)

Table 1. *Cont.*

Variables		Afghanistan % (N = 407) (n; SE)	Iraq % (N = 773) (n; SE)	PTSD % (N = 281) (n; SE)	Total % (N = 1180) (n; SE)
Got interpreter when needed	Never	18.6 (70)	13.9(102)	3.6 (10)	15.5 (172)
	Some of the time	35.4 (133)	26.0 (191)	22.4 (63)	29.1 (324)
	Most of the time	10.4 (39)	18. 5(136)	20.6 (58)	15.7 (175)
	Always	19.1 (72)	31.4 (231)	41.6 (117)	27.2 (303)
	Haven't needed	16.5 (62)	10.3 (76)	11.7 (33)	12.4 (138)
Use public transport	Would know very well	61.2 (226)	53.0 (376)	42.5 (117)	55.8 (602)
	Would know fairly well	19.0 (70)	21.9 (155)	26.2 (72)	20.9 (225)
	Would know a little	10.8 (40)	13.4 (95)	16.7 (46)	12.5 (135)
	Wouldn't know at all	8.9 (33)	11.7 (83)	14.5 (40)	10.8 (116)
Find gov. services	Would know very well	28.8 (106)	34.5 (244)	14.6 (40)	32.6 (350)
	Would know fairly well	19.8 (73)	21.5 (152)	23.4 (64)	20.9 (225)
	Would know a little	20.7 (76)	26.2 (185)	33.6 (92)	24.3 (261)
	Wouldn't know at all	30.7 (113)	17.8 (126)	28.5 (78)	22.2 (239)
Aus. Driver's Licence	Yes	84.1 (328)	76.7 (569)	73.5 (202)	79.2 (897)
	No	15.9 (62)	23.3 (173)	26.5 (73)	20.8 (235)
Acculturation Time between arrival and interview	2 years	3.7 (14)	3.8 (28)	2.1 (6)	3.7 (42)
	3 years	76.3 (289)	93.5 (695)	92.5 (260)	87.7 (984)
	4 or more	20.1 (76)	2.7 (20)	5.3 (15)	8.6 (96)
Community Support (own)	Yes	26.1 (94)	27.9 (205)	29.4 (82)	27.3 (299)
	Sometimes	29.4 (106)	21.4 (157)	23.3 (65)	24.0 (263)
	No	44.4 (160)	50.7 (372)	47.3 (132)	48.6 (532)
Community Support (other)	Yes	12.3 (43)	18.6 (135)	14.3 (39)	16.6 (178)
	Sometimes	14.8 (52)	13.7 (99)	15.8 (43)	14.0 (151)
	No	72.9 (256)	67.7 (490)	69.9 (190)	69.4 (746)
Friends in Australia	Mostly own ethnic/rel	43.9 (147)	39.2 (260)	43.3 (113)	40.7 (407)
	Mostly mixture/other comm	47.8 (160)	50.8 (337)	41.4 (108)	49.7 (497)
	No friends Aus yet	8.4 (28)	10.1 (67)	15.3 (40)	9.5 (95)
Source of stress-getting used to life in Australia	No selected	92.9 (312)	89.8 (624)	83.0 (224)	90.8 (938)
	Selected	7.1 (24)	10.2 (71)	17.0 (46)	9.2 (95)
Trust Privacy	Non response	16.7 (57)	9.9 (71)	9.5 (25)	9.8 (100)
	Yes	9.4 (32)	8.0 (57)	7.6 (20)	5.2 (53)
	No	56.3 (192)	74.3 (532)	69.7 (184)	70.6 (720)
	Haven't used gov. services	17.6 (60)	7.8 (56)	13.3 (35)	14.4 (147)
Discrimination Discrimination	No	91.5 (345)	93.3 (684)	86.7 (242)	92.7 (1029)
	Yes	8.5 (32)	6.7 (49)	13.3 (37)	7.3 (81)

N = number of observations in the entire sample; n = number of observations in each variable; % is percentage of participants; SE = standard error.

Afghan participants were significantly younger ($p < 0.001$), less educated ($p < 0.001$), and more likely to live in regional Australia ($p < 0.001$) compared to those from Iraq. No differences in English speaking proficiency or marital status were noted between groups. Participants from Afghanistan reported better self-rated health ($p < 0.001$), less psychological distress ($p < 0.001$), were less likely to have PTSD ($p < 0.001$) or a disability ($p < 0.001$), and experienced fewer traumatic events ($p < 0.001$) compared to participants from Iraq. In terms of structural barriers Afghan respondents had less knowledge about government services ($p < 0.001$) and were less likely to obtain an interpreter when needed ($p < 0.001$). However, fewer Iraqi refugees held a driver's licence ($p = 0.003$), and they faced more financial hardships ($p < 0.001$) than their Afghan counterparts. Moreover, despite Afghan refugees having resided in Australia for longer ($p < 0.001$), they were less likely to receive support outside of their own community compared to those from Iraq

($p = 0.030$). No other differences were noted between groups regarding support or friends. Refugees from Afghanistan reported more privacy concerns and were less likely to utilise government services in comparison to Iraqi refugees ($p < 0.001$). Differences in experiences of discrimination were non-significant between groups ($p = 0.274$).

Finally, 34.4% of refugees from Afghanistan (95% CI 31.74, 37.31) and 33.8% of refugees from Iraq (95% CI 30.55, 37.33) received professional help for emotional problems. Amongst those that met criteria for PTSD, 47.3% received professional help (95% CI 41.32, 53.49).

3.2. Multivariable Analysis

3.2.1. Afghan Sample

Within the block analysis, socio-demographic characteristics such as being female and older were positively associated with professional help-seeking, while those living in regional Australia were less likely to receive help. Refugees reporting poorer physical and mental health were more likely to have received professional help. In contrast, refugees facing fewer structural barriers were less likely to receive professional help. Specifically, having fewer financial hardships, not requiring interpreting assistance, having a driver's licence, and knowing how to find out about available government services were all associated with a lower likelihood of seeking help. Measures of acculturation, including not having any friends in Australia and finding the process of getting used to life in Australia stressful, were both associated with increased likelihood of receiving professional help. In the full model, only older age and higher psychological distress were positively associated with help-seeking. Refugees who lived in regional Australia did not require interpreting assistance and who were able to find out about available government services were less likely to receive help (Table 2).

Table 2. Multivariate analysis by country of birth, including the predictors in blocks (demographics, health, trauma exposure, structural barriers, acculturation, trust and discrimination and the criterion professional help-seeking) and the full model.

		Afghanistan				Iraq			
		Block Model		Full Model		Block Model		Full Model	
		OR	95% CI	OR	95% CI	OR	95% CI	OR	95% CI
Socio-demographics									
	Age	1.04 ***	[1.02,1.07]	1.04 *	[1.00,1.07]	1.02 **	[1.01,1.04]	1.01	[0.99,1.03]
Gender	Male (ref.)								
	Female	1.91 *	[1.17,3.12]	1.20	[0.65,2.23]	1.03	[0.77,1.38]	1.17	[0.83,1.65]
Married/Partnered	No (ref.)								
	Yes	0.79	[0.45,1.40]	-	-	1.11	[0.77,1.62]	-	-
Education level	Never attended School (ref.)								
	9 years or less	1.26	[0.76,2.09]	-	-	1.66	[0.72,3.82]	-	-
	10 years or less	1.16	[0.51,2.62]	-	-	1.74	[0.73,4.14]	-	-
	Post-school education	0.67	[0.10,4.59]	-	-	1.46	[0.59,3.61]	-	-
Location	Major cities (ref.)								
	Regional Australia	0.34 *	[0.14,0.79]	0.19 ***	[0.08,0.48]	1.00	[1.00,1.00]	-	-
English proficiency	Not at all (ref.)								
	Not well	0.79	[0.40,1.59]	1.47	[0.57,3.78]	0.63	[0.38,1.05]	0.62	[0.36,1.07]
	Well/Very well	0.71	[0.30,1.69]	2.56	[0.80,8.23]	0.46 *	[0.25,0.84]	0.55	[0.27,1.14]
N		373				728			
Health									
Self-rated health	Good (ref.)								
	Fair	2.09 *	[1.13,3.88]	1.89	[0.89,4.04]	1.54	[0.99,2.40]	1.49	[0.92,2.41]
	Poor	2.57 *	[1.22,5.40]	1.40	[0.54,3.64]	2.12 **	[1.24,3.62]	2.09 *	[1.15,3.79]
Kessler 6 Total Score		1.06 *	[1.01,1.12]	1.11 **	[1.04,1.19]	1.05 **	[1.02,1.09]	1.05 *	[1.01,1.09]
PTSD	No PTSD (ref.)								
	Probable PTSD	0.84	[0.38,1.87]	1.05	[0.41,2.68]	0.98	[0.63,1.51]	1.06	[0.66,1.70]
Long term illness or disability	No (ref.)								
	Yes	1.48	[0.80,2.73]	1.61	[0.80,3.23]	2.51 ***	[1.72,3.64]	2.31 ***	[1.51,3.55]
N		371				708			

Table 2. *Cont.*

		Afghanistan				Iraq			
		Block Model		Full Model		Block Model		Full Model	
		OR	95% CI	OR	95% CI	OR	95% CI	OR	95% CI
Trauma Exposure									
	1 (ref.)								
	2	1.04	[0.53,2.04]	-	-	1.85 *	[1.08,3.16]	-	-
	3	0.86	[0.36,2.08]	-	-	2.05 **	[1.23,3.43]	-	-
	4+	1.04	[0.55,1.93]	-	-	2.19 ***	[1.42,3.39]	-	-
	No response	0.72	[0.39,1.33]	-	-	1.53	[0.81,2.88]	-	-
N		361				703			
Structural Barriers									
Financial Hardship	4 or more (ref.)								
	0	0.60	[0.25,1.42]	1.37	[0.48,3.91]	0.27 **	[0.12,0.61]	0.41 *	[0.19,0.89]
	1	0.91	[0.32,2.54]	1.18	[0.39,3.57]	0.32 **	[0.14,0.73]	0.39 *	[0.18,0.85]
	2	1.23	[0.42,3.60]	1.98	[0.61,6.40]	0.21 **	[0.08,0.54]	0.21 ***	[0.08,0.52]
	3	0.31 *	[0.10,0.98]	0.49	[0.13,1.87]	0.83	[0.29,2.37]	0.90	[0.31,2.64]
Got interpreter when needed	Never (ref.)								
	Some of the time	1.53	[0.77,3.04]	1.28	[0.55,2.98]	2.20 *	[1.17,4.12]	1.24	[0.64,2.43]
	Most of the time	1.05	[0.38,2.88]	0.91	[0.28,3.01]	1.95	[0.95,3.97]	0.95	[0.41,2.18]
	Always	2.03	[0.93,4.43]	1.27	[0.45,3.58]	3.78 ***	[1.92,7.43]	1.44	[0.65,3.18]
	Haven't needed	0.31 *	[0.10,0.92]	0.28 *	[0.09,0.86]	1.47	[0.67,3.21]	1.29	[0.56,2.98]
Use public transport	Wouldn't know at all (ref.)								
	Would know very well	1.10	[0.44,2.78]	-	-	0.69	[0.35,1.35]	-	-
	Would know fairly well	1.38	[0.49,3.90]	-	-	0.67	[0.33,1.35]	-	-
	Would know a little	2.21	[0.80,6.13]	-	-	0.93	[0.46,1.86]	-	-
Find gov. services	Wouldn't know at all (ref.)								
	Would know very well	0.71	[0.35,1.47]	0.61	[0.27,1.38]	1.50	[0.82,2.74]	2.07 *	[1.15,3.75]
	Would know fairly well	0.46	[0.21,1.02]	0.33 **	[0.15,0.76]	1.48	[0.80,2.75]	1.81	[0.99,3.31]
	Would know a little	0.49 *	[0.25,0.96]	0.52	[0.24,1.15]	1.16	[0.67,2.01]	1.35	[0.78,2.35]
Aus. Driver's Licence	No (ref.)								
	Yes	0.53 *	[0.28,1.00]	-	-	0.78	[0.50,1.22]	-	-
N		362				691			
Acculturation									
Time btw. Arrival and interview	4 or more (ref.)								
	3 years	0.67	[0.36,1.26]	-	-	1.16	[0.33,4.09]	-	-
	2 years	0.37	[0.06,2.16]	-	-	1.76	[0.37,8.44]	-	-
Community Support (own)	No (ref.)								
	Sometimes	1.03	[0.55,1.91]	-	-	1.07	[0.64,1.79]	-	-
	Yes	0.84	[0.41,1.73]	-	-	0.82	[0.50,1.36]	-	-
Community Support (other)	No (ref.)								
	Sometimes	0.82	[0.37,1.83]	-	-	0.67	[0.37,1.22]	-	-
	Yes	0.44	[0.16,1.24]	-	-	1.04	[0.57,1.92]	-	-
Friends in Australia	Mostly mixture/ other comm. (ref.)								
	Mostly own ethnic/rel	1.52	[0.89,2.61]	-	-	1.39	[0.98,1.97]	-	-
	No friends Aus yet	3.09 **	[1.38,6.92]	-	-	1.43	[0.82,2.49]	-	-
Source of stress-getting used to life in Australia	Not selected (ref.)								
	Selected	3.14 *	[1.21,8.18]	2.31	[0.74,7.25]	1.44	[0.86,2.43]	0.87	[0.48,1.58]
N		277				646			
Trust									
Privacy	No (ref.)								
	Yes	0.94	[0.31,2.86]	-	-	1.78	[0.92,3.47]	-	-
	Nonresponse	1.20	[0.59,2.46]	-	-	1.46	[0.83,2.56]	-	-
	Haven't used gov. services	1.29	[0.73,2.29]	-	-	1.15	[0.70,1.88]	-	-
N		342				678			
Discrimination									
Discrimination	No (ref.)								
	Yes	0.67	[0.30,1.49]	-	-	1.14	[0.64,2.02]	-	-
N		377		331		733		686	

OR = odds ratio; 95% CI = 95% confidence interval; N = number of observations. Ref. = reference category. $p < 0.05$ *, $p < 0.01$ **, $p < 0.001$ ***.

3.2.2. Iraqi Sample

Within the Iraqi block analysis, older refugees were more likely to receive professional help while those with good English-speaking proficiency were less likely to receive help. Having a long-term disability or illness was also associated with increased likelihood of receiving professional help. Structural barriers such as having fewer financial hardships resulted in reduced professional help-seeking, while refugees that were able to receive an interpreter were more likely to seek professional help. Within the full model, poorer physical and mental health, alongside being able to find available government services, increased the likelihood of receiving help. In contrast, participants with fewer financial hardships were less likely to receive help (Table 2).

3.3. PTSD Sample

Amongst those with probable PTSD, having a disability or long-term illness was significantly associated with increased professional help-seeking, whereas having fewer financial hardships and living in regional Australia resulted in reduced help-seeking (Table 3).

Table 3. Full model displaying predictors of professional help-seeking within the PTSD sample.

Variables		OR	95% CI
Country of Birth	Iraq (ref.)		
	Afghanistan	1.89	[0.68,5.26]
Socio-demographic			
	Age	0.99	[0.96,1.02]
Gender	Male (ref.)		
	Female	1.35	[0.75,2.42]
English Proficiency	Not at all (ref.)		
	Not well	0.99	[0.44,2.25]
	Well/very well	0.75	[0.21,2.63]
Location	Major cities (ref.)		
	Regional Australia	0.15 *	[0.03,0.82]
Health			
Self-rated Health	Good (ref.)		
	Fair	1.78	[0.61,5.42]
	Poor	1.82	[0.61,5.42]
Kessler 6	Total score	1.05	[0.99,1.11]
Long Term Illness or Disability	No (ref.)		
	Yes	2.74 **	[1.35,5.59]
Structural Barriers			
Financial Hardship	4 or more (ref.)		
Financial Hardships	0	0.27 *	[0.08,0.92]
	1	0.34	[0.10,1.17]
	2	0.32	[0.09,1.24]
	3	0.69	[0.18,2.67]
Got interpreter when needed	Never (ref.)		
	Some of the time	3.35	[0.63,17.68]
	Most of the time	2.49	[0.39,15.67]
	Always	3.42	[0.57,20.70]
	Haven't needed	3.08	[0.57,16.83]
Find gov. services	Wouldn't know at all (ref.)		
	Would know very well	1.67	[0.57,4.88]
	Would know fairly well	0.87	[0.37,2.03]
	Would know a little	0.66	[0.31,1.44]
Source of stress- getting used to life in Australia	Not selected (ref.)		
	Selected	1.24	[0.57,2.68]
N	260		

OR = odds ratio; 95% CI = 95% confidence interval; N = number of observations. Ref. = reference category. $p < 0.05$ *, $p < 0.01$ **.

4. Discussion

This study sought to understand the factors associated with professional help-seeking for mental health problems within Iraqi and Afghan refugee populations in Australia, five years post-settlement. Factors of interest included socio-demographic characteristics, health, trauma exposure, structural barriers, acculturation, trust in government services, and experiences of discrimination, in line with Anderson's health care utilisation model [18]. The findings partially support the hypotheses, with differences noted between the two ethnic groups. Understanding these factors is crucial to developing suitable services tailored to the needs of refugees and enhancing their ability and willingness to access and engage with these services. Additionally, considering the increased rates of trauma-related mental illness amongst refugee populations, understanding the factors that promote professional help-seeking is critical in reducing the burden of mental health disorders on Australian communities [12,26].

Significant socio-demographic factors in the full model included age and living in regional Australia, albeit only in the Afghan sample. No associations were found between professional help-seeking and education level or being married. In the block analysis within the Afghan group, consistent with prior studies, older age and female gender were positively associated with professional help-seeking, while living in regional Australia held a negative association with help-seeking [15,25,50]. Similarly, amongst Iraqi refugees, being older was positively related to help-seeking; however, having good English-speaking proficiency resulted in a lower likelihood of seeking help. This finding contradicts previous research, which has suggested that refugees with poor English-speaking proficiency were less likely to receive professional help and have greater difficulties accessing services [28,51]. These results suggest that extra efforts are needed to promote mental health services amongst younger refugees and males, and additional mental health services targeting refugees in remote areas of Australia are needed. Further research in understanding why those with good English-speaking proficiency were not receiving professional help would be beneficial.

Amongst health and trauma related factors as hypothesised, within the full model, poorer self-rated health, greater psychological distress, and presence of a disability all increased the probability of seeking professional help while meeting criteria for PTSD held no association with help-seeking. Trauma exposure was significant at the block analysis level but only for the Iraqi sub-sample. Again, differences were noted between the two ethnic groups. Specifically, only psychological distress was consistently associated with professional help-seeking across both the Afghan and Iraqi refugee groups. Disability or presence of a long-term illness held no association with professional help-seeking amongst the Afghan sub-sample but was positively associated in the Iraqi group. These findings are aligned with Anderson's model (1995), which identified need as an important predictor of health care utilisation [18]. Interestingly, previous research on Afghan refugees found that higher rates of disability and better self-recognition of mental health symptoms were correlated with increased help-seeking from mental health professionals [16]. The association between physical health and professional help-seeking may be explained by the higher rates of somatic symptoms reported within refugee groups. These individuals may be seeking help for physical complaints and consequently receiving help for mental health problems [52]. The contrasting findings regarding disability in the Afghan sample could possibly be influenced by better overall health and lower rates of disability reported by Afghan participants compared to Iraqi participants. Finally, differences between ethnic groups in their help-seeking behaviours are consistent with previous research and highlight the importance of targeted mental health promotions that are culturally attuned to the characteristics of specific refugee groups [16]. Other clinical implications of these findings are that general practitioners may need specifically targeted training in recognising symptoms of poor mental health within this population and referral options to mental health specialists tailored to the needs of refugee groups.

The hypotheses related to structural barriers were also partly supported, and again, differences noted between the two groups. Specifically, amongst the Iraqi sub-sample in the full model, having fewer financial hardships was related to a decreased likelihood of receiving professional help, while, as hypothesised, knowing how to find out about available government services was associated with a greater likelihood of receiving professional help. In contrast, amongst the Afghan sub-sample, knowing fairly well how to find out about government services and not needing interpreting assistance was related to a lower likelihood of seeking professional help. Findings from the block analysis also suggested Afghan refugees with an Australian driver's license were less likely to receive professional help. No associations were found between knowing how to use public transport and professional help-seeking. These findings are contrary to previous research, which found financial hardship to be a significant barrier to help-seeking for most refugees as they were unable to pay for treatment or travel costs and often prioritised financial security over receiving help for mental health disorders [20]. A systematic review by Byrow et al. (2020) also found limited access to interpreters and understanding how to access available services was related to reduced help-seeking and longer durations of mental health disorders being left untreated [20]. A possible explanation for our contrasting results could be that refugees who were experiencing financial difficulties, language barriers, and difficulties navigating the new social systems were receiving support from other social services. It is possible that they were identified as needing psychological help in the context of other support services and had been linked with mental health professionals [53]. These findings imply that additional efforts are required to promote mental health services amongst refugees who are not in contact with other social services. They also again highlight the importance of targeted mental health promotion and services that focus on refugee groups separately based on cultural background.

When acculturative factors were taken into account in the full model, no factors were significantly associated with professional help-seeking. However, within the block model, contrary to predictions, those who found the acculturation process stressful and had no friends were more likely to seek professional help, albeit only in the Afghan sub-sample. No significant associations were found between time spent in Australia, receiving support from either one's own ethnic community or other communities and professional help-seeking. These findings are inconsistent with previous research, which has found that refugees who were more acculturated to the host culture were more likely to endorse seeking professional support for mental health problems [29]. However, previous studies have found that less acculturated refugees who experienced greater acculturative stress where more likely to have poorer mental health [53,54]. Therefore, it may be plausible in our study that those refugees who were less acculturated were experiencing poorer mental health and, thus, as suggested in Anderson's health care utilisation model, had a greater need for professional help [18]. These findings insinuate the need for additional services for refugees during the settlement period even five years post arrival to assist with adjusting to the host country and fostering social support. It is also important to mention that, given the study's design, time spent in Australia amongst our sample was highly homogenous. Future research incorporating a longer time span with greater sample variability is required to further examine the role of time in the host country as a predictor of help-seeking.

Both trusting that government services would keep information private and experiencing discrimination, were not significantly associated with receiving professional help. However, previous research on adolescent refugees in Australia found that lower trust in health professionals was related to fears that information would be disclosed to other community members, resulting in lower rates of professional help-seeking. Similarly, research has suggested that experiencing discrimination in the host country was associated with both poorer mental health and a reluctance to seek professional help [55,56]. Within our study, a very small number of participants reported experiencing discrimination; thus, this association may require further exploration with a larger sample size. Future studies could include open ended questions in order to develop a deeper understanding of refugees' experiences of discrimination and its influence on help-seeking.

Finally, amongst the sub-sample who met criteria for PTSD, only having a long term-disability or illness was positively related to receiving professional help. However, refugees with PTSD who had fewer financial hardships and lived in remote parts of Australia were less likely to receive professional help. These findings again highlight the possibility that refugees are being identified as needing help when they access other social services and health professionals and are then referred onto mental health professionals. The implications of these results are that more integrated and culturally informed services are required for this population. Additionally, it may be beneficial to promote mental health services amongst refugees who are performing well in other social and health domains apart from mental health. Help-seeking was lower among refugees with likely PTSD in regional areas, highlighting the need to improve availability and access to mental health services outside of major cities.

This study has a number of limitations. Firstly, as self-report measures were utilised, results may have been impacted by social desirability and recall bias [57]. Responses may have also been affected by issues around translation of surveys and transcultural bias [58]. A limitation of our quantitative design is that it is not clear whether participants fully understand subjective concepts, such as discrimination. Additionally, variables such as community support may have been influenced by perceptions of need for support rather than acculturation. Despite some limitations, the large sample size representative of the leading groups of refugees in Australia is a major strength of this study, as these results can be utilised to improve the resettlement outcomes of a large proportion of refugees in Australia. Future research may wish to extend these findings by utilising a more extensive measure of professional help-seeking. Future research including open-ended questions, or a mixed-method design would be beneficial. This would provide the opportunity to ask follow-up questions and, therefore, gain a better in-depth understanding of the reasons for selecting certain options. Additionally, incorporating qualitative methodologies would contribute to our understanding of the underlaying cultural characteristics that my influence help-seeking behaviors amongst these two populations.

5. Conclusions

This study was amongst the first to explore professional help-seeking for mental health problems five years post-settlement amongst two of the largest resettled groups of refugees in Australia. The findings showed significant differences between the two ethnic groups and suggested socio-demographic variables, poorer overall health and structural barriers all predicted professional help-seeking, albeit differently within the two refugee groups. These findings have significant implications for policy makers and service providers who aim to support this group during the resettlement period.

Author Contributions: Conceptualization, A.-M.T., S.S.-Y., R.N. and P.R.; formal analysis, A.-M.T. and P.R.; methodology, A.-M.T. and P.R.; supervision, S.S.-Y. and R.N.; writing—original draft, A.-M.T.; writing—review and editing, S.S.-Y., R.N. and P.R. All authors have read and agreed to the published version of the manuscript.

Funding: This research received no external funding.

Informed Consent Statement: Informed consent was obtained from all subjects involved in the BNLA study.

Data Availability Statement: Data used in this study are publicly available to approved researchers. Access is managed by the National Centre for Longitudinal Data on National Centre for Longitudinal Data Dataverse.

Acknowledgments: This paper uses unit record data from Building a New Life in Australia: the Longitudinal Study of Humanitarian Migrants (BNLA) conducted by the Australian Government Department of Social Services (DSS). The findings and views reported in this paper, however, are those of the authors and should not be attributed to the Australian Government, DSS, or any of DSS' contractors or partners. DOI: 10.26193/0AF6TZ.

Conflicts of Interest: S.S.-Y. is a guest editor of the Special Issue on Mental Health Promotion for Refugees and Other Culturally and/or Linguistically Diverse Migrant Populations. The authors declare no other conflicts of interest.

References

1. United Nations High Commissioner for Refugees (UNHCR). Mid-Year Trends 2020. Available online: https://www.unhcr.org/statistics/unhcrstats/5fc504d44/mid-year-trends-2020.html (accessed on 2 September 2021).
2. United Nations High Commissioner for Refugees (UNHCR). Refugee Statistics. 18 July 2021. Available online: https://www.unhcr.org/refugee-statistics/ (accessed on 2 September 2021).
3. Department of Home Affairs. Australia's Offshore Humanitarian Program: 2018–19. 2019. Available online: https://www.homeaffairs.gov.au/research-and-stats/files/australia-offshore-humanitarian-program-2018-19.pdf (accessed on 10 May 2021).
4. United Nations High Commissioner for Refugees (UNHCR). Convention and Protocol Relating to the Status of Refugees. 1951. Available online: https://www.unhcr.org/3b66c2aa10.html (accessed on 10 May 2021).
5. Department of Home Affairs. Afghanistan Update. 2021. Available online: https://www.homeaffairs.gov.au/help-and-support/afghanistan-update (accessed on 10 September 2021).
6. Bas-Sarmiento, P.; Saucedo-Moreno, M.J.; Fernández-Gutiérrez, M.; Poza-Méndez, M. Mental health in immigrants versus native population: A systematic review of the literature. *Arch. Psychiatr. Nurs.* **2017**, *31*, 111–121. [CrossRef] [PubMed]
7. Kartal, D.; Kiropoulos, L. Effects of acculturative stress on PTSD, depressive, and anxiety symptoms among refugees resettled in Australia and Austria. *Eur. J. Psychotraumatol.* **2016**, *7*, 1–11. [CrossRef]
8. Miller, K.E.; Rasmussen, A. The mental health of civilians displaced by armed conflict: An ecological model of refugee distress. *Epidemiol. Psychiatr. Sci.* **2017**, *26*, 129–138. [CrossRef]
9. Bogic, M.; Njoku, A.; Priebe, S. Long-term mental health of war-refugees: A systematic literature review. *BMC Int. Health Hum. Rights* **2015**, *15*, 1–41. [CrossRef] [PubMed]
10. Australian Bureau of Statistics. Mental Health, 2017–2018 Financial Year. 2018. Available online: https://www.abs.gov.au/statistics/health/health-conditions-and-risks/mental-health/latest-release (accessed on 10 May 2021).
11. McEvoy, P.M.; Grove, R.; Slade, T. Epidemiology of anxiety disorders in the Australian general population: Findings of the 2007 Australian national survey of mental health and wellbeing. *Aust. N. Z. J. Psychiatr.* **2011**, *45*, 957–967. [CrossRef]
12. Hamrah, M.S.; Hoang, H.; Mond, J.; Pahlavanzade, B.; Charkazi, A.; Auckland, S. The prevalence and correlates of symptoms of post-traumatic stress disorder (PTSD) among resettled Afghan refugees in a regional area of Australia. *J. Ment. Health* **2020**, *1*, 1–7. [CrossRef]
13. Rickwood, D.; Thomas, K. Conceptual measurement framework for help-seeking for mental health problems. *Psychol. Res. Behav. Manag.* **2012**, *5*, 173–183. [CrossRef] [PubMed]
14. Satinsky, E.; Fuhr, D.C.; Woodward, A.; Sondorp, E.; Roberts, B. Mental health care utilisation and access among refugees and asylum seekers in Europe: A systematic review. *Health Policy* **2019**, *123*, 851–863. [CrossRef]
15. Slewa-Younan, S.; Rioseco, P.; Guajardo, M.G.U.; Mond, J. Predictors of professional help-seeking for emotional problems in Afghan and Iraqi refugees in Australia: Findings from the Building a New Life in Australia Database. *BMC Public Health* **2019**, *19*, 1–11. [CrossRef]
16. Slewa-Younan, S.; Yaser, A.; Guajardo, M.G.U.; Mannan, H.; Smith, C.A.; Mond, J.M. The mental health and help-seeking behaviour of resettled Afghan refugees in Australia. *Int. J. Ment. Health Syst.* **2017**, *11*, 1–8. [CrossRef]
17. Whiteford, H.A.; Buckingham, W.J.; Harris, M.G.; Burgess, P.M.; Pirkis, J.E.; Barendregt, J.J.; Hall, W.D. Estimating treatment rates for mental disorders in Australia. *Aust. Health Rev.* **2014**, *38*, 80–85. [CrossRef]
18. Anderson, E.A. Measuring service quality at a university health clinic. *Int. J. Health Care Qual. Assur.* **1995**, *8*, 32–37. [CrossRef] [PubMed]
19. Azfredrick, E.C. Using Anderson's model of health service utilization to examine use of services by adolescent girls in South-Eastern Nigeria. *Int. J. Adolesc. Youth* **2016**, *21*, 523–529. [CrossRef]
20. Byrow, Y.; Pajak, R.; Specker, P.; Nickerson, A. Perceptions of mental health and perceived barriers to mental health help-seeking amongst refugees: A systematic review. *Clin. Psychol. Rev.* **2020**, *75*, 1–15. [CrossRef]
21. Kiselev, N.; Pfaltz, M.; Haas, F.; Schick, M.; Kappen, M.; Sijbrandij, M.; de Graaff, A.M.; Bird, M.; Hansen, P.; Ventevogel, P.; et al. Structural and socio-cultural barriers to accessing mental healthcare among Syrian refugees and asylum seekers in Switzerland. *Eur. J. Psychotraumatol.* **2020**, *11*, 1–16. [CrossRef]
22. Durbin, A.; Moineddin, R.; Lin, E.; Steele, L.S.; Glazier, R.H. Mental health service use by recent immigrants from different world regions and by non-immigrants in Ontario, Canada: A cross-sectional study. *BMC Health Serv. Res.* **2015**, *15*, 136–146. [CrossRef] [PubMed]

23. Mackenzie, C.S.; Scott, T.; Mather, A.; Sareen, J. Older adults' help-seeking attitudes and treatment beliefs concerning mental health problems. *Am. J. Geriatr. Psychiatr.* **2008**, *16*, 1010–1019. [CrossRef] [PubMed]
24. Marshall, G.N.; Berthold, S.M.; Schell, T.L.; Elliott, M.N.; Chun, C.A.; Hambarsoomians, K. Rates and correlates of seeking mental health services among Cambodian refugees. *Am. J. Public Health* **2006**, *96*, 1829–1835. [CrossRef]
25. Thikeo, M.; Florin, P.; Ng, C. Help seeking attitudes among Cambodian and Laotian refugees: Implications for public mental health approaches. *J. Immigr. Minority Health* **2015**, *17*, 1679–1686. [CrossRef]
26. Magaard, J.L.; Seeralan, T.; Schulz, H.; Brütt, A.L. Factors associated with help-seeking behaviour among individuals with major depression: A systematic review. *PLoS ONE* **2017**, *12*, e1–e17. [CrossRef]
27. Bauer, A.M.; Chen, C.N.; Alegría, M. English language proficiency and mental health service use among Latino and Asian Americans with mental disorders. *Med. Care* **2010**, *48*, 1097–1104. [CrossRef]
28. van der Boor, C.F.; White, R. Barriers to accessing and negotiating mental health services in asylum seeking and refugee populations: The application of the candidacy framework. *J. Immigr. Minority Health* **2019**, *22*, 156–174. [CrossRef] [PubMed]
29. Markova, V.; Sandal, G.M.; Pallesen, S. Immigration, acculturation, and preferred help-seeking sources for depression: Comparison of five ethnic groups. *BMC Health Serv. Research.* **2020**, *20*, 1–11. [CrossRef] [PubMed]
30. Schubert, C.C.; Punamäki, R.L.; Suvisaari, J.; Koponen, P.; Castaneda, A. Trauma, psychosocial factors, and help-seeking in three immigrant groups in Finland. *J. Behav. Health Serv. Res.* **2019**, *46*, 80–98. [CrossRef] [PubMed]
31. Salami, B.; Salma, J.; Hegadoren, K. Access and utilization of mental health services for immigrants and refugees: Perspectives of immigrant service providers. *Int. J. Ment. Health Nurs.* **2019**, *28*, 152–161. [CrossRef]
32. Zehetmair, C.; Zeyher, V.; Cranz, A.; Ditzen, B.; Herpertz, S.C.; Kohl, R.M.; Nikendei, C. A walk-in clinic for newly arrived mentally burdened refugees: The patient perspective. *Int. J. Environ. Res. Public Health* **2021**, *18*, 2275. [CrossRef]
33. Jorm, A.F.; Korten, A.E.; Jacomb, P.A.; Christensen, H.; Rodgers, B.; Pollitt, P. "Mental health literacy": A survey of the public's ability to recognise mental disorders and their beliefs about the effectiveness of treatment. *Med. J. Aust.* **1997**, *166*, 182–186. [CrossRef]
34. Lamb, C.F.; Smith, M. Problems refugees face when accessing health services. *N. S. W. Public Health Bull.* **2002**, *13*, 161–163. [CrossRef]
35. Tulli, M.; Salami, B.; Begashaw, L.; Meherali, S.; Yohani, S.; Hegadoren, K. Immigrant mothers' perspectives of barriers and facilitators in accessing mental health care for their children. *J. Transcult. Nurs.* **2020**, *31*, 598–605. [CrossRef]
36. Morris, M.D.; Popper, S.T.; Rodwell, T.C.; Brodine, S.K.; Brouwer, K.C. Healthcare barriers of refugees post-resettlement. *J. Community Health* **2009**, *34*, 529–538. [CrossRef]
37. Ziersch, A.; Due, C.; Walsh, M. Discrimination: A health hazard for people from refugee and asylum-seeking backgrounds resettled in Australia. *BMC Public Health* **2020**, *20*, 108–122. [CrossRef]
38. American Psychological Association. APA Dictionary of Psychology 2020. Available online: https://dictionary.apa.org/acculturation (accessed on 11 May 2021).
39. Beiser, M.; Simich, L.; Pandalangat, N. Community in distress: Mental health needs and help-seeking in the Tamil community in Toronto. *Int. Migr.* **2003**, *41*, 233–245. [CrossRef]
40. Dastjerdi, M.; Olson, K.; Ogilvie, L. A study of Iranian immigrants' experiences of accessing Canadian health care services: A grounded theory. *Int. J. Equity Health* **2012**, *11*, 55–70. [CrossRef]
41. Lincoln, A.K.; Lazarevic, V.; White, M.T.; Ellis, B.H. The impact of acculturation style and acculturative hassles on the mental health of Somali adolescent refugees. *J. Immigr. Minority Health* **2016**, *18*, 771–778. [CrossRef] [PubMed]
42. Berry, J.W. Immigration, acculturation, and adaptation. *Appl. Psychol.* **1997**, *46*, 5–34. [CrossRef]
43. Australian Institute of Family Studies. *Building a New Life in Australia: The Longitudinal Study of Humanitarian Migrants, Release 5 (Waves 1–5)*; ADA Dataverse, V4; Department of Social Services: Canberra, Australia, 2019. [CrossRef]
44. Hansen, M.; Andersen, T.E.; Armour, C.; Elklit, A.; Palic, S.; Mackrill, T. PTSD-8: A short PTSD inventory. *Clin. Prac. Epidem. Ment. Health* **2010**, *6*, 101–108. [CrossRef] [PubMed]
45. Kessler, R.C.; Barker, P.R.; Colpe, L.J.; Epstein, J.F.; Gfroerer, J.C.; Hiripi, E.; Howes, M.J.; Normand, S.L.T.; Manderscheid, R.W.; Walters, E.E.; et al. Screening for serious mental illness in the general population. *Arch. Gen. Psychiatr.* **2003**, *60*, 184–189. [CrossRef] [PubMed]
46. Kawakami, N.; Thi Thu Tran, T.; Watanabe, K.; Imamura, K.; Thanh Nguyen, H.; Sasaki, N.; Kuribayashi, K.; Sakuraya, A.; Thuy Nguyen, Q.; Thi Nguyen, N.; et al. Thi Huong Nguyen, G.; Minas, H.; Tsutsumi, A. Internal consistency reliability, construct validity, and item response characteristics of the Kessler 6 scale among hospital nurses in Vietnam. *PLoS ONE* **2020**, *15*, 1–15. [CrossRef]
47. Shoeb, M.; Weinstein, H.; Mollica, R. The Harvard trauma questionnaire: Adapting a cross-cultural instrument for measuring torture, trauma and posttraumatic stress disorder in Iraqi refugees. *Int. J. Soc. Psychiatry* **2007**, *53*, 447–463. [CrossRef] [PubMed]
48. Wu, S.; Renzaho, A.M.; Hall, B.J.; Shi, L.; Ling, L.; Chen, W. Time-varying associations of pre-migration and post-migration stressors in refugees' mental health during resettlement: A longitudinal study in Australia. *Lancet Psychiatr.* **2021**, *8*, 36–47. [CrossRef]
49. Seasholtz, M.B.; Kowalski, B. The parsimony principle applied to multivariate calibration. *Anal. Chim. Acta* **1993**, *277*, 165–177. [CrossRef]

50. Smith, L.; Hoang, H.; Reynish, T.; McLeod, K.; Hannah, C.; Auckland, S.; Slewa-Younan, S.; Mond, J. Factors shaping the lived experience of resettlement for former refugees in regional Australia. *Int. J. Environ. Res. Public Health* **2020**, *17*, 501. [CrossRef]
51. Dubus, N.; LeBoeuf, H.S. A qualitative study of the perceived effectiveness of refugee services among consumers, providers, and interpreters. *Transcult. Psychiatr.* **2019**, *56*, 827–844. [CrossRef] [PubMed]
52. Rometsch, C.; Denkinger, J.K.; Engelhardt, M.; Windthorst, P.; Graf, J.; Gibbons, N.; Pham, P.; Zipfel, S.; Junne, F. Pain, somatic complaints, and subjective concepts of illness in traumatized female refugees who experienced extreme violence by the "Islamic State" (IS). *J. Psychosom. Res.* **2020**, *130*, 1–9. [CrossRef]
53. Khawaja, N.G.; Hebbani, A.; Gallois, C.; MacKinnon, M. Predictors of employment status: A study of former refugee communities in Australia. *Aus. Psychol.* **2019**, *54*, 427–437. [CrossRef]
54. Song, Y.J.; Hofstetter, C.; Hovell, M.F.; Paik, H.Y.; Park, H.R.; Lee, J.; Irvin, V. Acculturation and health risk behaviors among Californians of Korean descent. *Prev. Med.* **2004**, *39*, 147–156. [CrossRef]
55. Hynie, M. The social determinants of refugee mental health in the post-migration context: A critical review. *Can. J. Psychiatr.* **2017**, *63*, 297–303. [CrossRef]
56. Spencer, M.S.; Chen, J.; Gee, G.C.; Fabian, C.G.; Takeuchi, D.T. Discrimination and mental health–related service use in a national study of Asian Americans. *Am. J. Public Health* **2010**, *100*, 2410–2417. [CrossRef]
57. Althubaiti, A. Information bias in health research: Definition, pitfalls, and adjustment methods. *J. Multidiscip. Health* **2016**, *9*, 211–217. [CrossRef]
58. Ogilvie, L.D.; Burgess-Pinto, E.; Caufield, C. Challenges and approaches to newcomer health research. *J. Transcult. Nurs.* **2008**, *19*, 64–73. [CrossRef] [PubMed]

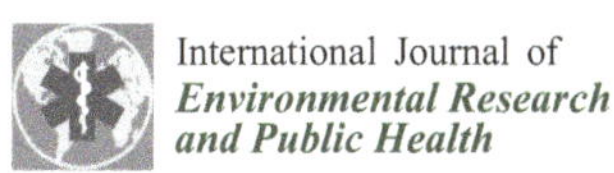

International Journal of
Environmental Research and Public Health

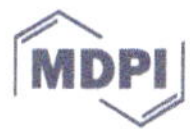

Brief Report

Screening for Posttraumatic Stress Symptoms in Young Refugees: Comparison of Questionnaire Data with and without Involvement of an Interpreter

Lauritz Rudolf Floribert Müller *,†, Johanna Unterhitzenberger †, Svenja Wintersohl, Rita Rosner and Julia König

Department of Psychology, Catholic University Eichstätt-Ingolstadt, Ostenstraße 25, 85072 Eichstätt, Germany; johanna.unterhitzenberger@ku.de (J.U.); svenja.wintersohl@gmx.de (S.W.); rita.rosner@ku.de (R.R.); julia.koenig@ku.de (J.K.)
* Correspondence: lauritz.mueller@ku.de; Tel.: +49-842-193-21265
† Joint first authors.

Abstract: Background: The substantial number of young refugees who have arrived in Europe since 2015 requires rapid screening to identify those in need of treatment. However, translated versions of screening measures are not always available, necessitating the support of interpreters. The Child and Adolescent Trauma Screen (CATS) is a validated questionnaire for posttraumatic stress symptoms. Here, we report on the psychometric properties of the CATS in a sample of young refugees as a function of interpreter involvement. **Methods:** A total of $N = 145$ ($M_{age} = 16.8$, $SD = 1.54$; 93% male) were assessed with the CATS, with half of the screenings conducted with and half without interpreters. Post hoc analyses included calculating internal consistency using Cronbach's α. We used confirmative factor analysis to investigate the factor structure. **Results:** The CATS total scale showed good reliability ($\alpha = 0.84$). Differences in psychometric properties between the interpreter vs. the no interpreter group were minor and tended to be in favor of the interpreter group. Results of a confirmatory factor analysis were acceptable after the exclusion of items with low item-scale correlations. **Conclusions:** The sample and the administration of the assessment represent the situation of young refugees in Germany, where resources are low and translated versions not always available. The CATS may be a helpful screening tool for clinicians working with young refugees, even when administered with an interpreter. Limitations include the post hoc design of the analysis without randomization of participants and the lack of a third comparison group using translated questionnaire versions.

Keywords: refugee; adolescent; assessment; screening; PTSD; interpreter

Citation: Müller, L.R.F.; Unterhitzenberger, J.; Wintersohl, S.; Rosner, R.; König, J. Screening for Posttraumatic Stress Symptoms in Young Refugees: Comparison of Questionnaire Data with and without Involvement of an Interpreter. *Int. J. Environ. Res. Public Health* **2021**, *18*, 6803. https://doi.org/10.3390/ijerph18136803

Academic Editor: Paul B. Tchounwou

Received: 30 April 2021
Accepted: 23 June 2021
Published: 24 June 2021

Publisher's Note: MDPI stays neutral with regard to jurisdictional claims in published maps and institutional affiliations.

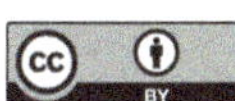

1. Introduction

Asylum-seeking youth, and especially unaccompanied asylum-seeking youth, have a high risk for posttraumatic stress disorder (PTSD; [1,2]). A brief and valid screening should constitute the first step of recently proposed stepped-care models to meet the psychological needs of young refugees, which are currently being tested in this group [3]. To this end, measures must be validated for culturally diverse samples. The Child and Adolescent Trauma Screen (CATS; [4]) is a short self-report questionnaire with items corresponding to PTSD criteria in the Diagnostic and Statistical Manual for Mental Disorders, 5th edition (DSM-5; [5]). It has been validated in an international (Western) sample with good reliability and validity and has since been used repeatedly with refugee youth [1,6,7].

However, self-report screening measures, including the CATS, are not available for all languages of interest in the refugee context, and, moreover, many asylum-seeking youth are illiterate and cannot use translated versions even when they exist [8]. Accordingly, in real-life care settings, screenings are often conducted with non-native language versions even when the respondents' language proficiency is low or must be supported by interpreters. In this context, untrained lay interpreters, who might be unfamiliar with mental health services, are often employed [9]. In principle, it is conceivable that the involvement of (lay) interpreters could change both screening results and therapeutic processes for a variety of reasons, including omission of cultural taboos in the translation process, role difficulties that might lead interpreters to take a directive rather than a neutral role, and lack of professional understanding regarding mental health services [10]. In terms of therapy effectiveness, the few existing post hoc findings on interpreter involvement present a mixed picture [11,12], whereby the latest study found that the group with interpreters involved showed poorer results than the comparison group without interpreters [12]. However, there are very few quantitative findings on the effects of employing an interpreter in mental health settings in general and, to our knowledge, no studies on the effects on screening or diagnostic results in particular.

Accordingly, this post hoc study aims (1) to investigate the internal consistency of the CATS in a sample of young refugees resettled to Germany using German language versions with vs. without the involvement of an interpreter; (2) to compare symptom severity, item values and item-scale correlations between the two groups; and (3) to examine the factor structure of the CATS in the total sample.

2. Materials and Methods

2.1. Procedure and Participants

Data from two studies were used with a total of $N = 145$. Study 1 assessed the mental health of $n = 98$ minor refugees resettled in southern Germany in an interview-like setting [1]. Study 2 was a pilot study [6] examining trauma-focused cognitive behavioral therapy [13] with $n = 47$ unaccompanied refugee minors. Overall, participants were, on average, $M = 16.73$ years of age ($SD = 1.54$). Most participants were unaccompanied ($n = 115, 78.8\%$) and boys ($n = 135, 93.1\%$), reflecting the population structure in Germany, where most unaccompanied refugee minors are male (for further sociodemographic information, see Supplementary Material Table S1).

Both studies were approved by the IRB of the Catholic University Eichstätt-Ingolstadt (2016/23 and 2015/02/16) and participants gave their written informed consent to participate in the respective study.

2.2. Measure

The Child and Adolescent Trauma Screen (CATS) assesses posttraumatic stress symptoms (PTSS) according to DSM-5 in youngsters aged 7 to 17 years [4]. Participants indicate whether they have experienced 15 potentially traumatic events (yes/no) and specify the currently most distressing event. Then, they rate 20 items on PTSS on a 4-point Likert scale (0—*never* to 3—*almost always*). The sum score is between 0 and 60, with scores ≥ 21 indicating clinically relevant PTSS. The four subscales—intrusion, avoidance, negative alterations in cognition and mood (NACM), and hyperarousal—can be formed, which refer to the PTSD diagnostic criteria in the DSM-5. The CATS has been validated in English, German, and Norwegian language versions. We used the German version. In half of the sample, $n = 72$ (50%), interpreters supported diagnostics (for one Study 1 participant, information on interpreter involvement was missing).

3. Data Analysis

We used SPSS version 25 (IBM, Armonk, USA) for all analyses. We examined descriptive statistics and internal consistency (Cronbach's α) for the CATS total score and symptom subscales, and for cases with and without involvement of an interpreter. We computed χ^2-statistics to examine differences in internal consistency between the two subgroups using cocron [14]. A confirmative factor analysis was applied to investigate the previously confirmed DSM-5 factor structure using AMOS for SPSS version 25. For RM-

SEA, values $\leq$ 0.06 (marginal: 0.07–0.08) [15] and for CFI and TLI, values $\geq$ 0.95 (marginal: 0.90–0.94) indicate a good fit [16].

4. Results

4.1. Internal Consistency

The CATS showed a good internal consistency with Cronbach's α = 0.84 in the total sample. Internal consistency was slightly, but not significantly, higher when assessed with an interpreter (n = 72; α = 0.85) than without one (n = 72; α = 0.82; $\chi^2(1)$ = 0.684, p = 0.408). The four symptom clusters differed in their internal consistency and showed rather poor results (see Table 1). Internal consistencies of the four subscales were consistently, but not significantly, lower in the group without an interpreter, with avoidance even having a negative value in this group.

Table 1. Internal consistencies (Cronbach's α) of the four subscales in the full sample and the two subsamples.

	Full Sample (n = 145)	Interpreter (n = 72)	No Interpreter (n = 72)	Group Difference $\chi^2(1)$	p
CATS total	0.838	0.852	0.818	0.684	0.408
Intrusion	0.727	0.748	0.699	0.370	0.543
Avoidance	0.310	0.432	−0.029	1.813 [a]	0.178
NACM	0.659	0.656	0.654	<0.001	0.983
Hyperarousal	0.585	0.606	0.580	0.052	0.821

Note. CATS = Child and Adolescent Trauma Screen. NACM = Negative alterations in cognition and mood. [a] As it was not possible to compute the comparison with a negative value of α, α = 0 was substituted in the group without interpreter.

4.2. Symptom Scores and Item Analyses

Participants from Study 1 had lower average CATS scores, M = 22.40, SD = 9.35, than participants from Study 2, M = 26.87, SD = 10.35, F (143) = 2.61, p = 0.010. CATS scores did not vary with interpreter involvement in either subsample. In Study 1, cases without interpreters had a mean CATS score of M = 21.56, SD = 9.07, and cases with interpreters of M = 23.91, SD = 9.78, T (96) = -1.200, p = 0.233, and in Study 2, cases without interpreters had a mean CATS score of M = 29.33, SD = 7.14 and with interpreters M = 26.51, SD = 11.03, T (44) = 0.727, p = 0.471.

Means and standard deviations, as well as corrected item-scale correlations of the 20 CATS items, are given in Table 2. Five items in the sample without interpreters, and three items in the sample with interpreters had item-scale correlations $\leq$ 0.30, resulting in five items (8, 10, 12, 16, and 17) in the overall sample with item-scale correlations $\leq$ 0.30.

4.3. Factorial Validity

The four-factor CFA model proposed by the DSM-5 and found by Sachser et al. (2017) did not show a very good fit. While RMSEA was good, at 0.06 (90% CI 0.04–0.07), the CFI was, at 0.86, below the acceptable range. Removing five items with item-scale correlations at or below r = 0.30 resulted in a slightly worse, but still acceptable, RMSEA of 0.07 (90% CI 0.05–0.09), and improved CFI to 0.89 (see Table 2).

Table 2. Item means, standard deviations and corrected item-scale correlations in the full sample and the two subsamples.

Item	Full Sample (n = 145)			Interpreter (n = 72)			No Interpreter (n = 72)		
	M	*SD*	ISC	*M*	*SD*	ISC	*M*	*SD*	ISC
1. Upsetting thoughts or pictures about what happened that pop into your head.	1.61	0.96	0.45	1.67	0.99	0.42	1.56	0.93	0.48
2. Bad dreams reminding you of what happened.	1.37	0.96	0.40	1.38	0.94	0.45	1.35	0.98	0.37
3. Feeling as if what happened is happening all over again.	0.99	1.05	0.47	1.19 [a]	1.11	0.50	0.81 [a]	0.96	0.41
4. Feeling very upset when you are reminded of what happened.	1.73	0.95	0.52	1.85	0.94	0.54	1.63	0.94	0.48
5. Strong feelings in your body when you are reminded of what happened (sweating, heart beating fast, upset stomach).	1.37	1.03	0.50	1.44	1.05	0.49	1.28	1.02	0.52
6. Trying not to think about what happened. Or to not have feelings about it.	2.00	0.90	0.37	2.14	0.92	0.52	1.88	0.85	**0.17**
7. Staying away from anything that reminds you of what happened (people, places, things, situations, talks).	1.05	1.11	0.38	1.32 [b]	1.17	0.33	0.79 [b]	0.99	0.40
8. Not being able to remember part of what happened.	0.70	0.89	**0.13**	0.74	0.87	**0.15**	0.67	0.92	**0.10**
9. Negative thoughts about yourself or others. Thoughts like I will not have a good life, no one can be trusted, the whole world is unsafe.	1.25	1.12	0.51	1.29	1.14	0.60	1.22	1.10	0.39
10. Blaming yourself for what happened. Or blaming someone else when it is not their fault.	0.67	0.87	**0.30**	0.69	0.87	0.33	0.65	0.87	**0.25**
11. Bad feelings (afraid, angry, guilty, ashamed) a lot of the time.	1.43	0.94	0.56	1.49	1.03	0.57	1.38	0.85	0.55
12. Not wanting to do things you used to do.	1.14	1.14	**0.30**	1.17	1.15	**0.27**	1.11	1.15	0.33
13. Not feeling close to people.	0.86	0.98	0.43	0.94	1.05	0.43	0.78	0.91	0.42
14. Not being able to have good or happy feelings.	1.15	1.00	0.57	1.24	1.05	0.61	1.07	0.95	0.52
15. Feeling mad. Having fits of anger and taking it out on others.	1.03	0.96	0.45	1.06	1.01	0.43	1.01	0.93	0.48
16. Doing unsafe things.	0.33	0.64	**0.29**	0.26	0.60	0.44	0.40	0.66	**0.16**
17. Being overly careful (checking to see who is around you).	1.23	1.12	**0.17**	1.19	1.11	**0.14**	1.26	1.14	**0.22**
18. Being jumpy.	1.11	1.05	0.43	1.03	1.01	0.39	1.19	1.10	0.52
19. Problems paying attention.	1.12	1.00	0.52	1.32 [c]	1.06	0.59	0.93 [c]	0.91	0.41
20. Trouble falling or staying asleep.	1.72	1.13	0.55	1.85	1.16	0.58	1.57	1.09	0.53

Note. The subscales are composed as follows: Intrusion (items 1, 2, 3, 4, 5), avoidance (items 6, 7), NACM (items 8, 9, 10, 11, 12, 13, 14), and hyperarousal (items 15, 16, 17, 18, 19, 20). *M* = mean; *SD* = standard deviation; ISC = item-scale correlations. ISCs ≤ 0.30 are in bold print. [a] significant difference between means, *T* (139.1) = −2.251, *p* = 0.026. [b] significant difference between means, *T* (138.1) = −2.915, *p* = 0.004. [c] significant difference between means, *T* (138.8) = −2.364, *p* = 0.019.

5. Discussion

We reported on the post hoc psychometric evaluation of the CATS as a function of interpreter involvement in a sample of severely traumatized refugee youngsters from 17 countries. The CATS previously showed good psychometric properties with translated versions and samples from Germany, Norway, and the US [4]. In our sample, the overall internal reliability was lower, but still good and did not differ between the subgroup that involved an interpreter and the one that did not. In our sample, however, avoidance, hyperarousal, and NACM showed questionable to very poor alphas, with a negative α for avoidance in the group without an interpreter. It must be kept in mind, however, that this subscale has only two items dealing with different forms of avoidance and is, therefore, not ideal to begin with from a factor analytic point of view [17]. Although the internal consistencies of the subscales tended to be consistently better in the group with interpreters, some of them were still outside the acceptable range. On the one hand, this could indicate that the young refugees were unfamiliar with psychological test formats [18], that language difficulties might have occurred, or that culturally divergent concepts were captured by the questionnaires. On the other hand, the sometimes low reliability even in the interpreter group may also stem from the difficulty of translating almost simultaneously in the screening situation and the resulting quality of translation for culturally disputable constructs. Accordingly, translated questionnaire versions, in which the translation process is more elaborate due to iterative improvements, could contribute to increasing the reliability in the recording of the subscales [19].

Five items had low corrected item-scale correlations of 0.30 or below, and this problem was more pronounced in the group not supported by an interpreter. The four-factor model showed an acceptable fit only after removing items with bad item characteristics and even then, fit indices were worse than those reported in the original study [4]. Given the heterogeneity of our sample including refugee youth from 17 countries, this deviation from the original study, which examined more homogeneous national samples, may not, however, be too surprising.

5.1. Limitations

A key limitation of this analysis is its retrospective nature and the fact that the variable of interest is difficult to manipulate experimentally. Study clinicians decided whether to employ an interpreter for screening according to their perception of participants' German language skills and preferences. However, most studies on the impact of interpreters on mental health services share this limitation. While sample 1 offered voluntary participation in a screening study, sample 2 was a service use sample, which might have resulted in selection biases affecting this analysis. Furthermore, a third group using translated versions was lacking and the subsamples were too small so as to conduct CFAs for both groups separately.

5.2. Implications

Overall, the psychometric differences between the two groups were small and tended to favor the assistance of interpreters (internal consistency, item-scale correlations). Considering the multilingual population of young refugees in Germany, where translated versions of screening measures are often lacking, the common practice to employ lay interpreters does not seem to be disadvantageous, at least in terms of reliability.

6. Conclusions

The CATS is a reliable screening instrument for PTSS in culturally diverse refugee youth samples, including its use with the involvement of interpreters, making it a feasible screening tool for professionals working in this field (available at https://ulmer-onlineklinik.de/course/view.php?id=1701, accessed on 24 June 2021). Assessments should be followed by a (semi-)structured interview to ascertain clinically relevant symptoms or diagnostic status. From a scientific point of view, these findings should be verified by means of a validation of the CATS with a gold standard clinical interview. Given the paucity of quantitative research findings on the influence of interpreters on processes in mental health services, which has been emphasized by a variety of research groups [10,20], this study can be understood as a starting point for further rigorous studies, despite the limitations due to the post hoc design.

Supplementary Materials: The following are available online at https://www.mdpi.com/article/10.3390/ijerph18136803/s1, Table S1: Characteristics of study sample.

Author Contributions: L.R.F.M. undertook the data collection in Study 1 and was responsible for drafting the manuscript. J.U. was principal investigator in both studies and was responsible for drafting the manuscript and analyzing the data. S.W. undertook the data collection in Study 2 and was responsible for the integration of datasets. R.R. supervised both studies and revised the manuscript. J.K. was involved in all issues with regard to data analysis and manuscript drafting. All authors have read and agreed to the published version of the manuscript.

Funding: This work was supported by the funding program proFor+ of the Catholic University Eichstätt-Ingolstadt (ID: 2316). Publication of this work was supported by the German Research Foundation (DFG) within the funding programme Open Access Publishing.

Institutional Review Board Statement: This is an additional analysis of two pre-studies. The studies were conducted according to the guidelines of the Declaration of Helsinki, and approved by the Institutional Review Board (or Ethics Committee) of the Catholic University Eichstätt-Ingolstadt (protocol code 2016/23 and 2015/02/16).

Informed Consent Statement: Informed consent was obtained from all subjects involved in the study. Written informed consent has been obtained from all participants to publish this paper.

Data availability statement: The datasets generated and analyzed during this study are not publicly available due to sensitive and potentially identifying participant information but are available from the corresponding author on reasonable request.

Acknowledgments: We would like to thank Margret Lang and Karl Büter and all participants.

Conflicts of Interest: The authors declare no conflict of interest. The sponsors had no role in the design, execution, interpretation, or writing of the study.

Abbreviations

CATS	Child and Adolescent Trauma Screen
CFA	Confirmatory factor analysis
CFI	Comparative fit index
DSM-5	Diagnostic and Statistical Manual for Mental Disorders, 5th edition
NACM	Negative alterations in cognition and mood
RMSEA	Root mean square error of approximation
PTSD	Post-traumatic stress disorder
PTSS	Post-traumatic stress symptoms
SPSS	Statistical Package for the Social Sciences
TLI	Tucker–Lewis index

References

1. Müller, L.R.F.; Büter, K.P.; Rosner, R.; Unterhitzenberger, J. Mental health and associated stress factors in accompanied and unaccompanied refugee minors resettled in Germany: A cross-sectional study. *Child Adolesc. Psychiatry Ment. Health* **2019**, *13*, 8. [CrossRef] [PubMed]
2. Von Werthern, M.; Grigorakis, G.; Vizard, E. The mental health and wellbeing of Unaccompanied Refugee Minors (URMs). *Child Abus. Negl.* **2019**, *98*, 104146. [CrossRef] [PubMed]
3. Rosner, R.; Sachser, C.; Hornfeck, F.; Kilian, R.; Kindler, H.; Muche, R. Improving mental health care for unaccompanied young refugees through a stepped-care approach versus usual care+: Study protocol of a cluster randomized controlled hybrid effectiveness implementation trial. *Trials* **2020**, *21*, 1–13. [CrossRef] [PubMed]
4. Sachser, C.; Berliner, L.; Holt, T.; Jensen, T.K.; Jungbluth, N.; Risch, E. International development and psychometric properties of the Child and Adolescent Trauma Screen (CATS). *J. Affect Disord.* **2017**, *210*, 189–195. [CrossRef] [PubMed]

5. American Psychiatric Association. *Diagnostic and Statistical Manual of Mental Disorders [DSM-5]*, 5th ed.; American Psychiatric Association: Washington, DC, USA, 2013. [CrossRef]
6. Unterhitzenberger, J.; Wintersohl, S.; Lang, M.; König, J.; Rosner, R. Providing manualized individual trauma-focused CBT to unaccompanied refugee minors with uncertain residence status: A pilot study. *Child Adolesc. Psychiatry Ment. Health* **2019**, *13*, 22. [CrossRef] [PubMed]
7. Pfeiffer, E.; Sukale, T.; Müller, L.R.F.; Plener, P.L.; Rosner, R.; Fegert, J.M. The symptom representation of posttraumatic stress disorder in a sample of unaccompanied and accompanied refugee minors in Germany: A network analysis. *Eur. J. Psychotraumatol.* **2019**, *10*, 1675990. [CrossRef] [PubMed]
8. Jakobsen, M.; Demott, M.A.M.; Heir, T. Prevalence of psychiatric disorders among unaccompanied asylum- seeking adolescents in Norway. *Clin. Pr. Epidemiol. Ment. Health* **2014**, *10*, 53–58. [CrossRef] [PubMed]
9. Gartley, T.; Due, C. The Interpreter Is Not an Invisible Being: A Thematic Analysis of the Impact of Interpreters in Mental Health Service Provision with Refugee Clients. *Aust. Psychol.* **2017**, *52*, 31–40. [CrossRef]
10. Rousseau, C.; Measham, T.; Moro, M.-R. Working with Interpreters in Child Mental Health. *Child Adolesc. Ment. Health* **2011**, *16*, 55–59. [CrossRef] [PubMed]
11. d'Ardenne, P.; Ruaro, L.; Cestari, L.; Fakhoury, W.; Priebe, S. Does Interpreter-Mediated CBT with Traumatized Refugee People Work? A Comparison of Patient Outcomes in East London. *Behav. Cogn. Psychother.* **2007**, *35*, 293–301. [CrossRef]
12. Sander, R.; Laugesen, H.; Skammeritz, S.; Mortensen, E.L.; Carlsson, J. Interpreter-mediated psychotherapy with trauma-affected refugees—A retrospective cohort study. *Psychiatry Res.* **2019**, *271*, 684–692. [CrossRef] [PubMed]
13. Cohen, J.A.; Mannarino, A.P.; Deblinger, E. *Treating Trauma and Traumatic Grief in Children and Adolescents*, 2nd ed.; Guilford Publications: New York, NY, USA, 2017.
14. Diedenhofen, B.; Musch, J. cocron: A Web Interface and R Package for the Statistical Comparison of Cronbach's Alpha Coefficients. *Int. J. Internet Sci.* **2016**, *11*, 51–60.
15. MacCallum, R.C.; Browne, M.W.; Sugawara, H.M. Power analysis and determination of sample size for covariance structure modeling. *Psychol. Methods* **1996**, *1*, 130–149. [CrossRef]
16. Hu, L.-T.; Bentler, P.M. Cutoff criteria for fit indexes in covariance structure analysis: Conventional criteria versus new alternatives. *Struct. Equ. Model* **1999**, *6*, 1–55. [CrossRef]
17. Kline, R.B. *Principles and Practice of Structural Equation Modeling*; Guilford Publications: New York, NY, USA, 2005.
18. Ehntholt, K.A.; Yule, W. Practitioner review: Assessment and treatment of refugee children and adolescents who have experienced war-related trauma. *J. Child Psychol. Psychiatry* **2006**, *47*, 1197–1210. [CrossRef] [PubMed]
19. Bhui, K.; Mohamud, S.; Warfa, N.; Craig, T.J.; Stansfeld, S.A. Cultural adaptation of mental health measures: Improving the quality of clinical practice and research. *Br. J. Psychiatry* **2003**, *183*, 184–186. [CrossRef] [PubMed]
20. Cecchet, S.J.; Calabrese, D. Interpreter-Mediated Therapy for Refugees: A Need for Awareness and Training. *Grad. Stud. J. Psychol.* **2011**, *13*, 12–16.

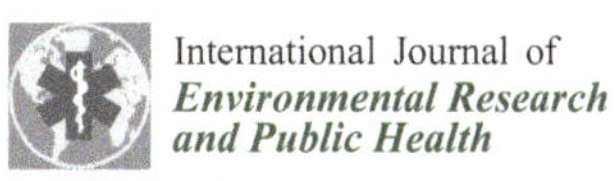

International Journal of
Environmental Research and Public Health

Article

Trauma, Post-Traumatic Stress Disorder, and Mental Health Care of Asylum Seekers

Rafael Youngmann [1,*], Rachel Bachner-Melman [1,2], Lilac Lev-Ari [1], Hadar Tzur [1], Ravit Hileli [3] and Ido Lurie [4,5]

1   Clinical Psychology Graduate Program, Ruppin Academic Center, Emek-Hefer 4015000, Israel; rachel.bachner@mail.huji.ac.il (R.B.-M.); ldlevari@gmail.com (L.L.-A.); hadartzur@gmail.com (H.T.)
2   School of Social Work and Social Welfare, Hebrew University of Jerusalem, Mount Scopus, Jerusalem 91905, Israel
3   Beer Ya'akov-Nez Tziona Mental Health Center, Beer Yaakov 70350, Israel; ravitkruvit@gmail.com
4   Department of Psychiatry, Sackler School of Medicine, Tel Aviv University, Tel Aviv 6812509, Israel; ido.lurie@gmail.com
5   Shalvata Mental Health Center, Hod Hasharon 69978, Israel
*   Correspondence: rafiyoung@ruppin.ac.il

Citation: Youngmann, R.; Bachner-Melman, R.; Lev-Ari, L.; Tzur, H.; Hileli, R.; Lurie, I. Trauma, Post-Traumatic Stress Disorder, and Mental Health Care of Asylum Seekers. *Int. J. Environ. Res. Public Health* **2021**, *18*, 10661. https://doi.org/10.3390/ijerph182010661

Academic Editor: Paul B. Tchounwou

Received: 16 August 2021
Accepted: 6 October 2021
Published: 12 October 2021

Publisher's Note: MDPI stays neutral with regard to jurisdictional claims in published maps and institutional affiliations.

Abstract: Asylum seekers in Israel from East Africa frequently experienced traumatic events along their journey, particularly in the Sinai Peninsula, where they were subjected to trafficking and torture. Exposure to trauma has implications for rights that are contingent on refugee status. This retrospective chart review aimed to characterize the types of traumas experienced by 219 asylum seekers (149 men) from Eritrea and Sudan who sought treatment at a specialized mental health clinic in Israel, and to compare the mental health of trauma victims ($n = 168$) with that of non-trauma victims ($n = 53$). About 76.7% of the asylum seekers had experienced at least one traumatic event, of whom 56.5% were diagnosed with post-traumatic stress disorder (PTSD). Most reported traumas were experienced en route in the Sinai, rather than in the country of origin or Israel. Few clinical differences were observed between trauma victims and non-trauma victims, or between trauma victims with and without a PTSD diagnosis. Our findings emphasize the importance of accessibility to mental and other health services for asylum seekers. Governmental policies and international conventions on the definition of human trafficking may need to be revised, as well as asylum seekers' rights and access to health services related to visa status.

Keywords: asylum seekers; Eritrea; Sudan; PTSD; trauma; mental health care

1. Introduction

The number of international migrants worldwide is growing, and currently exceeds 244 million [1]. Refugees and asylum seekers constitute one of the largest migratory movements, driven by violence, insecurity, and armed conflict [2]. Refugees are people who left their country of origin to avoid life-threatening circumstances or persecution for political, religious, or other reasons, and are recognized under the 1951 Convention on the Status of Refugees [3]. Asylum seekers have applied for but have not yet been granted refugee status. In 2020, there were 82.4 million refugees and 4.1 million asylum seekers worldwide [4].

As part of the global trend of migration, and in the wake of war and genocide in Darfur, and the political situation in Eritrea, the number of asylum seekers arriving in Israel from East Africa has increased significantly since 2006 [5,6]. Between 2006 and 2016, approximately 64,318 asylum seekers entered Israel, of whom 40,274 still resided there in 2016 [7]; 72% (29,014) from Eritrea, 20% (8002) from Sudan, 0.3% (121) from Ethiopia, 5.8% (2349) from other African countries and 2% (556) from elsewhere [7]. Based on the principle of non-refoulement, 91% of asylum seekers from Sudan and Eritrea have been granted group protection, including the right to remain in Israel until their home countries are deemed safe. The Israeli government has, however, adopted restrictive policies towards them, excluding them from full participation in Israel's social, political and health systems, with financial and psychological implications [6,8].

An estimated 7000 of the 52,961 asylum seekers who arrived in Israel between 2009 and 2013 [9] were exposed to kidnapping, torture, and human trafficking during their journey through the Sinai desert [6]. An estimated 4000 did not survive the journey [10]. Asylum seekers exploited in this way are defined by the UN conventions as "Smuggling Victims", "Torture Victims", or "Human Trafficking Victims" [11]. Only those recognized as "Trafficking Victims" or "Victims of Holding in Conditions of Slavery" by the State of Israel are legally entitled to shelter and rehabilitation services, including health insurance and a valid work permit, for one year [12], regardless of their physical and mental health status [13]. According to the UN Convention on the rights of refugees to health care [3], ratified by Israel in 1958 [14], asylum seekers who were victims of torture or human trafficking are entitled to recognition as refugees with rights to medical care and other services.

Asylum seekers living in Israel have very slim chances of receiving refugee status. In 2016, only 500 of the 37,016 asylum seekers from Sudan and Eritrea were officially recognized as "Trafficking Victims" or "Victims of Holding in Conditions of Slavery" [15]. These asylum seekers included 5000–7000 victims of torture, human trafficking and kidnapping in Sinai or their country of origin. No asylum seekers, however, were officially recognized as victims of human torture [15]. Of 13,764 asylum requests submitted by people from Sudan and Eritrea by July 2017, only ten had refugee status in 2018 [16], and therefore access to medical services. Others were granted access to health services in medical or psychiatric emergencies only [17]. Identifying victims of trafficking remains a major challenge due to the ambiguity of the international definition of exploitation [18], difficulties in defining types of victims in the Sinai desert [19,20], victims' lack of awareness of their rights [13], and restrictions imposed by the Israeli government on asylum seekers seeking recognition as trafficking victims [21].

The process of migration involves significant socio-psychological pressures that affect migrants' mental state. Asylum seekers and trafficking victims are particularly vulnerable to trauma-related disorders including post-traumatic stress disorder (PTSD), depression, somatic disorders, eating disorders, substance abuse (such as self-medication), self-injurious behavior, suicidality, and psychotic disorders [22–31]. As elsewhere, asylum seekers in Israel have high rates of emotional distress and psychiatric disorders [32,33]. Victims of torture experienced trauma directly or vicariously [6]. In addition, as a visible minority, African asylum seekers in Israel are vulnerable to racism and rejection by the local population [34,35]. Asylum seekers undoubtedly need social support, employment, and medical treatment to cope with post-migration challenges [36,37].

Most asylum seekers in Israel are not eligible for national health insurance, which provides psychiatric treatment [36,38]. One of their main options for psychiatric care is *Gesher* ("Bridge" in Hebrew), an adult (>18 years) psychiatric clinic established by the Ministry of Health in 2014 in Tel Aviv-Jaffa, for asylum seekers and other undocumented migrants [39]. The goal of the clinic is to deliver culturally competent and trauma-sensitive mental health treatment that includes the work of cultural brokers. A description of the clinic and its activities can be found elsewhere [40].

This study aimed to characterize asylum seekers mainly from Eritrea and Sudan who arrived in Israel through the Sinai Peninsula, between 2007 and 2013, including the types of traumas they experienced and the mental health care they received. These aims are of particular importance in Israel, where asylum seekers, referred to by the Ministry of the Interior as "infiltrators", have almost no access to mental health services.

We hypothesized that compared to asylum seekers who were not trauma victims, trauma victims would:

1. Be at greater risk for PTSD.
2. Have more consultations.
3. Receive psychiatric medication more frequently.
4. Report more drug/alcohol use.
5. Have more suicidal ideation.
6. Have more psychiatric hospitalizations.
7. Emotional support (operationalized by having a partner in Israel or by being employed) would be associated with a reduction in the risk for a PTSD diagnosis, number of clinic consultations, receiving psychiatric medications, drug and alcohol use, suicidal ideation, and psychiatric hospitalizations in Israel.

These outcomes have important implications for promoting the initiative to allow asylum seekers in Israel and elsewhere to benefit from health insurance and health services.

2. Materials and Methods

2.1. Measures

Demographic data were taken from patients' files: country of origin, age, gender, years of education, marital status, partner in Israel (yes/no/missing), full or partial employment, and religion (Muslim/Christian/other).

Categories of victims were defined as follows, based on international definitions [41] and the law in the State of Israel [8]:

- Trafficking victims had experienced recruitment, transportation, transfer, harboring, or receipt of persons using threat or force, coercion, abduction, fraud, deception or abuse of power, for exploitation [41].
- Torture victims had experienced repeated physical and mental violence, and suffered severe pain.
- Trafficking and torture victims had experienced both trafficking and torture.
- Sexual violence and torture victims had experienced both sexual violence and torture, involving severe physical or mental pain inflicted by others, from rape, inhuman, or degrading treatment [10].
- Smuggling victims had paid Bedouins in the Sinai Peninsula to be smuggled into Israel.
- Persecution victims had been imprisoned, almost killed, lost consciousness or forced to separate from family [42].
- Military trauma victims had experienced traumatic combat events in their country of origin.
- Civil trauma victims had experienced trauma of a criminal nature or an accident (work, car, etc.)

Place of trauma: country of origin; en route to Israel (Sinai); Israel.

PTSD was diagnosed by a mental health professional according to ICD-10 criteria (F43.1.) [43].

Number of consultations was the number of appointments with a mental health professional at the *Gesher* Clinic.

Additional variables: Psychiatric medications (yes/no); current drug abuse (yes/no); current alcohol use (yes/no); suicidal ideation (yes/no); and one or more psychiatric inpatient admissions in Israel (yes/no).

2.2. Procedure

The study was approved by the Internal Review Boards of the Abarbanel Mental Health Center and the Ruppin Academic Center [TASHAZ 26]. The data was collected and coded from the files by H.T. and R.H. Anonymity was strictly respected. Inter-rater reliability for variable coding between the coders for a random sample of 10 files, evaluated by H.T and I.L was 100%.

2.3. Data Analysis

Group comparisons were reported by the percentages within each group. Chi Square tests were conducted to compare between types of victimization in country of origin, en route in Sinai and in Israel with demographic variables. Chi Square tests were also conducted to assess if trauma victims would be at greater risk for PTSD than non-trauma victims. *t*-test analyses were conducted to assess the differences between trauma victims and non-trauma victims for the means of clinical consultations. Multiple *t*-test analyses were conducted, separately for trauma en route to Israel (Sinai), in Israel and in country of origin, and separately for types of trauma when warranted. Chi square analyses were also conducted to assess the frequencies of trauma victims' medication, hospitalization, and suicide ideation. Pearson correlations were used to assess relationships between variables. All statistical analyses were deemed significant at a $p < 0.05$ level. We built an index summing the locations where traumatic events were experienced. This Trauma Index ranged between 0 (no trauma) to 3 (trauma en route, trauma in Israel and trauma in country of origin).

SPSS version 23 (IBM, Amonk, NY, USA) was used for all analyses.

3. Results

3.1. Participants

This study is based on a retrospective chart review, based on medical records of 271 patients who were asylum seekers living in Israel and sought treatment at the *Gesher* Clinic from 2014–2016. The 52 patients who did not report whether they had been victims of trauma were excluded, so 219 asylum seekers (149 men, 68%) were included in the study. Their ages ranged from 20–61 (M = 32.7, SD = 7.65). Most (*n* = 134, 61.2%) were from Eritrea, 56 (25.6%) were from Sudan, 3 were from Ethiopia and 26 did not report their country of origin. Over half (*n* = 126, 57.5%) were unemployed. Of the 78 employed patients, 46 (21.0%) reported working full time. Most asylum seekers (*n* = 141, 64.4%) were Christian, 47 (21.5%) were Muslim and 31 (14.1%) did not report their religion. Participants reported receiving 0–20 years of education (M = 8.83, SD = 3.71) and had 0–9 children (M = 1.09, SD = 1.63), of whom 0–4 (M = 0.49, SD = 0.83) were born in Israel. Most (*n* = 125, 57.1%) were single, 78 (35.6%) were married, 11 divorced, and 3 widowed. Two of the single patients, 32 of those married, and one of those divorced had partners in Israel.

3.2. Traumatic Events in Country of Origin

Almost half (42.9%, *n* = 94) the asylum seekers reported having experienced traumatic events in their country of origin. Political persecution was reported by 38 (17.4%), physical or sexual violence by 24 (11.0%), military trauma by seven (3.2%), and civil trauma by 17 (7.8%). Table 1 shows demographic variables across different types of traumatic events in country of origin.

Significant differences were found for gender and country of origin. More men than women had suffered political persecution, military trauma and civil trauma. Asylum seekers from Eritrea suffered more traumatic events than those from Sudan, except for civil war.

3.3. Traumatic Events en Route to Israel

There were significant differences for gender and country of origin across asylum seekers who experienced different types of trauma en route to Israel (in the Sinai Peninsula). Only about one quarter of the non-victims were women, and almost two-thirds from Eritrea. Most smuggling, torture and trafficking victims were men, whereas most sexual violence and torture victims were women. Approximately three-quarters of the torture victims and the trafficking and torture victims, and over 80% of the sexual violence victims were from Eritrea. There were no significant between-group differences for family status, religion, employment or partner in Israel (see Table 2).

Table 1. Demographic variables across different types of traumatic events in country of origin.

Type of Victim	Gender: Men n (%)	Spouse in Israel n (%)	Family Status n (%)			Country of Origin n (%)			Religion n (%)	Employed (%)
			Single	Married	Other	Ethiopia	Eritrea	Sudan	Muslim	Yes
No traumatic events $n = 125$	80 (64.5)	24 (20.2)	72 (57.6)	45 (36.0)	8 (6.4)	1 (0.9)	83 (76.9)	24 (22.2)	23 (21.5)	45 (38.1)
Political persecution $n = 38$	32 (88.9)	3 (8.8)	22 (59.5)	13 (35.1)	2 (5.4)	0 (0)	24 (68.6)	11 (31.4)	8 (25.0)	9 (25.0)
Physical/sexual violence $n = 24$	12 (52.2)	4 (18.2)	12 (52.2)	9 (39.1)	2 (8.7)	1 (5.0)	13 (65.0)	6 (30.0)	3 (15.8)	10 (50.0)
Military trauma $n = 7$	6 (85.7)	0 (0)	5 (71.4)	2 (28.6)	0 (0)	0	6 (100)	0 (0)	1 (16.7)	3 (42.9)
Civil trauma $n = 17$	14 (82.4)	2 (12.5)	11 (64.7)	4 (23.5)	2 (11.8)	(0)	5 (31.3)	11 (68.8)	8 (50.0)	7 (43.8)
Significance	$\chi^2_{(4)} = 13.3$ $p = 0.01$	NS	NS			$\chi^2_{(8)} = 21.00$ $p = 0.007$			NS	NS

Table 2. Demographic variables of asylum seekers who experienced different types of trauma in the Sinai Peninsula, and non-trauma victims.

Table	Gender: Men n (%)	Spouse in Israel n (%)	Family Status n (%)			Country of Origin ** n (%)			Religion n (%)	Employed n (%)
			Single	Married	Other	Ethiopia	Eritrea	Sudan	Muslim	Yes
Non-victims * $n = 105$	74 (71.8)	82 (84.5)	57 (54.8)	39 (37.5)	8 (7.7)	1 * (1.2)	53 (63.1)	30 (35.7)	25 (30.8)	42 (43.8)
Trafficking $n = 4$	0	2 (50.0)	2 (50.0)	1 (25.0)	1 (25.0)	1 (50.0)	1 (50.0)	0 (0)	0	1 (25.0)
Torture $n = 62$	50 (83.3)	48 (84.2)	38 (62.3)	20 (32.8)	3 (4.9)	0 (0)	45 (75.0)	15 (25.0)	12 (22.2)	19 (33.3)
Trafficking & torture $n = 14$	9 (64.3)	12 (92.3)	11 (78.6)	3 (21.4)	0 (0)	0 (0)	10 (76.9)	3 (23.1)	3 (27.3)	5 (38.5)
Sexual violence & torture $n = 23$	7 (30.4)	16 (69.6)	10 (43.5)	11 (47.8)	1 (4.3)	1 (4.3)	19 (82.6)	3 (13.0)	0 (0)	9 (39.1)
Smuggling $n = 11$	9 (81.8)	10 (90.9)	7 (63.6)	4 (36.4)	0 (0)	0 (0)	6 (54.5)	5 (45.5)	4 (40.0)	2 (18.2)
Significance	$\chi^2_{(5)} = 32.2$ $p < 0.001$	NS	NS			$\chi^2_{(10)} = 40.04$ $p < 0.001$			NS	NS

* Only 84 non-victims reported their country of origin. ** Included in the table are only participants for whom we had data concerning country of origin and type of victimization.

3.4. Traumatic Events in Israel

Only 23 (10.5%) of the asylum seekers reported experiencing traumatic events in Israel. Eleven (~48%) were from Eritrea and 13 (~57%) were Christian. Nine (4.1%) reported having experienced sexual or physical violence in Israel. Fourteen (6.4%) of the asylum seekers reported having experienced civil trauma in Israel. Ten (71.4%) were male, 12 (85.7%) had no partner in Israel, half were married, and 7 (58.3%) were from Eritrea. Half were Muslim and most ($n = 10$, 71.4%) were unemployed.

Hypothesis 1 (H1). *Trauma victims would be at greater risk for PTSD than non-trauma victims.*

To assess differences between trauma victims and non-trauma victims for PTSD diagnosis, multiple chi square analyses were conducted, separately for trauma en route to Israel (Sinai), in Israel, and in country of origin, and then separately for types of trauma in each location.

A PTSD diagnosis was given to 96 (43.8%) of the asylum seekers. Trauma was experienced by 114 (52.1%) asylum seekers in Sinai, 23 (10.5%) in Israel and 94 (42.9%) in their country of origin. Asylum seekers who experienced trauma in Sinai were more likely to be diagnosed with PTSD than those who did not, and asylum seekers who experienced trauma in their country of origin were more likely to be diagnosed with PTSD than those who did not (see Figure 1). The number of asylum seekers who reported traumatic events in Israel was insufficient for statistical analysis (e.g., 4.1% [9] were victims of physical/sexual violence, and 6.4% [14] were victims of civil trauma). It was not possible to perform statistical analyses between groups, because the expected cells in chi square were in some cases less than 5.

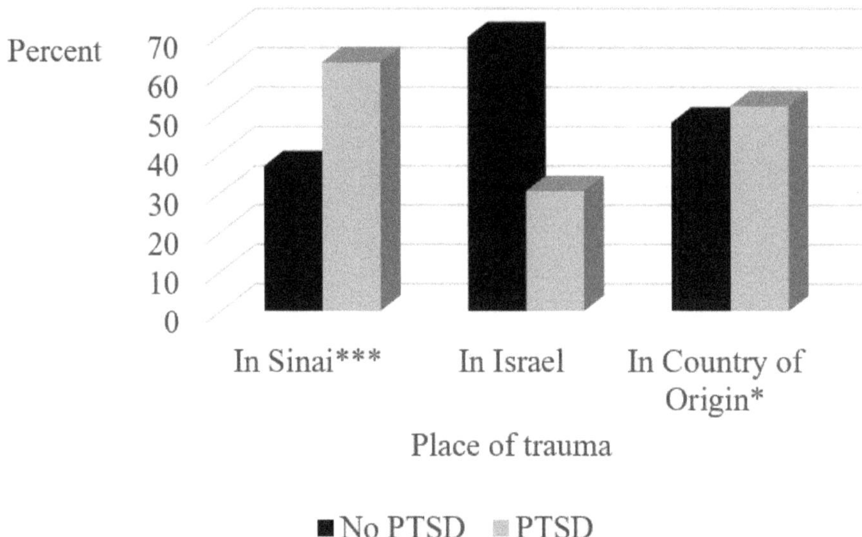

Figure 1. Percentage of asylum seekers with PTSD across place of trauma. *** Significant at $p < 0.001$, * Significant at $p < 0.05$. PTSD = Post-traumatic stress disorder.

Fifty-one (23.3%) asylum seekers reported no trauma, one of whom received a PTSD diagnosis. Approximately half (111, 50.7%) experienced trauma at one location, 51 (23.3%) at two locations and 6 (2.7%) at all three places of trauma. The Trauma Index of asylum seekers with a PTSD diagnosis (M = 1.33, SD = 0.54) was significantly higher than that of those without a PTSD diagnosis (M = 0.84, SD = 0.83; $t(217) = -5.07$, $p < 0.001$).

Victims of any kind of torture en route to Israel (torture, trafficking and torture/sexual violence and torture) were more likely to receive a diagnosis of PTSD than those who did not experience torture en route to Israel ($X^2(5) = 57.89$, $p < 0.001$; see Figure 2). The vast majority of smuggling victims had no PTSD diagnosis.

No significant differences were observed in the frequency of PTSD diagnoses across different types of trauma in Israel. Victims of political persecution or physical/sexual trauma in their country of origin were significantly more likely to receive a PTSD diagnosis than non-victims of political persecution or physical/sexual trauma ($X^2(4) = 15.07$, $p = 0.005$; see Figure 3).

The number of clinical consultations ranged from 1–45 (M = 9.29, SD = 9.21). To assess differences between trauma victims and non-trauma victims for clinical consultations, multiple t-test analyses were conducted, separately for trauma en route to Israel (Sinai), in Israel and in country of origin, and separately for types of trauma when warranted.

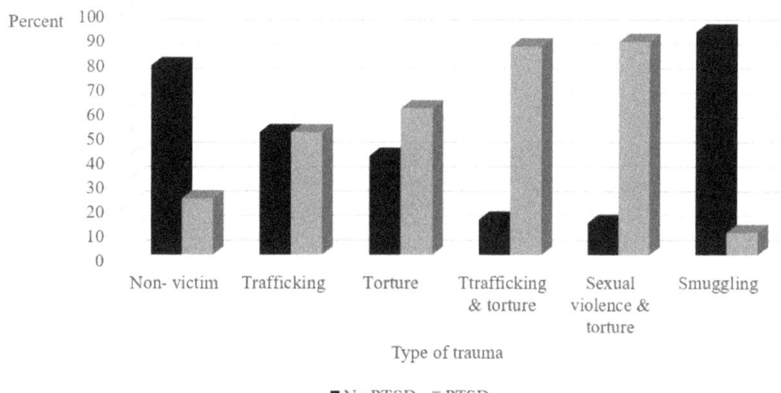

Figure 2. Percentage of asylum seekers who experienced trauma en route to Israel, with and without PTSD as a function type of trauma. PTSD = Post-traumatic stress disorder.

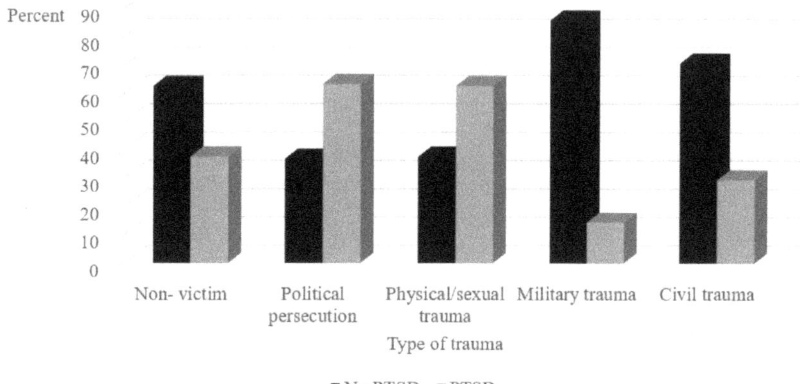

Figure 3. Percentage of asylum seekers with and without PTSD across different types of trauma in country of origin. PTSD = Post-traumatic stress disorder.

Hypothesis 2 (H2). *Trauma victims would have more clinical consultations than non-trauma victims.*

There was no significant difference in the number of clinical consultations between asylum seekers who experienced trauma en route to Israel and those who did not, or between those who experienced trauma in Israel and those who did not. However, the 94 asylum seekers who experienced trauma in their country of origin had significantly more clinical consultations (M = 11.82, SD = 10.27) than the 125 who did not (M = 0.49, SD = 0.73, $p < 0.001$). Asylum seekers who suffered civil trauma in their country of origin had the highest number of consultations (M = 13.27, SD = 12.53), followed by victims of physical/sexual trauma (M = 11.29, SD = 8.96), political persecution (M = 11.00, SD = 10.15), military trauma (M = 9.14, SD = 8.21), and non-trauma victims (M = 7.49, SD = 7.95; F (4193) = 2.52, $p = 0.04$). There was a positive, significant association between the Trauma Index and number of clinical consultations (r = 0.25, $p < 0.001$).

Hypothesis 3 (H3). *Trauma victims would be prescribed more psychiatric medication than non-trauma victims.*

Most participants (n = 190, 86.8%) were prescribed psychiatric medication. To compare trauma victims with non-trauma victims, multiple chi square analyses were conducted. No significant between-group differences emerged for different locations or types of traumas. However, participants who were prescribed psychiatric medication had a higher number of clinic consultations (M = 9.82, SD = 9.19) than those who did not (M = 6.52, SD = 9.11, $t(200)$ = −1.68, p = 0.045).

Hypothesis 4 (H4). *Trauma victims would report more drug and alcohol use than non-trauma victims.*

Only 18 (8.2%) of the asylum seekers reported using alcohol and 10 (4.6%) reported using drugs. To assess differences between trauma victims and non-trauma victims for alcohol and drug use, multiple chi square analyses were conducted. No between-group differences for alcohol or drug use were observed for type or place of trauma or for the Trauma Index.

Hypothesis 5 (H5). *Trauma victims would report more suicide ideation than non-trauma victims.*

Only 15 (6.8%) of the asylum seekers reported suicidal ideation. To assess differences between trauma victims and non-trauma victims for suicidal ideation, multiple chi square analyses were conducted, for place of trauma and then for types of trauma. No significant between-group differences were found for trauma en route to Israel or in country of origin, and no significant association was found between suicide ideation and the Trauma Index. However, significantly more asylum seekers who suffered trauma in Israel experienced suicidal ideation (n = 7, 33.3%) than those who did not (n = 8, 4.7%; $X^2_{(1)}$ = 21.48, p < 0.001). As can be seen in Figure 4, fully 75% of asylum seekers who suffered physical or sexual violence in Israel reported suicidal ideation.

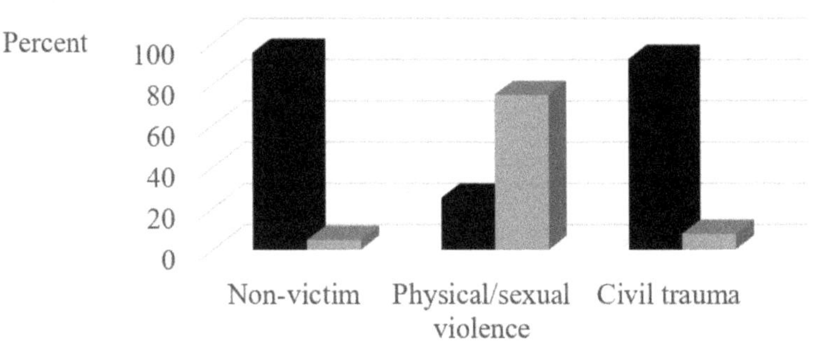

Figure 4. Percentage of asylum seekers with and without suicide ideation as a function type of trauma in Israel (n = 193).

Hypothesis 6 (H6). *Trauma victims would have more psychiatric hospitalizations than non-trauma victims.*

Twenty-seven (12.3%) of the asylum seekers had been hospitalized in psychiatric units in Israel. To assess differences between trauma victims and non-trauma victims for psychiatric hospitalization, multiple chi square analyses were conducted, separately for place of trauma and then for type of trauma. No significant difference was found for trauma in Israel or in country of origin. However, significantly fewer asylum seekers who had suffered trauma en route to Israel ($n = 6$, 5.5%) reported a history of psychiatric hospitalizations than those who had not ($n = 21$, 21.4%; $X^2_{(1)} = 11.54$, $p < 0.001$). This finding was in the opposite direction to our hypothesis.

Hypothesis 7 (H7). *Emotional support (i.e., having a partner in Israel or being employed) would be associated with fewer PTSD diagnoses, clinic consultations, psychiatric medication prescriptions, drug and alcohol use, suicidal ideation, and psychiatric hospitalizations.*

Chi-square analyses were conducted to assess whether having a partner in Israel (yes/no) and/or being employed (yes/no) were related to PTSD diagnoses, number of consultations, psychiatric medication, drug and alcohol use, suicidal ideation and/or psychiatric hospitalizations. No significant differences were found between having a partner in Israel and the other variables. A significant association was observed between employment status and alcohol use. More currently employed participants ($n = 11$, 14.7%) abused alcohol than currently unemployed participants ($n = 7$, 5.7%; $X^2_{(1)} = 4.52$, $p = 0.03$). This finding was in the opposite direction to our hypothesis.

4. Discussion

This study aimed to examine the psychiatric status and mental health care of asylum seekers in Israel, mostly from Eritrea and Sudan, who received psychiatric treatment at the *Gesher* Clinic in Israel between 2014 and 2016. We compared the profiles of those who had experienced traumatic events with those who had not, since this distinction has policy implications in Israel.

Only asylum seekers whom the State of Israel recognizes as victims of trafficking and slavery are entitled to medical care and rehabilitation services, yet even these are limited in duration [21] The most surprising finding was, perhaps, that in contrast to our hypotheses, there were few significant differences in the psychiatric characteristics that differentiated between trauma victims and non-trauma victims, and between asylum seekers with and without PTSD. Those with PTSD were no more likely than those without PTSD to take psychiatric medications, use psychoactive drugs and alcohol, have suicide ideation, and report a history of psychiatric hospitalizations. All asylum seekers included in this study were in mental distress, whether or not they reported having experienced a traumatic event or were diagnosed with PTSD. All had turned to a psychiatric clinic for help, and it, therefore, seems arbitrary to restrict access to psychiatric care to the few whom the State of Israel has recognized as refugees, or victims of human trafficking or slavery.

The high prevalence of PTSD among trauma victims is in line with previous studies highlighting the vulnerability of asylum seekers and refugees to cumulative trauma [25,31,44,45]. Traumatic experiences occur in asylum seekers' countries of origin, along migratory routes, and in their post-migratory environment.

Among asylum seekers who were victim of trauma, the highest prevalence of PTSD was observed among those who experienced trauma in the Sinai Peninsula en route to Israel. This supports previous findings that asylum seekers who crossed the Sinai desert were victims of a wide range of traumas [6]. They were found to be at high risk for mental health problems [46], and prolonged exposure to traumatic events greatly increased their risk of developing PTSD [47]. Similar risk was found in asylum seekers from various countries in Switzerland, who had experienced or witnessed torture [48]. The low rate of PTSD observed among victims of smuggling may stem from the complicated relationship between smuggling and trafficking—some incidents of smuggling turn into trafficking and some incidents of trafficking turn into smuggling [10]. It may be that being smuggled may scar the souls of asylum seekers less than previous or subsequent traumatic experiences.

Political persecution and physical/sexual trauma in the asylum seekers' country of origin were risk factors for PTSD. Cumulative documentation from victims of political persecution and physical or sexual violence in Eritrea and Sudan corroborates the depth of their vulnerability from these forms of trauma [49–51]. Asylum seekers who had experienced trauma in their country of origin also had more clinical consultations than those who did not, underscoring the heavy residue of trauma in their country of origin.

No specific trauma in the host country, Israel, was found to be associated with PTSD. This may be due to the small number of asylum seekers who reported experiencing trauma in Israel. In addition, many asylum seekers may experience high distress due to post-migration difficulties, whether or not they experienced traumatic events on their migratory path [6,37,52]. Such post-migration difficulties include socioeconomic, social, and interpersonal factors, asylum-related bureaucracy, immigration policy [53], and perceived threat of detention and deportation [54]. Future research should examine the relative impact of specific postmigration stressors on PTSD and mental health.

Asylum seekers who were victims of trauma and diagnosed with PTSD had experienced traumas in more places than those without PTSD. Traumatic events were most experienced in the Sinai Peninsula, followed by country of origin. This supports previous findings that experiencing trauma in more than one location increases risk for PTSD and other disorders among asylum seekers [55,56]. Experiencing a traumatic event in the Sinai desert conferred risk for PTSD, underscoring the severe and prolonged injuries suffered by the asylum seekers in Sinai [6,47]. However, experiencing an additional traumatic event elsewhere along the asylum seekers' journey did not increase this risk further. This suggests that the asylum seekers' overall subjective experience of having been traumatized, regardless of the number of their traumatic experiences, confers risk for developing PTSD [57].

Whereas both men and women commonly experience torture, trafficking and sexual violence during their migratory journeys, particularly in Africa [19,58], certain traumas appear to be gender-based. Most torture, trafficking and smuggling victims in our study were men, whereas most sexual violence and torture victims were women. Similar findings were reported in other studies on this population [6,59], and asylum seekers in other Western countries [60–62].

Fully 43 (8%) of the trauma victims in our study received a PTSD diagnosis, underscoring the devastating effects of trauma such as torture, trafficking, and physical and sexual violence [6,28]. However, 37% did not. Whereas resilience is a possible explanation, it is important to keep in mind that all participants were in treatment for mental problems at the *Gesher* Clinic. One non-trauma victim was diagnosed with PTSD. She may have omitted to report a traumatic event or been misdiagnosed, possibly due to cross-cultural variation in the presentation of posttraumatic symptoms [63]. Similarly, at least some of the non-trauma victims may not have reported traumatic events they experienced.

In contrast to our hypothesis, a similar percentage of trauma and non-trauma victims were prescribed psychiatric medications. This was no doubt because they were prescribed to the vast majority of asylum seekers. Medications may have been needed, available, convenient, and over-prescribed. We unfortunately had no access to reliable information on the patients referred to individual or group psychotherapy; however, these may be under-used and regarded with mistrust because of differences in cultural attitudes [36,64].

Number of clinical appointments does not necessarily indicate a need for treatment or a level of distress [64]. Prescriptions for psychiatric medications require monitoring, which may explain the association between the number of clinical consultations and the prescription of psychiatric medications. In Israel, at the time of the study, the movement of asylum seekers was restricted and the renewal of medical prescriptions was a common pretext for freedom of movement [65].

Notably, no differences in alcohol or drug use were found between asylum seekers with and without PTSD, which can perhaps be attributed to low rates of report and self-disclosure. Low rates of substance and alcohol abuse were also reported among Russian, Somali and Kurdish migrants in Finland [66], and refugees from former Yugoslavia and the Middle East in Sweden [67]. Although some studies have observed massive drug use in some ethnic minorities in the US [68], Muslim refugees may be protected against substance use and misuse [29]. In this study, employed asylum seekers reported using more alcohol than the unemployed, possibly because they could pay for them.

Suicide ideation was not reported more frequently by asylum seekers who were victims of trauma and those who were non-trauma victims, whether in the country of origin or en route to Israel. Suicide ideation may have been underreported in our study, since there are high rates of suicidality among asylum seekers in Australia [23] and the U.S. [69], among moderate and severe levels of distress among Afghanistan and Syrian asylum seekers in Sweden [70], and detention can increase the risk for suicide ideation in asylum seekers [71]. Yet, most (75%) of victims of physical/sexual violence in Israel reported suicidal ideation. Post-resettlement violence was found to have a larger association with mental health symptoms than pre-resettlement exposure, among Somali refugees in the US and Canada [72]. Trauma-affected refugees in Germany who experienced an additional stressful life event during treatment had more severe symptoms of PTSD, anxiety, and depression than those without a renewed event [73]. Experiencing a new trauma, especially physical or sexual violence in the "land of refuge", a place that had offered hope for a better future, may lead to despair to the point of wanting to die. Whereas physical/sexual violence experienced in one's country of origin or en route is traumatic, it may still leave hope for a better future.

Asylum seekers with and without PTSD had similar numbers of psychiatric hospitalizations in Israel. Surprisingly, victims of trauma in Sinai with PTSD reported fewer hospitalizations than those without PTSD. This may suggest resilience, although factors such as socio-demographic and ecological variations in their post-migratory environment, possible alternatives to psychiatric admission, like the Open Clinic of Physicians for Human Rights [47], and traditional healers and religious leaders [36,74] may explain this finding.

Previous research found that emotional support from a partner [75,76] and employment [77,78] in the host country was protective against PTSD. However, we did not find having a partner in Israel or being employed to be associated with lower risk for PTSD, psychiatric medications, clinical consultations, alcohol abuse, suicide ideation, or psychiatric inpatient admissions. A study examining the association between perceived social support and posttraumatic symptoms among Eritrean and Sudanese male asylum seekers in Israel found a significant negative link between the two, but only for men who reported low exposure to traumatic events [36]. In our study, 76.7% of the asylum seekers reported experiencing at least one traumatic event at some point along their process of migration, which may explain why having a partner was not connected to lower distress levels. It is known that the levels of torture experience in the Sinai Desert by trauma victims from Eritrea and Sudan are extreme [10,59].

The lack of association between PTSD diagnosis and employment may be explained by the fact that over half the participants (57.5%) were unemployed and almost 80% of the employed worked part-time, presumably not out of choice. Economic opportunities such as the right to work and access to full employment have been found to have a linear relationship with mental health among refugees and asylum seekers [78]. However, earnings from part-time employment in Israel are not high and does not generally provide economic security in Israel. Part-time employment may even render asylum seekers in Israel vulnerable to trafficking and abuse. Employment may not have been protective of PTSD in this study because most asylum seekers were employed part-time. Moreover, a residence permit is a precondition for asylum seekers to obtain a work permit in Israel. Residence permits are temporary and must be periodically renewed at the Ministry of the Interior [21], which adds to the burden and stress of employed asylum seekers.

This study has several limitations. First, given the cross-sectional nature of the data, causality cannot be determined. Second, the findings are based on a clinical sample of asylum seekers who sought psychiatric help at a specific clinic. It is therefore unclear whether the findings can be generalized to a broader population of asylum seekers. Third, the asylum seekers were assessed by different mental health workers and the inter-judge reliability of diagnoses and other information recorded in the files was not assessed.

Professionals based their assessments on patients' self-report so some information may have been biased or omitted.

5. Conclusions

Although this is a clinical sample, with a relatively small number of participants, the findings of this study add to our knowledge about the psychiatric status of asylum seekers seeking mental health care in Israel. The study examined differences between trauma victims and non-trauma victims, and between trauma victims with and without PTSD. Although trauma victims received more PTSD diagnoses than non-victims, no differences were observed between the psychiatric status and mental health care of victims versus non-victims of trauma among asylum seekers in Israel from East Africa. Asylum seekers are a vulnerable population, and it is vital to understand that the risks and hazards they face before, during, and after their migration journey increase the risk for physical and mental problems among trauma victims and non-trauma victims alike. It may be of value to integrate cultural and societal-structural approaches such as the Socio-Cultural Formulation [79] into the psychiatric assessment of asylum seekers. This could help make it clear that they are vulnerable and deserving of psychiatric treatment and psychological support. In any case, clinicians should examine the mental health status of asylum seekers and victims of human trafficking with thoroughness and dignity, and ensure that they receive the help warranted by their experiences and needs.

From a clinical perspective, the lack of difference between the psychiatric status and mental health care of victims versus non-victims in this study strongly support a recent initiative of the Israel Ministry of Health [80]. According to this initiative, the Israeli government would provide health insurance for asylum seekers [80] and abandon the narrow interpretation of the Refugee Convention [3] adopted to date in the field of health. The results of our study strengthen the case for establishing organized, coordinated, sustainable mental health services that serve the needs of the community of asylum seekers in Israel. It would seem to be appropriate for the Ministry of Health or a Health Maintenance Organization to extend tailored services to meet the needs of the community.

The few clinical differences we observed between asylum seekers who were victims of human trafficking, torture, and other atrocities and asylum seekers who were non-trauma victims challenges the narrow interpretation currently given by the State of Israel to the international conventions it ratified. The Refugee Convention [3] and the Palermo Protocol [41], for example, enable Israel to recognize only 0.06% of all asylum seekers' applications for refugee status [80]. This stance joins local and international voices calling for a review of the Palermo Protocol [41] and the definition of human trafficking [81–83], so as to " … protect and assist the victims of such trafficking, with full respect for their human rights" ([41]; Article 2(b)), and help asylum seekers gain access to appropriate services, regardless of their visa status.

Author Contributions: R.Y.—conceived the study (with I.L.), supervised H.T. in the fieldwork (along with R.B.-M.) and wrote most of the paper. R.B.-M. guided the fieldwork, contributed significantly to conceptualization, methodology, and writing the manuscript. L.L.-A. analyzed the data and wrote the Results section. H.T. conducted the fieldwork, collect the raw data, contributed significantly to the statistical analyses. R.H. collect the raw data. I.L. conceived the study, contributed significantly to ensure the reliability of the data, and commented on all sections of the manuscript. All authors have read and agreed to the published version of the manuscript.

Funding: This research received no external funding.

Institutional Review Board Statement: The study was conducted according to the guidelines of the Declaration of Helsinki and approved by the Institutional Review Board of Abarbanel Mental Health Center, Israel. Protocol code 123; 1 March 2015.

Informed Consent Statement: Informed consent was waived since the study was a retrospective chart review. Anonymity was kept during all stages of data processing.

Data Availability Statement: The data is available on demand from the corresponding author.

Acknowledgments: The authors would like to thank Tehila Jouchovitzky and Era Ben Yehoyada for their support of the clinic's work and data collection.

Conflicts of Interest: The authors declare no conflict of interest.

References

1. McAuliffe, M.; Ruhs, M. World Migration Report 2018. Geneva: International Organization for Migration. 2017. Available online: https://publications.iom.int/fr/system/files/pdf/wmr_2018_en_chapter7.pdf (accessed on 25 June 2021).
2. United Nations Population Division, Department of Economic and Social Affairs. 2019. Available online: https://population.un.org/wpp/Publications/Files/WPP2019_10KeyFindings.pdf (accessed on 21 July 2019).
3. United Nations High Commission for Refugees. Convention and Protocol Relating to the Status of Refugees. 2010. Available online: https://www.unhcr.org/3b66c2aa10 (accessed on 12 June 2021).
4. Refugee Statistics. USA for UNHCR 2020. Available online: https://www.unrefugees.org/refugee-facts/statistics/ (accessed on 17 September 2021).
5. Paz, Y. Ordered Disorder: African Asylum Seekers in Israel and Discursive Challenges to an Emerging Refugee Regime. Geneva, Switzerland: UNHCR, Policy Development and Evaluation Service. 2011. Available online: https://www.refworld.org/pdfid/4d7e19ab2.pdf (accessed on 10 July 2021).
6. Nakash, O.; Langer, B.; Nagar, M.; Shoham, S.; Lurie, I.; Davidovitch, N. Exposure to traumatic experiences among asylum seekers from Eritrea and Sudan during migration to Israel. *J. Immigr. Minor. Health* **2015**, *17*, 1280–1286. [CrossRef]
7. Israel Population and Migration Authority. Foreigners' Data in Israel. 2016. Available online: https://www.unhcr.org/il/wp-content/uploads/sites/6/2020/07/PIBA-2016-Summary-English-stats.pdf (accessed on 21 September 2021).
8. Israel Book of Laws. Foreign Workers Act. 1991. Available online: https://www.refworld.org/docid/4c36ed992.html (accessed on 30 July 2021).
9. Israel Population and Migration Authority. Foreigners' Data in Israel. 2014. Available online: https://www.gov.il/BlobFolder/reports/foreigners_summary_2013/he/2013_summary_foreignworkers_report.pdf (accessed on 4 July 2021).
10. van Reisen, M.; Estefanos, M.; Rijken, C. *Human Trafficking in the Sinai: Refugees between Life and Death*; Wolf Legal Publishers: Oisterwijk, The Netherlands, 2012; Available online: http://humantraffickingsearch.org/wp-content/uploads/2017/06/report_Human_Trafficking_in_the_Sinai_20120927.pdf (accessed on 15 August 2021).
11. United Nations High Commission for Refugees. Refugee Interwiki Protection and Human Trafficking. Selected Legal Reference Materials. 2008. Available online: https://www.refworld.org/pdfid/498705862.pdf (accessed on 31 July 2021).
12. Israel Ministry of Justice. Anti Human-Trafficking law: Legislation Amendment, 2006; Article 375a of the Penal Law. 1977. Available online: https://www.justice.gov.il/En/Units/Trafficking/MainDocs/israeltraffickinglawexplained.pdf (accessed on 15 August 2021).
13. Hacker, D.; Cohen, O. The Shelters in Israel for Survivors of Human Trafficking. 2012. Available online: https://m.tau.ac.il/sites/law-english.tau.ac.il/files/media_server/Law/faculty%20members/Daphna%20Hacker/The%20Shelters%20in%20Israel.pdf (accessed on 30 July 2021).
14. See, H.; Jamahiriya, L.A. States parties to the 1954 convention relating to the status of stateless persons. *Refug. Surv. Q.* **1997**, *16*, 189.
15. Gutzeit, Z.; Physicians for Human Rights–Israel (PHRI), Tel Aviv, Israel. Personal communication, 2019.
16. Jewish Federation. Illegal Migrants & Refugees in Israel Major Trends and Background Information. 2018. Available online: https://cdn.fedweb.org/fed-42/2212/Migrants%2520to%2520Israel%2520-%2520Full%2520Background%2520Briefing%2520February%25209%25202018.pdf (accessed on 6 August 2019).
17. Israel Ministry of Foreign Affairs, National Health Insurance. 1995. Available online: https://www.mfa.gov.il/mfa/mfa-archive/1990-1995/pages/national%20health%20insurance.aspx (accessed on 30 July 2021).
18. Bassiouni, C.M.; Rothenberg, D.; Higonnet, E.; Farenga, C.; Invictus, A.S. Addressing international human trafficking in women and children for commercial sexual exploitation in the 21st century. *Rev. Int. de Droit Pénal* **2010**, *81*, 417–491. [CrossRef]
19. Van Reisen, M.; Rijken, C. Sinai trafficking: Origin and definition of a new form of human trafficking. *Soc. Incl.* **2015**, *3*, 113–124. [CrossRef]
20. Van Reisen, M.; Rijken, C.; Estefanos, M. *The Human Trafficking Cycle: Sinai and Beyond*; Wolf Legal Publishers: Brussels, Belgium, 2014.
21. Aid Organization for Refugees and Asylum Seekers in Israel—ASAF. State Department 2019 Annual Trafficking in Persons (TIP) Report—Input from ASSAF. 2019. Available online: https://assaf.org.il/en/sites/default/files/Annual%20Trafficking%20in%20Persons%20-%20ASSAF%202019.pdf (accessed on 14 August 2021).
22. Gargiulo, A.; Tessitore, F.; Le Grottaglie, F.; Margherita, G. Self-harming behaviours of asylum seekers and refugees in Europe: A systematic review. *Int J. Psychol.* **2021**, *56*, 189–198. [CrossRef]
23. Procter, N.; Posselt, M.; Ferguson, M.; McIntyre, H.; Kenny, M.A.; Curtis, R.; Loughhead, M.; Clement, N.; Mau, V. An evaluation of suicide prevention education for people working with refugees and asylum seekers: Improvements in competence, attitudes, and confidence. *Crisis J. Crisis Interv. Suicide Prev.* **2021**. [CrossRef]
24. Giacco, D.; Laxhman, N.; Priebe, S. Prevalence of and risk factors for mental disorders in refugees. *Semin. Cell Dev. Biol.* **2018**, *77*, 144–152. [CrossRef] [PubMed]

25. Turrini, G.; Purgato, M.; Ballette, F.; Nosè, M.; Ostuzzi, G.; Barbui, C. Common mental disorders in asylum seekers and refugees: Umbrella review of prevalence and intervention studies. *Int. J. Ment. Health Syst.* **2017**, *11*, 1–14. [CrossRef] [PubMed]
26. Lindert, J.; von Ehrenstein, O.S.; Priebe, S.; Mielck, A.; Brähler, E. Depression and anxiety in labor migrants and refugees—A systematic review and meta-analysis. *Soc. Sci. Med.* **2009**, *69*, 246–257. [CrossRef]
27. Tsutsumi, A.; Izutsu, T.; Poudyal, A.K.; Kato, S.; Marui, E. Mental health of female survivors of human trafficking in Nepal. *Soc. Sci. Med.* **2008**, *66*, 1841–1847. [CrossRef] [PubMed]
28. Zimmerman, C.; Hossain, M.; Yun, K.; Gajdadziev, V.; Guzun, N.; Tchomarova, M.; Ciarrocchi, R.A.; Johansson, A.; Kefurtova, A.; Scodanibbio, S.; et al. The health of trafficked women: A survey of women entering posttrafficking services in Europe. *Am. J. Public Health* **2008**, *98*, 55–59. [CrossRef] [PubMed]
29. Dupont, H.J.; Kaplan, C.D.; Verbraeck, H.T.; Braam, R.V.; van de Wijngaart, G.F. Killing time: Drug and alcohol problems among asylum seekers in the Netherlands. *Int. J. Drug Policy* **2005**, *16*, 27–36. [CrossRef]
30. Fazel, M.; Wheeler, J.; Danesh, J. Prevalence of serious mental disorder in 7000 refugees resettled in western countries: A systematic review. *Lancet* **2005**, *365*, 1309–1314. [CrossRef]
31. Hollander, A.-C.; Dal, H.; Lewis, G.; Magnusson, C.; Kirkbride, J.; Dalman, C. Refugee migration and risk of schizophrenia and other non-affective psychoses: Cohort study of 1.3 million people in Sweden. *BMJ* **2016**, *352*, i1030. [CrossRef] [PubMed]
32. Dick, M.; Fennig, S.; Lurie, I. Identification of emotional distress among asylum seekers and migrant workers by primary care physicians: A brief report. *Isr. J. Psychiatry Relat. Sci.* **2015**, *52*, 14. [PubMed]
33. Nakash, O.; Nagar, M.; Lurie, I. The Association Between Postnatal Depression, Acculturation and Mother–Infant Bond Among Eritrean Asylum Seekers in Israel. *J. Immigr. Minor. Health* **2016**, *18*, 1232–1236. [CrossRef] [PubMed]
34. Duman, Y.H. Infiltrators Go Home! Explaining Xenophobic Mobilization Against Asylum Seekers in Israel. *J. Int. Migr. Integr.* **2015**, *16*, 1231–1254. [CrossRef]
35. Lurie, I.; Nakash, O. Exposure to trauma and forced migration: Mental health and acculturation patterns among asylum seekers in Israel. In *Trauma and Migration*; Springer: Cham, Switzerland, 2015; pp. 139–156.
36. Nakash, O.; Nagar, M.; Shoshani, A.; Lurie, I. The association between perceived social support and posttraumatic stress symptoms among Eritrean and Sudanese male asylum seekers in Israel. *Int. J. Cult. Ment. Health* **2017**, *10*, 261–275. [CrossRef]
37. Slonim-Nevo, V.; Lavie-Ajayi, M. Refugees and asylum seekers from Darfur: The escape and life in Israel. *Int. Soc. Work.* **2017**, *60*, 568–587. [CrossRef]
38. Meltzer, E.; Elkayam, O. Caring for illegal immigrants within the public hospital: The need for an urgent solution. *Harefuah* **2003**, *142*, 402–404, 488.
39. Rubin, L.; Belmaker, I.; Somekh, E.; Urkin, J.; Rudolf, M.; Honovich, M.; Bilenko, N.; Grossman, Z. Maternal and child health in Israel: Building lives. *Lancet* **2017**, *389*, 2514–2530. [CrossRef]
40. Hileli, R.; Strous, R.; Lewis, Y.D.; Lurie, I. Building the bridge: Psychiatric treatment for asylum-seekers and survivors of human trafficking in Israel: The experience of the Gesher Clinic, 2014–2015. *Isr. J. Psychiatry* **2021**, *58*, 30–37. Available online: http://medicalmagazines.co.il/issue68/index.html?r=34 (accessed on 15 August 2021).
41. UN General Assembly. Protocol to Prevent, Suppress and Punish Trafficking in Persons, Especially Women and Children, Sup-Plementing the United Nations Convention Against Transnational Organized Crime. 2000. Available online: http://www.unhcr.org/refworld/docid/3ae6b3a94.html (accessed on 30 July 2021).
42. Silove, D.; Steel, Z.; McGorry, P.; Miles, V.; Drobny, J. The impact of torture on post-traumatic stress symptoms in war-affected Tamil refugees and immigrants. *Compr. Psychiatry* **2002**, *43*, 49–55. [CrossRef] [PubMed]
43. World Health Organization. *The ICD-10 Classification of Mental and Behavioral Disorders: Clinical Descriptions and Diagnostic Guidelines*; World Health Organization: Geneva, Switzerland, 1992.
44. Barbieri, A.; Visco-Comandini, F.; Fegatelli, D.A.; Dessì, A.; Cannella, G.; Stellacci, A.; Pirchio, S. Patterns and predictors of PTSD in treatment-seeking African refugees and asylum seekers: A latent class analysis. *Int. J. Soc. Psychiatry* **2021**, *67*, 386–396. [CrossRef]
45. Steel, Z.; Chey, T.; Silove, D.; Marnane, C.; Bryant, R.; Van Ommeren, M. Association of torture and other potentially traumatic events with mental health outcomes among populations exposed to mass conflict and displacement. *JAMA* **2009**, *302*, 537–549. [CrossRef]
46. Lijnders, L. Caught in the borderlands: Torture experienced, expressed, and remembered by Eritrean asylum seekers in Israel. *Oxf. Monit. Forced Migr.* **2012**, *2*, 64–76.
47. Siman-Tov, M.; Bodas, M.; Wang, A.; Alkan, M.; Adini, B. Impact of traumatic events incurred by asylum-seekers on mental health and utilization of medical services. *Scand. J. Trauma Resusc. Emerg. Med.* **2019**, *27*, 85. [CrossRef] [PubMed]
48. Le, L.; Morina, N.; Schnyder, U.; Schick, M.; Bryant, R.A.; Nickerson, A. The effects of perceived torture controllability on symptom severity of posttraumatic stress, depression and anger in refugees and asylum seekers: A path analysis. *Psychiatry Res.* **2018**, *264*, 143–150. [CrossRef]
49. Human Rights Watch, World Report 2020. Available online: https://www.hrw.org/world-report/2020# (accessed on 14 August 2021).
50. Tronvoll, K.; Mekonnen, D.R. *African Garrison State: Human Rights and Political Development in Eritrea*; Boydell & Brewer Ltd.: New York, NY, USA, 2014; Chapter 7; pp. 92–106.
51. Connell, D. Escaping Eritrea—Why they flee and what they face. *Middle East Rep.* **2012**, *264*, 2–9.

52. Jannesari, S.; Hatch, S.; Prina, M.; Oram, S. Post-migration social–environmental factors associated with mental health problems among asylum seekers: A systematic review. *J. Immigr. Minor. Health* **2020**, *22*, 1055–1064. [CrossRef]
53. Li, S.S.Y.; Liddell, B.; Nickerson, A. The relationship between post-migration stress and psychological disorders in refugees and asylum seekers. *Curr. Psychiatry Rep.* **2016**, *18*, 82. [CrossRef] [PubMed]
54. Yaron, H.; Hashimshony-Yaffe, N.; Campbell, J. "Infiltrators" or refugees? An analysis of Israel's policy towards African asylum-seekers. *Int. Migr.* **2013**, *51*, 144–157. [CrossRef]
55. Bruhn, M.; Rees, S.; Mohsin, M.; Silove, D.; Carlsson, J. The range and impact of postmigration stressors during treatment of trauma-affected refugees. *J. Nerv. Ment. Dis.* **2018**, *206*, 61–68. [CrossRef] [PubMed]
56. Beiser, M.; Simich, L.; Pandalangat, N.; Nowakowski, M.; Tian, F. Stresses of passage, balms of resettlement, and posttraumatic stress disorder among Sri Lankan Tamils in Canada. *Can. J. Psychiatry* **2011**, *56*, 333–340. [CrossRef]
57. Palgi, Y.; Avidor, S.; Shrira, A.; Bodner, E.; Ben-Ezra, M.; Zaslavsky, O.; Hoffman, Y. Perception counts: The relationships of inner perceptions of Trauma and PTSD symptoms across time. *Psychiatry* **2018**, *81*, 361–375. [CrossRef]
58. Araujo, J.D.O.; De Souza, F.M.; Proença, R.; Bastos, M.L.; Trajman, A.; Faerstein, E. Prevalence of sexual violence among refugees: A systematic review. *Rev. Saúde Pública* **2019**, *53*, 78. [CrossRef] [PubMed]
59. Gebreyesus, T.; Sultan, Z.; Ghebrezghiabher, H.M.; Singh, N.; Tol, W.A.; Winch, P.J.; Davidovitch, N.; Surkan, P.J. Violence en route: Eritrean women asylum-seekers experiences of sexual violence while migrating to Israel. *Health Care Women Int.* **2019**, *40*, 721–743. [CrossRef] [PubMed]
60. Aguirre, N.G.; Milewski, A.R.; Shin, J.; Ottenheimer, D. Gender-based violence experienced by women seeking asylum in the United State: A lifetime of multiple traumas inflicted by multiple perpetrators. *J. Forensic Leg. Med.* **2020**, *72*, 101959. [CrossRef]
61. Belanteri, R.A.; Hinderaker, S.G.; Wilkinson, E.; Episkopou, M.; Timire, C.; De Plecker, E.; Mabhala, M.; Takarinda, K.C.; Bergh, R.V.D. Sexual violence against migrants and asylum seekers. The experience of the MSF clinic on Lesvos Island, Greece. *PLoS ONE* **2020**, *15*, e0239187. [CrossRef]
62. Mundy, S.S.; Foss, S.L.W.; Poulsen, S.; Hjorthøj, C.; Carlsson, J. Sex differences in trauma exposure and symptomatology in trauma-affected refugees. *Psychiatry Res.* **2020**, *293*, 113445. [CrossRef]
63. Hinton, D.E.; Lewis-Fernández, R. The cross-cultural validity of posttraumatic stress disorder: Implications for DSM-5. *Depression Anxiety* **2010**, *28*, 783–801. [CrossRef] [PubMed]
64. Bäärnhielm, S.; Laban, K.; Schouler-Ocak, M.; Rousseau, C.; Kirmayer, L.J. Mental health for refugees, asylum seekers and displaced persons: A call for a humanitarian agenda. *Transcult. Psychiatry* **2017**, *54*, 565–574. [CrossRef]
65. Physicians for Human Rights. Managing the despair. Monitoring report: Asylum seekers at the Holot facility, April–September 2014. Available online: https://il.boell.org/sites/default/files/managing-the-despair-eng-5.11.14.pdf (accessed on 12 June 2021).
66. Salama, E.; Niemelä, S.; Suvisaari, J.; Laatikainen, T.; Koponen, P.; Castaneda, A.E. The prevalence of substance use among Russian, Somali and Kurdish migrants in Finland: A population-based study. *BMC Public Health* **2018**, *18*, 651. [CrossRef] [PubMed]
67. Manhica, H.; Gauffin, K.; Almquist, Y.B.; Rostila, M.; Berg, L.; de Cortázar, A.R.G.; Hjern, A. Hospital admissions due to alcohol related disorders among young adult refugees who arrived in Sweden as teenagers—A national cohort study. *BMC Public Health* **2017**, *17*, 644. [CrossRef] [PubMed]
68. James, W.H.; Kim, G.K.; Armijo, E. The influence of ethnic identity on drug use among ethnic minority adolescents. *J. Drug Educ.* **2000**, *30*, 265–280. [CrossRef]
69. Taylor, S.; Charura, D.; Williams, G.; Shaw, M.; Allan, J.; Cohen, E.; Meth, F.; O'Dwyer, L. Loss, grief, and growth: An interpretative phenomenological analysis of experiences of trauma in asylum seekers and refugees. *Traumatol.* **2020**. [CrossRef]
70. Leiler, A.; Hollifield, M.; Wasteson, E.; Bjärtå, A. Suicidal Ideation and Severity of Distress among Refugees Residing in Asylum Accommodations in Sweden. *Int. J. Environ. Res. Public Health* **2019**, *16*, 2751. [CrossRef] [PubMed]
71. Robjant, K.; Hassan, R.; Katona, C. Mental health implications of detaining asylum seekers: Systematic review. *Br. J. Psychiatry* **2009**, *194*, 306–312. [CrossRef] [PubMed]
72. Salhi, C.; Scoglio, A.A.J.; Ellis, H.; Issa, O.; Lincoln, A. The relationship of pre- and post-resettlement violence exposure to mental health among refugees: A multi-site panel survey of somalis in the US and Canada. *Soc. Psychiatry Psychiatr. Epidemiol.* **2021**, *56*, 1015–1023. [CrossRef]
73. Schock, K.; Böttche, M.; Rosner, R.; Wenk-Ansohn, M.; Knaevelsrud, C. Impact of new traumatic or stressful life events on pre-existing PTSD in traumatized refugees: Results of a longitudinal study. *Eur. J. Psychotraumatology* **2016**, *7*, 32106. [CrossRef]
74. Sabar, G. In the holy land everyone is legal. It's different in Israel: The religious arena (Christian) of African asylum seekers in Israel. In *Where Levinsky Meets Asmara: Social and Legal Aspects of Israeli Asylum Policy*; Kritzman-Amir, T., Ed.; Hakibbutz Hameuhad: Tel Aviv, Israel, 2015; pp. 289–340. (In Hebrew)
75. Schweitzer, R.; Melville, F.; Steel, Z.; Lacherez, P. Trauma, post-migration living difficulties, and social support as predictors of psychological adjustment in resettled sudanese refugees. *Aust. N. Z. J. Psychiatry* **2006**, *40*, 179–187. [CrossRef] [PubMed]
76. Beiser, M. Personal and social forms of resilience: Research with Southeast Asian and Sri Lankan Tamil refugees in Canada. In *Refuge and Resilience: International Perspectives on Migration*; Simich, L., Andermann, L., Eds.; Springer: Dordrecht, The Netherlands, 2014; pp. 73–90.
77. Sonne, C.; Carlsson, J.; Bech, P.; Vindbjerg, E.; Mortensen, E.L.; Elklit, A. Psychosocial predictors of treatment outcome for trauma-affected refugees. *Eur. J. Psychotraumatology* **2016**, *7*, 30907. [CrossRef]

78. Porter, M.; Haslam, N. Predisplacement and postdisplacement factors associated with mental health of refugees and internally displaced persons. *JAMA* **2005**, *294*, 602–612. [CrossRef] [PubMed]
79. Weiss, M.G.; Aggarwal, N.K.; Gómez-Carrillo, A.; Kohrt, B.; Kirmayer, L.J.; Bhui, K.S.; Like, R.; Kopelowicz, A.; Lu, F.; Farías, P.J.; et al. Culture and social structure in comprehensive case formulation. *J. Nerv. Ment. Dis.* **2021**, *209*, 465–466. [CrossRef] [PubMed]
80. Pelg, B. Israeli Government Nearing Plan to Give Health Insurance for Asylum Seekers. Haaretz Israeli News. 19 July 2021. Available online: https://www.haaretz.com/israel-news/.premium-israeli-government-nearing-plan-to-give-health-insurance-for-asylum-seekers-1.10011286 (accessed on 1 August 2021).
81. Zuker, G.; Avigal, N. The Numbers Speak for Themselves: The Israeli Asylum Process. Hebrew Immigrant Aid Society (HIAS). 2020. Available online: https://drive.google.com/file/d/1Pjyg6tFs1TgkNkTLfYagNDof5UtWh8A6/view (accessed on 2 August 2021).
82. Goździak, E.M.; Vogel, K.M. Palermo at 20: A retrospective and prospective. *J. Hum. Traffick.* **2020**, *6*, 109–118. [CrossRef]
83. Shamir, H. A labor paradigm for human trafficking. *UCLA Law Rev.* **2012**, *60*, 76–136. Available online: https://www.uclalawreview.org/a-labor-paradigm-for-human-trafficking-2/ (accessed on 11 August 2021).

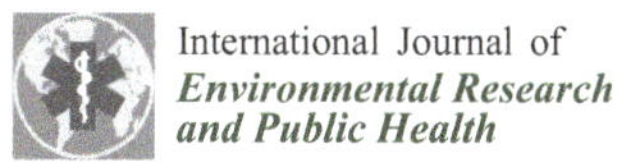

International Journal of
*Environmental Research
and Public Health*

MDPI

Review

Refugee Women with a History of Trauma: Gender Vulnerability in Relation to Post-Traumatic Stress Disorder

Macarena Vallejo-Martín [1,*], Ana Sánchez Sancha [2] and Jesús M. Canto [1]

1   Department of Social Psychology, Social Work, Social Anthropology and East Asia Studies, Faculty of Psychology and Speech Therapy, University of Malaga, 29016 Malaga, Spain; jcanto@uma.es

2   Department of Personality, Assessment and Psychological Treatment, Faculty of Psychology and Speech Therapy, University of Malaga, 29016 Malaga, Spain; sanchezsanchaana@gmail.com

*   Correspondence: mvallejo@uma.es

Abstract: Refugees represent a population whose living conditions have a strong impact on their mental health. High rates of post-traumatic stress disorder (PTSD), more than other mental disorders, have been found in this group, with women having the highest incidence. The objective of the present systematic review was to identify and examine studies from the last fifteen years on the relationship between the impact of traumatic experiences and PTSD psychopathology in refugee women. Twelve studies were included, from which the overall results approved this relation. In addition, six of these studies show that exposure to sexual trauma in refugee women is associated with the high odds of being at risk for PTSD. These findings suggest that gender-related traumatic experiences can explain the high rate of PTSD in refugee women and highlight the unmet need for psychosocial health care in this population.

Keywords: refugee women; post-traumatic stress disorder (PTSD); traumatic experiences; sexual violence; systematic review

Citation: Vallejo-Martín, M.; Sánchez Sancha, A.; Canto, J.M. Refugee Women with a History of Trauma: Gender Vulnerability in Relation to Post-Traumatic Stress Disorder. *Int. J. Environ. Res. Public Health* **2021**, *18*, 4806. https://doi.org/10.3390/ijerph18094806

Academic Editors: Shameran Slewa-Younan and Greg Armstrong

Received: 30 March 2021
Accepted: 29 April 2021
Published: 30 April 2021

Publisher's Note: MDPI stays neutral with regard to jurisdictional claims in published maps and institutional affiliations.

1. Introduction

At present, we are in the midst of a humanitarian crisis that is causing millions of people to be displaced, for reasons of war, violence and the precarious situations in their countries of origin. Specifically, the UNHCR [1] estimates that 70.8 million people are forcefully displaced all over the world, resulting in 25.9 million refugees, half of whom are under the age of 18. The circumstances in which refugees often flee cause them to experience mental health problems and a significant deterioration in their psychological well-being [2,3]. Mental disorders and psychosocial problems are much more frequent in individuals that have had to confront these types of adversities, such as being exposed to a humanitarian crisis [4] or experiencing different types of discrimination [5]. In this sense, it was confirmed that refugees have a rate of mental disorders that is twice than that identified in migrant workers [6].

The traumatic events experienced before and during displacement cause refugees to suffer from psychological manifestations related to loss of persons or places with symptoms of grief, traumatic reactions and even dissociative symptoms or acute stress disorders [7]. Situations of uncertainty and problems of adaptation also arise, since refugees grapple with unpredictable and difficult changes [1]. As a consequence of this exposure to stressful and traumatizing factors, the majority of uprooted persons experience suffering and diverse emotional problems [8]. Among the different disorders and mental health problems that can affect refugees, post-traumatic stress disorder (PTSD) and depression are the most frequent [9–11].

1.1. Post-Traumatic Stress Disorder in Refugees

PTSD is considered to be the mental disorder most specific to refugees and it is associated with circumstances involving political and social repression, war and armed conflict, as well as violence and torture, to which they are subjected in their countries of origin [12]. Although post-traumatic stress symptoms can be different in diverse cultures, there is abundant historical and transcultural evidence indicating that exposure to extreme traumatic experiences can activate extreme psychological stress [13]. When individuals suffer from a traumatic experience and do not have the capacity to integrate it by themselves with their cognitive and emotional schemes, a dissociation mechanism may appear as a defense strategy, allowing them to continue living with their previous mental schemes while wiping out the painful part of the experience from their consciousness [14]. This disassociation mechanism can be understood as "a memory phobia" that prevents integration of traumatic events and disassociates these memories from the consciousness [15]. The continued use of disassociation as a way of coping with stress interferes with memory and psychological functioning, hindering the integration of associated memories and causing an inability to provide a coherent narrative of events [16,17]. Furthermore, sharing these negative experiences can cause shame, guilt and a high degree of distress, which very significantly impacts self-image and sense of personal worth, leading to a tendency to avoid and repress these issues [18].

The most widely known consequence of exposure to traumatic events is PTSD. PTSD was officially categorized as a mental disorder in the 1980 edition of the Diagnostic and Statistical Manual of Mental Disorder (DSM) [19]. An individual is diagnosed as suffering from PTSD when the symptoms caused by the trauma are severe and prolonged and interfere with their social and/or occupational functioning [20]. In the DSM-5 [21], PTSD is characterized by the presence of multiple symptoms that can be grouped into four clusters: (1) intrusive symptoms (for example, nightmares), (2) persistent avoidance of stimuli associated with the trauma, (3) negative alterations in cognition and mood associated with the traumatic event (for example, difficulty concentrating, guilt, etc.), and (4) alterations in arousal and reactivation associated with the traumatic event (for example, difficulty sleeping).

According to Weinstein, Khabbaz and Legate [22] "becoming a refugee is a powerful risk factor for indicators of psychological disorders such as stress, generalized stress and posttraumatic stress disorder (PTSD)". Between 10 and 40% of refugees suffer from mental disorders after having experienced grave traumatic events in their countries of origin [9]. At the same time, different studies [11,23] have determined that among refugees, the rate of PTSD is higher than any other mental disorder. In addition, this group is ten times more likely to experience PTSD than the general population [24]. In the same vein, the study by Priebe, Giacco, and El-Nagib [25] points to a higher prevalence of PTSD and depression among refugees compared with the general population. Furthermore, refugees that have been submitted to torture and/or rape have the highest rates of PTSD [26]. For example, in a research on refugees from North Korea, significantly higher rates of suicidal thoughts and alcohol consumption after experiencing rape were found in comparison with refugees who had not undergone such types of traumatic experiences [27].

1.2. Gender Differences and PTSD: Traumatic Experiences in Refugee Women

According to Tolin and Foa [28], women are twice as likely as men to meet the criteria for PTSD, despite the fact that men usually experience greater overall exposure to traumatic events throughout their lifetimes. For Griffin, Resick and Mechanic [29], the dissociative response seems to be more common in individuals who have suffered sexual aggression. Along these lines, Norris [30] points out the survivors of rape are more prone to manifesting PTSD than victims of car accidents, robbery, physical assault, combat, fire, events involving deaths, and natural disasters. As such, it can be said that rape is the event most strongly linked to PTSD [31,32].

Wolfe and Kimerling [33] observed that the high incidence of sexual assault among women and the extremely high rates of PTSD in survivors of sexual assault contribute to the idea that being female is a risk factor for PTSD. According to different studies [30,31,34], throughout their lives, women contend with sexual assault and rape to a greater degree than men do. Accordingly, the most gender-based type of trauma is sexual violence. This gender difference in the risk of sexual victimization has clear implications for PTSD [35]. As such, in any study analyzing differences between men and women and PTSD, a significant role should be given to sexual-based trauma, since it is strongly linked to gender [35].

According to the UNHCR [36], refugee women often experience gender-based trauma, described as sexual violence that includes rape, forced impregnation, forced abortion, sexual trafficking, sexual slavery and the intentional spreading of sexually transmitted diseases, including HIV. Along these lines, Ward and Vann [37] establish that displaced women and girls are vulnerable to suffering from sexual violence, including forced sex/rape, sexual abuse by an intimate partner, child sexual abuse, coerced sex and sex trafficking in settings of humanitarian conflicts. For that reason, this population group presents a profile that is especially harmed and vulnerable and that often display symptoms of complex trauma [38]. However, studies focusing on the mental health status of refugee women are scarce [39]. This fact could be due to different reasons. First, upon interviewing extremely traumatized women, there is a serious risk that the questions may act to trigger traumatic content, which could be destabilizing, causing retraumatization and hindering recovery [40]. On the other hand, highly traumatized individuals can have difficulties concentrating long enough so as to complete extensive questionnaires [41]. At the same time, the language barrier can represent another obstacle to communicating with these individuals [42]. Additionally, women who have been the object of sexual assault might be rejected by their community and family and on many occasions, they are not able to make any sort of revelations in their interviews for asylum [43]. Likewise, in many cultures, rape and sexual assault are taboo subjects, for example, in Somali culture [44].

The aforementioned factors may be some of the reasons why few studies have examined specific violence in refugee women (suffered both in the fleeing phases in their countries of origin and in the experiences in the country of asylum where violence may persist) [45] and the effects it has on their mental health. The objective of this study is to present a systematic review that analyzes the relation between the impact of traumatic experiences in refugee women and developing PTSD. We consider this comprehensive review of the available research to date is original, innovative, and essential to understanding trauma in refugee women. Moreover, it is important for several reasons. Firstly, because of the need for attention that the refugee and asylum-seeking population have with respect to their mental health, which in most cases is affected by the experiences they have undergone. Secondly, it is essential to carry out this analysis from a gender perspective, determining the role that certain specific factors or traumatic events suffered by women, such as sexual violence understood in a broad sense, have on the deterioration of their psychological well-being and in the triggering of different disorders. Thirdly, so that the conclusions drawn from this study can be incorporated into resettlement or community integration programs for refugees, especially women, giving mental health a special relevance for the reconstruction of their lives.

2. Method

Literature Search and Study Selection

A systematic review of published studies on the incidence of PTSD in refugee women was made. This search was carried out through four research platforms: PsycInfo, Pubmed, Science Direct and Scopus, being limited to articles published between April 2005 and December 2020. In order to obtain a specific search, result from the terms "post-traumatic stress" and "female refugees" or "refugee women" were used. We followed the Preferred Reporting Items for Systematic Reviews and Meta-Analysis (PRISMA) guidelines for our study search and selection [46,47].

With the purpose of establishing uniform selection standards, the following inclusion criteria were applied: (a) publications of studies and clinical trials; (b) type of study: cohort studies or case-control studies; (c) language: Spanish or English; (d) population group: refugee women with a history of trauma; (e) diagnosis: PTSD by means of internationally accepted assessments instruments, including interviews that apply criteria from the Diagnostic and Statistical Manual of Mental Health Disorders (DSM) or the International Classification for Diseases (CIE); (f) published during the period 2005–2020; (g) journals with a high impact factor indexed in the Journal Citation Reports (JCR).

In addition, the following exclusion criteria were established: (a) narrative accounts, qualitative systematic reviews, and case studies; (b) subjects without a past history of trauma or PTSD diagnosis; (c) studies that used non-standardized tests; (d) studies whose data duplicates another study or that are not original; (e) articles in a language other than Spanish or English; (f) studies prior to 2005; (g) journals not having a high impact factor or not JCR-indexed.

The database search generated 82 results, which were classified in the Mendeley Desktop program. Two additional studies were identified, after reviewing articles from the bibliographic references of the research studies chosen. A total of 21 duplicated articles were excluded, so 63 articles were revised by title and abstract. Of these, 51 were excluded for not meeting the inclusion criteria, obtaining 12 articles that were read in their entirety and which were all chosen to be included in the results of our review. The search strategy results are summarized in Figure 1.

Unfortunately, a meta-analysis was not feasible given the diversity of the methodology used in the studies and the different co-variables dealt with in each one of them [48]. Accordingly, a narrative analysis was used, which enabled us to improve our understanding of PTSD in refugee women and help us to identify issues of importance to take into account in future paths for socio-healthcare intervention in this group.

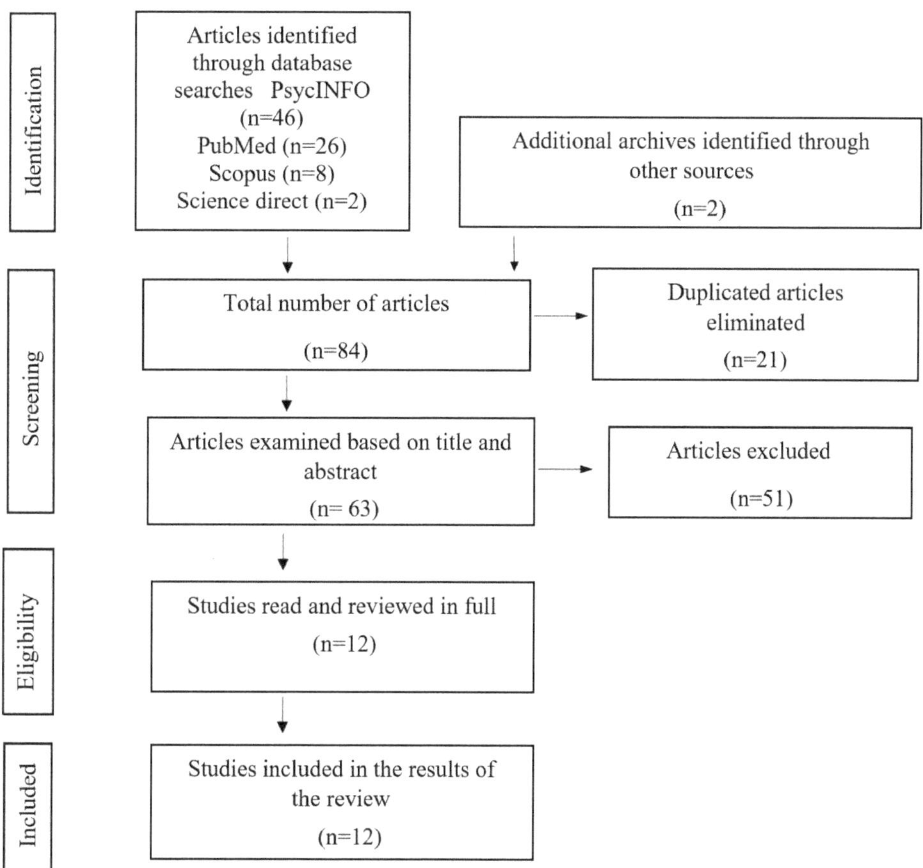

Figure 1. Preferred Reporting Items for Systematic Reviews and Meta-Analysis (PRISMA) flow diagram of each stage of the study selection.

3. Results

A critical reading was performed and a synthesis made of the 12 selected articles. These articles provided original data on PTSD in refugee women. Table 1 shows the main results of the studies considered.

In general, the chosen studies include participants from different countries, especially those who are in a situation of displacement (highlighting the Democratic Republic of the Congo and Somalia). The studies were carried out among adolescents and adults in different countries: The United States of America (1, 3), Canada (2), the Democratic Republic of the Congo (4, 5), the Republic of Uganda (6, 7), Germany (8, 11), Turkey (9), Australia (10), and the Republic of South Africa (12). Participants included both refugees and asylum seekers. The age of participants ranged between 13 and 85. The research was of a transversal nature, with the exception of study 3, for which a longitudinal follow-up took place at three and a half years of resettlement.

Table 1. Main results and characteristics of selected studies.

ID-Article	Authors and Year	Sample	Origin of Study	Assessment Objective	Instruments	Results
1.	Robertson C.L., Halcon L., Savik K., Johnson D., (2006) [49]	N = 458 (M = 200; F = 258)	Somalia and South Central Ethiopia	PTSD (Trauma and Torture)	PCL-C	High levels of PTSD symptoms were found in women with many children.
2.	Reedwood-Campbell L., Thind H., Howard M., (2008) [50]	N = 85 F	Kosovo	PTSD	HTQ	A fourth of the population scored high in PTSD.
3.	Vojvoda D., Weine S.M., McGlashan T. (2008) [51]	N = 21 (M = 12; F = 9)	Bosnia	PTSD	PSS	Scores for PTSD severity were higher in women. A significant difference was observed at the three-and-a-half-year follow-up point.
4.	Johnson K., Scott J., Rughita B. (2010) [52]	N = 998 (405 M; 593 F)	Democratic Republic of Congo	PTSD (Sexual violence)	PSS-I	The results showed that 50.1% of the population met the criteria of PTSD, with the highest scores being among women, and 70.2% of them met criteria based on experiences of sexual violence, with scores being higher among women.
5.	Schalinski L., Elbert T., Schauer M. (2011) [53]	N = 53 F	Democratic Republic of Congo	PTSD and disassociation	PSS-I	Thirty-six subjects met all the criteria for PTSD and sexual assault was the most frequent traumatic event. The greater the disassociation and the higher the number of traumatic events, the greater the severity of PTSD.
6.	Ssenyonga J., Owens V., Olema D.K. (2012) [54]	N = 89 (M = 33; F = 56)	Democratic Republic of Congo	PTSD	PSD	Forty-four subjects suffered PTSD, of which 33 were women who scored higher than men in intrusion, evasion, and hyper-activation symptoms and in general severity of PTSD.
7.	Morof D.F., Sami S., Mangeni M (2014) [55]	N= 117 F	Democratic Republic of Congo and Somalia	PTSD (sexual and/or physical violence)	HTQ	Eighty-three women had PTSD symptoms (71% of the population).
8.	Schalinski I., Moran J., Schauer M … (2014) [56]	N = 50 F (PTSD = 33; NO PTSD = 17)	Far and Middle East, The Balkans, Africa and India	PTSD and Disassociation	CAPS; Shut- D; IAPS.	Patients with PTSD displayed intrusive memories, while the control group (NO PTSD) did not report having such memories. The women with the most severe PTSD symptoms displayed greater disassociation.
9.	Alpak G., Unal A. Bulbul F., (2015) [57]	N = 352 (M = 179; F = 173)	Syria and Turkey	PTSD	DSM-IV-TR	One hundred and eighteen of the participants were diagnosed with PTSD. Eleven of them suffered from acute PTSD, 105 from chronic PTSD and 2 from late onset PTSD.
10.	Haldane J, Nickerson A. (2016) [58]	N = 91 (M = 60; F = 31)	Iran, Sri Lanka; Afghanistan and Iraq	PTSD (impact of gender in interpersonal non-interpersonal traumatic experiences)	HTQ	A significant relation was found between non-interpersonal trauma and symptoms of PTSD. In women, a relation was observed between PTSD symptoms and traumatic interpersonal events, while in men the significant association was between PTSD symptoms and non-interpersonal traumatic events.

Table 1. *Cont.*

ID-Article	Authors and Year	Sample	Origin of Study	Assessment Objective	Instruments	Results
11.	Rometsch-Ogioun C., Denkinger J.K., Windthorst P., ... (2018) [42]	-	Northern Iraq (Yazidí women)	Factors related with past histories of trauma.	Questionnaire designed by psychologists and psychologists	The psychological symptoms identified as particularly significant were nightmares, insomnia and depression.
12.	Mhlongo M.D., Tomita A., Thela L. (2018) [59]	N = 157	Burundi, Democratic Republic of Congo, Ghana, Mozambique, Ruanda, Uganda, Malawi and Zimbabwe.	Relation between experience of traumatic event and PTSD.	LEC; HTQ	Exposure to a higher number of traumatic events was associated with a higher likelihood to be at risk for PTSD. Exposure to sexual trauma was associated with a higher likelihood to be at risk for PTSD in women.

All of the studies evaluated PTSD, except number 11, which based its research on factors associated with the history of trauma measured by a questionnaire designed by psychologists and psychiatrists. In addition, some of the studies assessed dissociative symptoms (5, 8), sexual violence (4), sexual and/or physical violence (7), the impact of gender on traumatic experiences (10) and trauma and torture (1). With respect to sexual violence, the different studies operationalized it in a broad sense, including: forced marriages, individual and gang rapes, molestation, abuse, forced to undress, sexual slavery, forced to perform sexual acts with another person, stripped of clothing, forced abortions and touching.

3.1. PTSD and Other Mental Health Problems in Refugee Women

Of the twelve selected articles, five of them based their sample solely on female refugees (2, 5, 7, 8, and 11) and four specifically reported data regarding the prevalence of PTSD in this population group. Three of them showed similar and significant results in relation to the presence of PTSD symptoms in refugee women, with the percentage ranging from 66% to 71% [50,55,56], only 25.9% of the women had a score that indicated the presence of PTSD. At the same time, study 11 [42] was the only one that did not assess PTSD itself, but rather psychological symptoms through scores given by healthcare professionals. The most noteworthy symptoms related to trauma were nightmares, followed by insomnia and depression. The subjects also suffered from somatic ailments such as aches and pains, dizziness, and gastrointestinal issues.

In different studies (4, 5, 7 and 8) PTSD in refugee women was linked with other mental health problems, such as dissociative symptoms and depression. In Study 5, disassociation was pointed out as a predictor of PTSD severity in women with traumatic experiences, since the female participants that suffered from greater disassociation had a higher PTSD score. At the same time, study 8 [56] revealed that women patients with a higher degree of PTSD displayed greater disassociation and this correlated with symptoms of depression. Specifically, in this study, it was shown that the severity of PTSD in refugee women was linked to disassociation and severity of depression, being very closely interrelated. Other research studies also pointed to the relationship between depression and PTSD. For example, in study 5 [53] and study 7 [55] there was a high prevalence of depression (almost 95%), and in study 4 [52] it was observed that 40.5% of the sample met the criteria of having a major depressive disorder.

Study 1 [49] carried out a comparative analysis among three groups of women: women without children, women who had between one and six children and women with more than six children. It was found that the female refugees who were mothers with more than six children had undergone a higher number of torture and traumatic events, for which they had much more significant scores in PTSD than women who had fewer than six children or none. They also had higher rates of illiteracy, limited knowledge of spoken English, were caring for the children on their own, and were less likely to be working. At the same time, almost half of the women reported taking medication to calm themselves down, and nearly one in ten reported having seen a physician for their health problems. The majority used prayer to combat stress. The accounts involving greater exposure to trauma were highly correlated with more social, psychological and physical problems, and higher PTSD scores. Furthermore, 89% of women with large families reported having had to do things in order to survive that still bothered them, and almost two thirds (64%) of these women stated that they had been exposed to various types of torture, including rape.

3.2. Differences in PTSD between Male and Female Refugees

Seven of the studies carried out a differential analysis of the presence of PTSD symptoms among male and female refugees (1, 3, 4, 6, 9, 10, and 12). Similar results were obtained in all of them. In general, the women were more exposed to traumatic events and scored higher in psychological problems, including PTSD, than men. For example, study 6 [54] found that 75% of female refugees had PTSD compared with 25% of the men. Furthermore, women obtained higher scores than men in intrusive symptoms, evasion symptoms, hyper-activation symptoms and overall PTSD severity. Along these same lines are the results of study 9 [57], which pointed out that the likelihood of having PTSD is much higher in women than in men. On the other hand, studies 1 [49], 4 [52] and 10 [58] showed that, even although there were no differences in the presence of PTSD among men and women, the scores for the latter were higher. These higher scores in women for PTSD also seem to become exacerbated over time. According to study 3 [51], the scores for PTSD severity were higher in women than in men at the three moments of assessment (baseline, after one year, and after three and a half years) but the differences were only statistically significant at the three-and-a-half-year follow-up.

At the same time, with regard to traumatic events, study 5 [53] analyzed the differences between a traumatic event experienced firsthand and one that was witnessed. The traumatic self-experienced event referred to whether the participant had been the victim of a traumatic event and witnessed ones, to whether the participant was the witness who observed the traumatic event involving another person. The results indicated that the number of traumatic self-experienced events significantly predicted the severity of PTSD. Furthermore, study 6 [54] revealed that the experienced traumatic load made up the most significant contributing factor to PTSD and that it was higher in refugee women.

Study 10 [58], on the other hand, assessed the effect of two types of trauma: interpersonal and non-interpersonal. The first type is conceived as a traumatic event that is perpetrated by another person with the intention of harming or threatening an individual; for example, rape or sexual abuse, torture, brainwashing, imprisonment, witnessing the murder of family members or friends, etc. Non-interpersonal trauma is not based on a relationship with others, and encompasses, for example, lack of food or water, being in poor health without access to medical care, lack of shelter, forced isolation, etc. The results of this study showed that in female refugees a link could be observed between PTSD symptoms and six of the eight traumatic interpersonal events: imprisonment, serious injuries, combat situations, brainwashing, rape or sexual abuse, and torture. On the contrary, for men, none of the subtypes of interpersonal trauma produced a significant effect in relation to PTSD symptoms. Three of the eight subtypes of non-interpersonal trauma did have an effect, however: lack of food or water, being near death and in poor health without access to medical care. In the case of women, none of the subtypes of non-interpersonal trauma produced significant effects in relation to PTSD symptoms.

3.3. Traumatic Experiences in Refugee Women: The Importance of Rape and Sexual Abuse

The importance of violence and sexual abuse in refugee women in relation to the presence of PTSD symptoms is reflected in six studies (4, 5, 6, 7, 10, and 12). In general, all of them reveal that refugee women suffer more sexual assault and forced sex than men do, and that these traumatic experiences are associated with a greater risk of having PTSD. For example, in study 4 [52], the rate of sexual violence reported by women was 39.7%

compared to 23.6% in men, which significantly increased the presence of PTSD. In addition, according to study 5 [53], the firsthand traumatic event most often experienced among refugees is sexual assault (96.2% for this case). In study 7 [55], it was found that 87.2% of those surveyed reported having been subjected to some type of physical or sexual violence during their lives, of which 84.6% reported physical violence and 71.8% sexual violence. At the same time, the weighted prevalence of forced sex was 48.8% and attempted rape was 58.3%.

In study 6 [54], significant correlations were found between sexual assault and other types of violence by a family member or an acquaintance and PTSD. Furthermore, a relation was established between having had sexual contact before the age of 18 with an individual five or more years older and PTSD, with PTSD significantly higher in women than in men. Along these lines are studies 10 [58] and 12 [59], whose results showed a relation between rape, sexual abuse and exposure to sexual traumas, and PTSD symptoms in refugee women.

3.4. PTSD over Time

In the longitudinal study 3 [51], rates of PTSD were assessed in male as well as female refugees at three different moments: baseline, after one year and after three and a half years. At the beginning of the assessment, 76% met the diagnostic criteria of PTSD, 33% did so at one year, and at three and a half years, 24% of the subjects did. An inverse correlation was found between the global assessment of functioning (GAF) scores and PTSD severity scores. Although the severity of the PTSD symptoms diminished with time, the majority of the refugees continued having at least one or more symptoms related to traumas after three and a half years. In addition, the refugee women who did not speak the language of the host country seemed to be more vulnerable to the persistence of effects stemming from the trauma.

4. Discussion

Upon reviewing the existing literature to determine the relation between refugee women and PTSD, twelve studies dealing with this subject were identified. In these studies, important evidence was found for a high prevalence of PTSD in refugee women [55,56]. Furthermore, the presence of PTSD and its severity seems to be linked to other mental health problems, such as dissociative symptoms [56] and depression [52,53,55].

With respect to the differences between men and women, the majority of the studies pointed out that the incidence of PTSD is significantly higher in women than in men [54,57] Other studies reported that although there are no differences between the presence of PTSD in men and women, there are in fact differences with respect to its severity, as it is higher among the latter [49,52,58]. In addition, according to the study by Vojvoda et al. [51], these differences become sharper with time, finding a greater degree of severity in refugee women than in men three and half years after resettlement.

Likewise, women are more vulnerable to displaying PTSD symptoms from interpersonal-type traumatic experiences (for example, sexual abuse or torture), while men are more prone to suffering PTSD as a result of traumatic experiences of a non-interpersonal type (such as lack of food or lack of water) [58]. Additionally, refugees could suffer from PTSD if the violence incurred is carried out by a family member or an acquaintance, and in this sense, women experience it to a greater degree than men do [54]. At the same time, according to the study by Schalinski et al. [53], the severity of PTSD is determined depending on whether the traumatic event of the refugees is self-experienced or if, on the contrary, it is witnessed, with firsthand experience resulting in a greater degree of severity. For the authors, women are more likely to live through a traumatic experience firsthand than are men, for which the severity of PTSD is greater.

After a review of the different studies, it seems clear that the higher predominance and severity of PTSD in refugee women is related to gender-based traumatic experiences, such as rape, sexual assault and abuse, or genital mutilation, among others [52–55,58,59]. As stated by the World Health Organization (WHO), situations of conflict and displacement can exacerbate gender violence already existing in families and communities and bring about new forms of violence (for example, sexual slavery) against women and girls [60]. In this sense, the meta-analysis carried out by Tolin and Foa [28] on gender differences and the risk of suffering traumatic experiences and having PTSD, had observed that women are more likely than men to meet the criteria of PTSD, in spite of having a lower overall likelihood of having a traumatic experience. As such, in accordance with this review, men are more likely than women to experiences accidents, non-sexual assault, combat or war, fire or natural disaster, serious illness or non-specific injury. However, women are more likely than men to report sexual assault and child sexual abuse. Furthermore, according to the study by Schalinski et al. [53], the most common traumatic event experienced firsthand in refugees is sexual assault.

The results obtained from this review of the different studies are in line with the theory of situational vulnerability to trauma with respect to the symptoms of PTSD formulated by Pimlott-Kubiak and Cortina [34]. According to this theory, being a woman raises the risk of sexual victimization throughout an individual's lifetime and this victimization increases the risk of suffering from PTSD [35]. Thus, the source of the main risk resides not in the female gender itself, but in the adjacent situation. For Pimlott-Kubiak and Cortina [34], female vulnerability to PTSD is simply a product of exposure to gender-based trauma and not to any attributes that women have.

In today's world, the relation between gender-based traumatic experiences, the psychological difficulties of refugee women and possible intervention programs are an emerging topic of interest [61] and they are not reliable [62]. In fact, according to the UNHCR [63], sexual violence among female refugees is often unknown, due to different factors. On one hand, this is due to the social stigma and shame associated with rape that weighs upon the women, and on the other, due to fear of possible reprisals (rejection, blame, isolation, criminalization, increased gender inequality and punishment by other forms of violence, among others). Furthermore, as pointed out by Robbers and Morgan [61], it is likely that refugee women who are victims of sexual violence do not know how to act or where to go, are terrorized by their family members, and mistrust official procedures and authorities, since they might be immersed a circle of systematic violence. This leads to survivors often avoiding communication of their traumatic experiences, which makes us suppose that data on the presence of PTSD is not entirely accurate. This results in possible erroneous interpretations and unawareness of the psycho-socio healthcare needs of this population group [64]. This review sheds light on the relation between posttraumatic stress disorder and refugee women, especially if they have suffered a traumatic experience linked to sexual violence in any of its manifestations, which we hope will serve as a starting point for future work.

Limitations and Future Research Lines

The main obstacle encountered in this study is the scant literature and lack of research on PTSD and the mental health of refugee women. This represented a challenge in gathering the most information possible, while also highlighting the need to analyze results found until now, aimed at gathering coherent data to promote research, create awareness among the general population, and promote social and healthcare actions in this group with their pronounced need for multidisciplinary care and intervention, particularly with respect to sexual violence. In this sense, the review undertaken by Robbers and Morgan [61] points out that sexual violence against refugee women is a complex public health concern, which requires a multicomponent solution and cultural sensitivity.

On the other hand, as observed in the study by Redwood-Campbell et al. [50], in which slightly more than one-fourth of the refugee women obtained a score indicating the presence of PTSD, these women can unconsciously block or feel uncomfortable about revealing intimate and painful experiences of sexual nature, due to religious and cultural issues, or they may be facing other barriers such as language or illiteracy. Due to these factors, the results of this study and other similar ones must be approached with caution, taking into account the numerous interferences that could arise in making a diagnosis of the mental health problems in refugees, particularly in women. In this sense, some of the studies included in this review [42,56] found numerous somatic ailments in women with histories of trauma. For socio-healthcare professionals, it is very important to take into account this expression of PTSD, because, in many instances, physical pain is more obvious and easier to detect than psychological issues. As various authors have pointed out [65–68], trauma, especially when it involves the body, stays in the body, and although possible associated emotions tend to be avoided, the body responds to the pain of the unconscious memory through somatization. For this reason, it is essential that the socio-healthcare teams who attend to this population group be aware of the involvement of PTSD or traumatic experiences in a patient's physical symptoms and ailments, with the aim of ensuring effective treatment.

It would also be favorable to target the research to better assess symptoms of disassociation in refugee women, since it is a reaction to trauma that cannot be concealed. Work by Schalinski et al. [53] revealed that the self-experienced traumatic event most frequently reported is sexual assault, which was related with higher scores for PTSD severity that at the same time was diagnosed by disassociation, and for which it could be concluded that the disassociated response seems most common in individuals who have been sexually assaulted [29]. This finding invites us to direct possible future research lines to examine the presence of dissociative symptoms in refugee women, aimed at studying its relation to traumatic experiences of a sexual nature.

5. Conclusions

As a final conclusion, we would like to underline that mental health disorders are to a large extent determined by social and cultural factors and they must be taken into consideration for their analysis and intervention in refugees. In this sense, with respect to the differences between men and women, as established by the WHO [60] (p. 3), "gender determines the power differential and control that men and woman have over socioeconomic determinants in their lives and their mental health, their position, social condition, the way that they are treated in society and their susceptibility and exposure to specific risks to their mental health". Accordingly, to understand the impact of traumatic experiences on mental health and deterioration of psychological wellbeing in refugee women, analysis from the perspective of gender is necessary, with attention paid to power relations between men and women, focusing on the significant emotional impact for women that these relations can entail, linked to having experienced traumatic events of sexual violence.

In a similar vein, this gender analysis has implications for intervention strategies aimed at survivors. Gender violence and sexual abuse must be a vital component in treatment programs and social reconstruction for refugees, particularly women. Thus, prevention and the response to sexual violence must include the active participation of refugee women in the design as well as in the implementation of prevention measures [61]. Prevention programs must hence be focused on increasing their empowerment, training and education in order to reduce sexual violence [69,70], involve the entire community [71] and transform gender norms, reinforcing community responsibility [72].

Author Contributions: Conceptualization, M.V.-M. and A.S.S.; methodology, M.V.-M. and A.S.S.; writing—original draft preparation, M.V.-M. and A.S.S.; writing—review and editing, M.V.-M.; supervision, J.M.C.; funding acquisition, J.M.C. All authors have read and agreed to the published version of the manuscript.

Funding: This research has been funded by the University of Malaga research project "The role of stereotypes in intergroup relationships in the multicultural context of the province of Malaga" (Reference Number 18-B3-02).

Institutional Review Board Statement: Not applicable.

Informed Consent Statement: Not applicable.

Data Availability Statement: Not applicable.

Conflicts of Interest: The authors declare that there are no potential conflicts of interest with respect to the research, authorship and/or publication of the article.

References

1. United Nations High Commissioner for Refugees (UNHCR). *Refugee Population Statistics*; UNHCR: Geneva, Switzerland, 2020; Available online: https://www.unhcr.org/refugee-statistics/ (accessed on 17 February 2021).
2. Ellis, B.H.; Murray, K.; Barrett, C. Understanding the mental health of refugees: Trauma, stress, and the cultural context. In *Current Clinical Psychiatry. The Massachusetts General Hospital Textbook on Diversity and Cultural Sensitivity in Mental Health*; Parekh, R., Ed.; Human Press: Totowa, NJ, USA, 2014; pp. 165–187. [CrossRef]
3. Führer, A.; Eichner, F.; Stang, A. Morbidity of asylum seekers in a medium-sized German city. *Eur. J. Epidemiol.* **2016**, *31*, 703–706. [CrossRef]
4. Horwitz, A.V. Distinguishing distress from disorders psychological outcomes of stressful social arrangements. *Health Interdiscip. J. Soc. Study Health Illn. Med.* **2007**, *11*, 273–289. [CrossRef]
5. Vargas, S.M.; Huey, S.J., Jr.; Miranda, J. A critical review of current evidence on multiple types of discrimination and mental health. *Am. J. Orthopsychiatry* **2020**, *90*, 374–390. [CrossRef]
6. Koch, T.; Liedl, A.; Ehring, T. Emotion regulation as a transdiagnostic factor in Afghan refugees. *Psychol. Trauma Theory Res. Pract. Policy* **2020**, *12*, 235–243. [CrossRef] [PubMed]
7. Angora, R.A. Trauma y estrés en población refugiada en tránsito hacia Europa. *Clín. Contemp.* **2016**, *7*, 125–136. [CrossRef]
8. Sleijpen, M.; June ter Heide, F.J.; Mooren, T.; Boeije, H.R.; Kleber, R.J. Bouncing forward of young refugees: A perspective on resilience research directions. *Eur. J. Psychotraumatol.* **2013**, *4*, 20124. [CrossRef] [PubMed]
9. Lindert, J.; von Ehrenstein, O.S.; Priebe, S.; Mielck, A.; Brähler, E. Depression and anxiety in labor migrants and refugees–a systematic review and meta-analysis. *Soc. Sci. Med.* **2009**, *69*, 246–257. [CrossRef] [PubMed]
10. Nesterko, Y.; Jäckle, D.; Friedrich, M.; Holzapfel, L.; Glaesmer, H. Health care needs among recently arrived refugees in Germany: A cross-sectional, epidemiological study. *Int. J. Public Health* **2020**, *65*, 811–821. [CrossRef]
11. Reavell, J.; Fazil, Q. The epidemiology of PTSD and depression in refugee minors who have resettled in developed countries. *J. Ment. Health* **2017**, *26*, 74–83. [CrossRef]
12. Gorst-Unsworth, C.; Goldenberg, E. Psychological sequelae of torture and organised violence suffered by refugees from Iraq: Trauma-related factors compared with social factors in exile. *Br. J. Psychiatry* **1998**, *172*, 90–94. [CrossRef]
13. Brewin, C.R.; Dalgleish, T.; Joseph, S. A dual representation theory of posttraumatic stress disorder. *Psychol. Rev.* **1996**, *103*, 670–686. [CrossRef] [PubMed]
14. Van der Kolk, B.A. The body keeps the score: Memory and the evolving psychobiology of posttraumatic stress. *Harv. Rev. Psychiatry* **1994**, *1*, 253–265. [CrossRef]
15. Van der Kolk, B.A.; Van der Hart, O. The intrusive past: The flexibility of memory and the engraving of trauma. *Am. Imago* **1991**, *48*, 425–454.
16. Van der Kolk, B.A. Psychobiology of posttraumatic stress disorder. In *Textbook of Biological Psychiatry*; Panksepp, J., Ed.; Wiley-Liss: New York, NY, USA, 2004; pp. 319–344. [CrossRef]
17. Van der Kolk, B.A. Developmental Trauma Disorder: Toward a rational diagnosis for children with complex trauma histories. *Psychiatr. Ann.* **2005**, *35*, 401–408. [CrossRef]
18. Tankink, M.; Richters, A. Silence as a coping strategy: The case of refugee women in the Netherlands from South-Sudan who experienced sexual violence in the context of war. In *Voices of Trauma*; Drožđek, B., Wilson, J.P., Eds.; Springer: Boston, MA, USA, 2007; pp. 191–210. [CrossRef]
19. Spitzer, R.L.; First, M.B.; Wakefield, J.C. Saving PTSD from itself in DSM-V. *J. Anxiety Disord.* **2007**, *21*, 233–241. [CrossRef] [PubMed]
20. Muldoon, O.T.; Haslam, S.A.; Haslam, C.; Cruwys, T.; Kearns, M.; Jetten, J. The social psychology of responses to trauma: Social identity pathway associate with divergent traumatic responses. *Eur. Rev. Soc. Psychol.* **2019**, *30*, 311–348. [CrossRef]
21. American Psychiatric Association (APA). *Diagnostic and Statistical Manual of Mental Disorders (DSM-5)*; American Psychiatric Pub: Washington, DC, USA, 2013. [CrossRef]
22. Weinstein, N.; Khabbaz, F.; Legate, N. Enhancing need satisfaction to reduce psychological distress in Syrian refugees. *J. Consult. Clin. Psychol.* **2016**, *84*, 645–650. [CrossRef] [PubMed]
23. Doctors Without Borders. Asylum Seekers in Italy: An Analysis of Mental HEALTH distress and Access to Healthcare. Available online: https://www.msf.org/italy-mental-health-disorders-asylum-seekers-and-migrants-overlooked-inadequate-reception-system (accessed on 11 December 2020).
24. Crumlish, N.; O'Rourke, K. A systematic review of treatments for post-traumatic stress disorder among refugees and asylum-seekers. *J. Nerv. Ment. Dis.* **2010**, *198*, 237–251. [CrossRef] [PubMed]

25. Priebe, S.; Giacco, D.; El-Nagib, R. Public health aspects of mental health among migrants and refugees: A review of the evidence on mental health care for refugees, asylum seekers and irregular migrants in the WHO European Region. In *Health Evidence Network Synthesis Report*; WHO Regional Office for Europe: Copenhagen, Denmark, 2016. Available online: https://www.ncbi.nlm.nih.gov/books/NBK391045/ (accessed on 18 January 2021).

26. Steel, Z.; Chey, T.; Silove, D.; Marnane, C.; Bryant, R.A.; Van Ommeren, M. Association of torture and other potentially traumatic events with mental health outcomes among populations exposed to mass conflict and displacement: A systematic review and meta-analysis. *J. Am. Med Assoc.* **2009**, *302*, 537–549. [CrossRef]

27. McFarlane, A.C.; Atchison, M.; Rafalowicz, E.; Papay, P. Physical symptoms in post-traumatic stress disorder. *J. Psychosom. Res.* **1994**, *38*, 715–726. [CrossRef]

28. Tolin, D.F.; Foa, E.B. Sex differences in trauma and posttraumatic stress disorder: A quantitative review of 25 years of research. *Psychol. Bull.* **2006**, *132*, 959–992. [CrossRef] [PubMed]

29. Griffin, M.G.; Resick, P.A.; Mechanic, M.B. Objective assessment of peritraumatic dissociation: Psychophysiological indicators. *Am. J. Psychiatry* **1997**, *154*, 1081–1088. [CrossRef] [PubMed]

30. Norris, F.H. Epidemiology of trauma: Frequency and impact of different potentially traumatic events on different demographic groups. *J. Consult. Clin. Psychol.* **1992**, *60*, 409–418. [CrossRef]

31. Kessler, R.C.; Sonnega, A.; Bromet, E.; Hughes, M.; Nelson, C.B. Posttraumatic stress disorder in the National Comorbidity Survey. *Arch. Gen. Psychiatry* **1995**, *52*, 1048–1060. [CrossRef]

32. Norris, F.H.; Murphy, A.D.; Baker, C.K.; Perilla, J.L.; Rodríguez, F.G.; Rodríguez, J.D.J.G. Epidemiology of trauma and posttraumatic stress disorder in Mexico. *J. Abnorm. Psychol.* **2003**, *112*, 646–656. [CrossRef]

33. Wolfe, J.; Kimerling, R. Gender issues in the assessment of posttraumatic stress disorder. In *Assessing Psychological Trauma and PTSD*; Wilson, J.P., Keane, T.M., Eds.; The Guilford Press: New York, NY, USA, 1997; pp. 192–238.

34. Pimlott-Kubiak, S.; Cortina, L.M. Gender, victimization, and outcomes: Reconceptualizing risk. *J. Consult. Clin. Psychol.* **2003**, *71*, 528–539. [CrossRef] [PubMed]

35. Cortina, L.M.; Kubiak, S.P. Gender and posttraumatic stress: Sexual violence as an explanation for women's increased risk. *J. Abnorm. Psychol.* **2006**, *115*, 753–759. [CrossRef]

36. United Nations High Commissioner for Refugees (UNHCR). *Chin Women from Myanmar Find Help Down a Winding Lane in Delhi*; UNHCR: Geneva, Switzerland, 2009. Available online: http://www.unhcr.org/4a76f7466.html (accessed on 1 March 2021).

37. Ward, J.; Vann, B. Gender-based violence in refugee settings. *Lancet* **2002**, *360*, 13–14. [CrossRef]

38. Comisión Española de Ayuda al Refugiado (CEAR). Informe 2020: Las Personas Refugiadas en España y Europa. Available online: https://www.cear.es/wp-content/uploads/2020/06/Informe-Anual_CEAR_2020_.pdf (accessed on 22 January 2021).

39. Quercetti, F.; Ventosa, N. Crisis de refugiados: Un análisis de las concepciones presentes en los estudios sobre la salud mental de las personas refugiadas y solicitantes de asilo. In *VIII Congreso Internacional de Investigación y Práctica Profesional en Psicología XXIII. Jornadas de Investigación XII Encuentro de Investigadores en Psicología del MERCOSUR*; Acta Académica: Buenos Aires, Argentina, 2016; Available online: https://www.aacademica.org/000-044/280 (accessed on 8 January 2021).

40. Buckley-Zistel, S.; Krause, U. *Gender, Violence, Refugees*; Berghahn Books: New York, NY, USA, 2017.

41. Montgomery, E. Long-term effects of organized violence on young Middle Eastern refugees' mental health. *Soc. Sci. Med.* **2008**, *67*, 1596–1603. [CrossRef] [PubMed]

42. Rometsch-Ogioun El Sount, C.; Denkinger, J.K.; Windthorst, P.; Nikendei, C.; Kindermann, D.; Renner, V.; Ringwald, J.; Brucker, S.; Tran, V.M.; Zipfel, S.; et al. Psychological Burden in Female, Iraqi Refugees Who Suffered Extreme Violence by the "Islamic State": The Perspective of Care Providers. *Front. Psychiatry* **2018**, *9*, 562. [CrossRef] [PubMed]

43. Burnett, A. Asylum seekers and refugees in Britain: Health needs of asylum seekers and refugees. *BMJ* **2001**, *322*, 544–547. [CrossRef]

44. Bokore, N. Suffering in silence: A Canadian-Somali case study. *J. Soc. Work Pract.* **2013**, *27*, 95–113. [CrossRef]

45. Alexander, A.J.; Arnett, J.J.; Jena, S.P.K. Experiences of Burmese Chin refugee women: Trauma and survival from pre-to postflight. *Int. Perspect. Psychol. Res. Pract. Consult.* **2017**, *6*, 101–114. [CrossRef]

46. Shamseer, L.; Moher, D.; Clarke, M.; Ghersi, D.; Liberati, A.; Petticrew, M.; Shekelle, P.; Stewart, L.A. Preferred reporting items for systematic review and meta-analysis protocols (PRISMA-P) 2015: Elaboration and explanation. *BMJ* **2015**, *350*, g7647. [CrossRef] [PubMed]

47. Liberati, A.; Altman, D.G.; Tetzlaff, J.; Mulrow, C.; Gøtzsche, P.C.; Ioannidis, J.P.A.; Clarke, M.; Devereaux, P.J.; Kleijnen, J.; Moher, D. The PRISMA statement for reporting systematic reviews and meta-analyses of studies that evaluate health care interventions: Explanation and elaboration. *J. Clin. Epidemiol.* **2009**, *62*, 1–34. [CrossRef] [PubMed]

48. Borenstein, M.; Hedges, L.V.; Higgins, J.P.T.; Rothstein, H.R. *Introduction to Meta-Analysis*; John Wiley & Sons, Ltd.: Chichester, NY, USA, 2009.

49. Robertson, C.L.; Halcon, L.; Savik, K.; Johnson, D.; Spring, M.; Butcher, J.; Westermeyer, J.; Jaranson, J. Somali and Oromo refugee women: Trauma and associated factors. *J. Adv. Nurs.* **2006**, *56*, 577–587. [CrossRef]

50. Redwood-Campbell, L.; Thind, H.; Howard, M.; Koteles, J.; Fowler, N.; Kaczorowski, J. Understanding the health of refugee women in host countries: Lessons from the Kosovar re-settlement in Canada. *Prehospital Disaster Med.* **2008**, *23*, 322–327. [CrossRef]

51. Vojvoda, D.; Weine, S.M.; McGlashan, T.; Becker, D.F.; Southwick, S.M. Posttraumatic stress disorder symptoms in Bosnian refugees 3 1/2 years after resettlement. *J. Rehabil. Res. Dev.* **2008**, *45*, 421–426. [CrossRef] [PubMed]
52. Johnson, K.; Scott, J.; Rughita, B.; Kisielewski, M.; Asher, J.; Ong, R.; Lawry, L. Association of sexual violence and human rights violations with physical and mental health in territories of the Eastern Democratic Republic of the Congo. *J. Am. Med. Assoc.* **2010**, *304*, 553–562. [CrossRef]
53. Schalinski, I.; Elbert, T.; Schauer, M. Female dissociative responding to extreme sexual violence in a chronic crisis setting: The case of Eastern Congo. *J. Trauma. Stress* **2011**, *24*, 235–238. [CrossRef] [PubMed]
54. Ssenyonga, J.; Owens, V.; Olema, D.K. Traumatic experiences and PTSD among adolescent Congolese Refugees in Uganda: A preliminary study. *J. Psychol. Afr.* **2012**, *22*, 629–632. [CrossRef]
55. Morof, D.F.; Sami, S.; Mangeni, M.; Blanton, C.; Cardozo, B.L.; Tomczyk, B. A cross-sectional survey on gender-based violence and mental health among female urban refugees and asylum seekers in Kampala, Uganda. *Int. J. Gynecol. Obstet.* **2014**, *127*, 138–143. [CrossRef]
56. Schalinski, I.; Moran, J.; Schauer, M.; Elbert, T. Rapid emotional processing in relation to trauma-related symptoms as revealed by magnetic source imaging. *BMC Psychiatry* **2014**, *14*, 193. [CrossRef]
57. Alpak, G.; Unal, A.; Bulbul, F.; Sagaltici, E.; Bez, Y.; Altindag, A.; Dalkilic, A.; Savas, H.A. Post-traumatic stress disorder among Syrian refugees in Turkey: A cross-sectional study. *Int. J. Psychiatry Clin. Pract.* **2014**, *19*, 45–50. [CrossRef]
58. Haldane, J.; Nickerson, A. The impact of interpersonal and noninterpersonal trauma on psychological symptoms in refugees: The moderating role of gender and trauma type. *J. Trauma. Stress* **2016**, *29*, 457–465. [CrossRef] [PubMed]
59. Mhlongo, M.D.; Tomita, A.; Thela, L.; Maharaj, V.; Burns, J.K. Sexual trauma and post-traumatic stress among African female refugees and migrants in South Africa. *S. Afr. J. Psychiatry* **2018**, *24*, 1208.
60. World Health Organization. WHO Multi-Country Study on Women's Health and Domestic Violence Against Women: Initial Results on Prevalence, Health Outcomes and Women's Responses. 2005. Available online: https://www.who.int/reproductivehealth/publications/violence/24159358X/en/ (accessed on 25 February 2021).
61. Robbers, G.M.L.; Morgan, A. Potencial de programas para la prevención y respuesta a la violencia sexual contra mujeres refugiadas: Una revisión de la literatura. *Reprod. Health Matters* **2018**, *25*, 69–89. [CrossRef] [PubMed]
62. Vu, A.; Adam, A.; Wirtz, A.; Pham, K.; Rubenstein, L.; Glass, N.; Beyrer, C.; Singh, S. The Prevalence of Sexual Violence among Female Refugees in Complex Humanitarian Emergencies: A Systematic Review and Meta-analysis. *PLoS Curr.* **2014**, *6*, 6. [CrossRef]
63. United Nations High Commissioner for Refugees (UNHCR). *Sexual and Gender-Based Violence Against Refugees, Returnees, and Internally Displaced Persons*; UNHCR: Geneva, Switzerland, 2003. Available online: https://www.unhcr.org/protection/women/3f696bcc4/sexual-gender-based-violence-against-refugees-returnees-internally-displaced.html (accessed on 3 March 2021).
64. United Nations High Commissioner for Refugees. *Working with Men and Boy Survivors of Sexual and Gender-BASED Violence in Forced Displacement*; UNHCR: Geneva, Switzerland, 2012. Available online: https://www.refworld.org/pdfid/5006aa262.pdf (accessed on 15 February 2021).
65. Gupta, M.A. Review of somatic symptoms in post-traumatic stress disorder. *Int. Rev. Psychiatry* **2013**, *25*, 86–99. [CrossRef]
66. Hoge, C.W.; Terhakopian, A.; Castro, C.A.; Messer, S.C.; Engel, C.C. Association of posttraumatic stress disorder with somatic symptoms, health care visits, and absenteeism among Iraq war veterans. *Am. J. Psychiatry* **2007**, *164*, 150–153. [CrossRef]
67. Pribor, E.F.; Yutzy, S.H.; Dean, J.T.; Wetzel, R.D. Briquet's syndrome, dissociation, and abuse. *Am. J. Psychiatry* **1993**, *150*, 1507–1511. [CrossRef] [PubMed]
68. Scaer, R.C. *The Body Bears the Burden: Trauma, Dissociation and Disease*; The Haworth Medical Press: New York, NY, USA, 2001.
69. Spangaro, J.; Adogu, C.; Zwi, A.B.; Ranmuthugala, G.; Davies, G.P. Mechanisms underpinning interventions to reduce sexual violence in armed conflict: A realist-informed systematic review. *Confl. Health* **2015**, *9*, 1–14. [CrossRef] [PubMed]
70. Tappis, H.; Freeman, J.; Glass, N.; Doocy, S. Effectiveness of Interventions, Programs and Strategies for Gender-based Violence Prevention in Refugee Populations: An Integrative Review. *PLoS Curr.* **2016**, *19*, 8. [CrossRef]
71. Hossain, M.; Zimmerman, C.; Watss, C. Preventing violence against women and girls in conflict. *Lancet* **2014**, *383*, 2021–2022. [CrossRef]
72. Gurman, T.A.; Trappler, R.M.; Acosta, A.; McCray, P.A.; Cooper, C.M.; Goodsmith, L. "By seeing with our own eyes, it can remain in our mind": Qualitative evaluation findings suggest the ability of participatory video to reduce gender-based violence in conflict-affected settings. *Health Educ. Res.* **2014**, *29*, 690–701. [CrossRef] [PubMed]

MDPI
St. Alban-Anlage 66
4052 Basel
Switzerland
Tel. +41 61 683 77 34
Fax +41 61 302 89 18
www.mdpi.com

International Journal of Environmental Research and Public Health Editorial Office
E-mail: ijerph@mdpi.com
www.mdpi.com/journal/ijerph

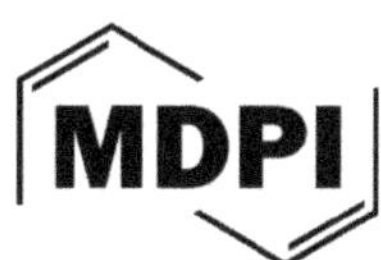

9 783036 547145